2-9-00

D1233810

FROM SOUND TO SYNAPSE

FROM SOUND
TO SYNAPSE

Physiology of The Mammalian Ear

C. Daniel Geisler
Department of Neurophysiology
and
Department of Electrical and Computer Engineering
University of Wisconsin-Madison

New York   Oxford
Oxford University Press
1998

Oxford University Press

Oxford   New York
Athens   Auckland   Bangkok   Bombay   Buenos Aires
Calcutta   Cape Town   Dar es Salaam   Delhi
Florence   Hong Kong   Istanbul   Karachi
Kuala Lumpur   Madras   Madrid   Melbourne
Mexico City   Nairobi   Paris   Singapore
Taipei   Tokyo   Toronto   Warsaw

and associated companies in

Berlin   Ibadan

Copyright © 1998 by C. Daniel Geisler

Published by Oxford University Press, Inc.
198 Madison Avenue, New York, New York 10016

Oxford is a registered trademark of Oxford University Press

Library of Congress Cataloging-in-Publication Data

Geisler, C. Daniel.
From sound to synapse : physiology of the mammalian ear /
C. Daniel Geisler.
p.   cm.   Includes bibliographical references and index.
ISBN 0-19-510025-5
1. Ear — Physiology.   2. Hearing.   I. Title.
QP461.G26   1998
573.8′919 — dc21   97-13565

1 3 5 7 9 8 6 4 2

Printed in the United States of America
on acid-free paper

. . . for I am fearfully and wonderfully made. Marvelous are your works.

Psalm 139:14

PREFACE

Since the mid-1980s there have been rapid advances in our understanding of how the ear works. Our shop talk now centers on "cochlear amplifiers" and motile sensory cells, concepts that barely existed 10 years ago. The advances have been so great and on so broad a scale that we now have a pretty good picture of how the ear transforms acoustic signals into neural pulses. It is to communicate this picture that the book was written.

There are other books in this same vein, but most tend to be technical or specialized (or both). This volume complements those books, presenting a broad overview of the mammalian ear in as nontechnical a manner as seems consistent with supplying a theoretical basis for understanding the various processes involved. These theoretical explanations are mostly qualitative, with equations used sparingly. Nevertheless, an effort has been made to ensure that these explanations, as far as they go, are accurate. References for more complete statements of these theories, and sometimes competing ones as well, are given for those who wish to pursue them.

My experience has shown that it is particularly important for those interested in the functioning of the ear to understand the concepts behind the extensive (often implicit) use of repetitive, sinusoidally shaped waveforms (i.e. pure tones) as acoustic stimuli. For those readers whose appreciation of this technique is limited or rusty, three appendices introduce the formal definition of sinusoidal waveforms and illustrate their usefulness in the analysis of temporal signals and system behavior. The material in these appendices, especially Appendix A, is therefore important for understanding the book as a whole, and it should be studied by readers unfamiliar with (or forgetful of) that material. Written with a minimum of mathematics, the appendices make considerable use of examples and analogies.

The figures in the book reprinted from the literature have been selected as those most clearly presenting the effects discussed in the text. The caption of each of these figures includes the explanatory material and then, if permission was needed, an asterisk, which indicates that there is a notation of the copyright holder in the reference list under the particular article or book from which the illustration was borrowed.

The bibliography is of necessity limited to a tiny fraction of what has been published in the field. My intent was to give some of the latest references on each topic, reviews if available, and some of the seminal papers.

C. D. G.

Madison, Wis.
April 1997

ACKNOWLEDGMENTS

I am greatly indebted to many people for their personal assistance in the creation of this book. Many contributions are indirect, the result of provocative discussions carried on with colleagues around the world. I am particularly indebted to my compatriots here at the University of Wisconsin in Madison—faculty, students, staff—who have provided me with a wonderfully supportive and stimulating environment for more than 30 years.

I especially thank Donata Oertel for suggesting the book and for providing an important early review. The penetrating critique of the initial manuscript by Richard Lyon is also greatly appreciated, as are the reviews of William Rhode and Nigel Cooper. Individual chapters benefited from the insightful reviews and suggestions of John Brugge, Robert Fettiplace, John Guinan, Veronica Heide, Joseph Hind, Keith Kluender, Mark Pyle, and Robert Wickesberg. Their input has been most helpful and is much appreciated.

Further thanks are due to John Brugge for making the animations produced under his direction available for viewing on the Department of Neurophysiology's World Wide Web site (see Fig. 1.1). Thanks also to Ravi Kochhar for his creation and maintenance of that Web site.

My very special thanks to Carol Dizack for creating all of the drawn figures, some more than once, and for preparing the reproductions of contributed and previously published figures. Thanks also to Jeffrey House of Oxford University Press for his support and advice.

It should be acknowledged that most of the contributions to the field of ear research in the United States have been supported by the National Institute of Deafness and Other Communication Disorders (NIH). As is shown herein, that support is proving to be a wise investment. Support by the University of Wisconsin—Madison for my own work is also gratefully recognized, as is the access to the fascinating world of audition provided for me by Walter Rosenblith, my former major Professor.

I am also grateful for the support and suggestions of my family and friends, notably Alvin Y. Yoshinaga and Janet Schrieber.

Finally, a heartfelt tribute goes to my wife, Peg, for her unfailing support and encouragement throughout this task and throughout my entire career.

CONTENTS

1. Introduction   3
   Task of the Ear   3
   Characteristics of Transformations by the Ear   4
   General Organization of this Book   5
   Entrée   7

I MECHANISMS OF THE EAR

2. Sound Waves   11
   Propagation of Sound Waves   12
   Amplitudes   14
   Waveforms   17
   Frequency–Pressure Range of Human Perception   20

3. External Ear   23
   Acoustic Considerations   23
   Physical Mechanisms of Interaural Sound Differences   28
   Functional Usage of Interaural Differences   33
   Implications Regarding Performance of the Auditory System   35

4. Middle Ear   37
   Reptilian Middle Ear   37
   Mammalian Middle Ear   40
   Middle Ear Muscles   49
   Diagnostic Tests Involving the Middle Ear   52
   Recapitulation   53

5.   Sound-Induced Vibrations in the Inner Ear   55
        Basic Anatomy   55
        Sound Propagation in the Inner Ear   56
        Mechanical Measurements in Dead Cochleas   57
        Model of Cochlear Partition Vibrations   60
        Mechanical Measurements in Living Cochleas   64
        Response Patterns to Complex Sounds   69
        A Look Ahead   70
6.   Transfer of Sound-Induced Vibrations to Sensing Cells   72
        Functional Anatomy   72
        Basic Mechanical Motions   80
        Chemical and Electrical Milieu of the Organ of Corti   85

II   HAIR CELL FUNCTIONS

7.   Transduction Processes in Hair Cells   91
        Structural Anatomy   92
        Transduction of Ciliary Rotations into Cell Potentials   94
        Mechanisms of Hair Cell Frequency Selectivity   101
8.   Hair Cells of the Mammalian Cochlea   109
        Structural Anatomy   109
        Ion Flows Through Plasma Membranes   111
        Basic Electrophysiology   112
        Transduction Potentials   114
        Motility of Outer Hair Cells (''Reverse Transduction'')   118
9.   Cochlear Amplifier   125
        Historical Background   125
        Role of Outer Hair Cells in Cochlear Partition Vibrations   127
        Cochlear Model   133
        Another Possible Amplification Process   137
        Summary   138
10.   Nonlinear Responses of the Cochlear Partition:
      Suppressions and Otoacoustic Emissions   139
        Review of Linear Systems   140
        ''Two-Tone'' Suppressions   140
        Otoacoustic Emissions   152
        Summary of Nonlinear Phenomena   164

III   NEURAL RESPONSES

11.   Afferent Innervation   169
        Synaptic Transmission Between Hair Cells and
            Afferent Neurons   170
        Neural Activity in the Absence of Deliberate
            Acoustic Stimulation   175
12.   Responses of Primary Auditory Neurons to
      Single Tones   183
        General Pattern of Responses   184
        Properties of Discharge Rate Responses   187
        Temporal Synchronization of Discharges to
            Stimulus Waveforms   197

13. Responses of Primary Auditory Neurons to Other
    Basic Sounds   204
        Relations Between Time and Frequency   204
        Responses to Clicks   206
        Responses to Random Noise   208
        Responses to Modulated Tones   211
        Responses to Pairs of Tones   216
        Coda   227

14. Responses of Primary Auditory Neurons to
    Speech Sounds   229
        Speech Acoustics   230
        Responses to Vowel Sounds   233
        Responses to Certain "Voiceless" Consonants   237
        Class of Useful Models   238
        Responses to Consonant–Vowel Combinations (Syllables)   239
        Responses to Syllables in Noise   244
        Summary   247

15. Feedback from the Central Nervous System   249
        Anatomy   250
        Responses of Single Efferent Neurons   253
        Cochlear Responses to Efferent System Activation   256
        Neurotransmitters of the Efferent Systems   264
        Model of MOC Efferent Activity   265
        Functions of the Cochlear Efferent Systems   268
        Roles of Efferents in other Acousticolateralis Systems   271
        Synopsis   272

IV DAMAGE AND TREATMENT

16. Damage to the Ear and Hearing Impairment   275
        Threats to the Sense of Hearing   275
        Defects in the External and Middle Ears ("Conductive"
            Hearing Losses)   277
        Defects in the Inner Ear ("Sensory" and "Strial" Losses)   280
        Defects in Primary Auditory Neurons (Neural Pathology)   291
        Tinnitus   292
        Summary   294

17. Treatments for Damaged Ears   295
        Procedures and Prostheses for Treating Middle Ear Disorders   296
        Aids for Treating Inner Ear Disorders   297
        Treatments for Tinnitus   311
        Repair and Regrowth of the Damaged Cochlea   312
        Curtain   315

Appendix A: Fourier Theory: Representation of Continuous
Waveforms with Sinusoids   318
        Sinusoids (Sines and Cosines)   318
        Usefulness of Sinusoids   320
        Harmonic Relations   321
        Fourier Series   322
        Fast Fourier Transform   325
        Aperiodic Signals   326
        Other Analysis Techniques   327

Appendix B: Acoustic Resonances   328

Appendix C: Impedance   330
    Responses of Linear (Time-Invariant) Systems   330
    Impedance Calculations   331

References   339
Index   371

FROM SOUND TO SYNAPSE

1

INTRODUCTION

TASK OF THE EAR

The auditory sense in mammals is capable of almost unbelievable feats. Barn owls, for instance, can successfully hunt in total darkness, guided by the slight sounds made by their prey. Many bats are able to detect, track, and capture a moth using only reflected sound pulses within a few tenths of a second, even though the moth hears the bat's sonar pulses and takes evasive action. The temporal sensitivity of the sonar system that underlies this ability is estimated to be as fine as 10 nanoseconds ($1/100$th of a microsecond). Although the temporal sensitivity of humans is not as precise, our hearing capabilities are such that we can recognize a familiar voice with the utterance of a single word. Cat hearing is so sensitive your pet can detect sounds not much stronger than those made by air molecules bumping against each other.

The first stage in any auditory system is sound detection. In some systems, such as an electronic sound recorder, the detector has a relatively simple job. It must transduce the sound signal into an electrical signal whose wave shape is, as far as possible, an exact replica of the incoming acoustic wave shape. In mammals, however, indeed everywhere in the vertebrate kingdom, the sound detector has a much more complex function. It must work between two arenas with extremely different characteristics. In the external arena, a single continuous acoustic waveform forms its input, while in the internal arena its output is a barrage of neural pulses traveling concurrently on a group of nerve axons that may number many thousands. Thus the ear, during the process of detecting and encoding the acoustic signal, accomplishes a large degree of *transformation*.

After decades of work by legions of dedicated workers, we now have a broad-brush picture of just how this remarkable acoustic-to-neural transformation occurs in the mammalian ear. It is the purpose of this book to present that overview. Delving into this complicated system, we must consider separately the workings of many of its constituent parts, even of some individual cells. Lest we lose sight of the forest for the trees, three fundamental, interrelated characteristics of the ear can serve as a framework around which to organize the pieces of the puzzle.

CHARACTERISTICS OF TRANSFORMATIONS BY THE EAR

First and foremost, the ear seems devoted to *preserving the temporal structure* of the incoming signal. To meet this demand with the often brief and rapidly changing acoustic waveforms that occur in nature, the entire ear is mechanically and biochemically fine-tuned for ultra-fast reactions (often the fastest in the body). Consequently it has a short ''attention span.'' That is, acoustic events that occurred more than a few milliseconds before the present instant are generally ignored, except for setting the ear's ''attention'' at a certain stimulus level. The neural output of the ear, then, is generally a moment-by-moment reflection of the always changing acoustic environment.

The second general feature of the ear is that *changes in stimulus intensity* seem far more important than the absolute intensity levels themselves. Like the eye, the ear adapts to the general intensity level of the incoming signal. In particular, the portion of the ear's machinery that encodes the auditory signal into neural pulses is devoted largely to registering accurately, even emphasizing, the *shape* of the incoming acoustic waveform, not its size.

The third and closely related feature is that the ear, again like the eye, performs an enormous amount of *amplitude compression* during the process of its signal transformations. The amplitudes of incoming sound waves can vary by seven orders of magnitude, from a pin dropping to explosions; their neural representations must be squeezed down to fit within the few hundred pulses per second that characterize the maximum discharge rates of the neurons serving the ear. To accomplish this Herculean task, the sizes of the responses are systematically compressed during virtually every stage of the ear's transduction process. Impressively, the overall compression is done with such finesse that the signal's wave *shape* is well preserved at all but the highest intensity levels.

GENERAL ORGANIZATION OF THIS BOOK

This book is organized to lead the reader, stage by stage, through the ear along the same pathway an acoustic signal would take: collection by the outer ear, conduction through the middle ear, and introduction into the inner ear where it travels down a long, thin duct, setting up a train of individualized mechanical vibrations as it progresses. These individual vibrations are then sensed by highly specialized detectors and encoded into patterns of neural signals that are rapidly conducted to the brain stem. Signals from the central nervous system are fed back to the ear at numerous points along this pathway, and their roles are considered herein at appropriate places. The book's journey ends with a consideration of ear impairments and the treatments and aids presently available for their amelioration.

For purposes of clarification, current models of various stages of sound processing are included at various points in the text. To be sure, many types and levels of models exist. Some are little more than compact descriptions of the data. Let us say, for example, that the vibrations of a particular structure within the ear were found to vary in size in a manner that was inversely proportional to the frequency of an incoming tone. At one level, this relation could be represented (modeled) with the simple equation: amplitude = (C/frequency), where C is an arbitrary constant chosen to fit the equation to the data most closely. A summary relation is thus obtained, but it provides no insight into the mechanisms involved.

On another, much deeper level, this same mathematical equation could be the final product of an explicit theory. In the case at hand, let us theorize that the observed inverse relation is due solely to frictional forces housed within the structure being measured. To test this theory we take the above equation, which is known to describe the idealized action of frictional forces alone, measure the strengths of the structure's internal friction processes, and use those strengths to estimate the value of the constant C in the equation. If the equation's output were to compare well with the physiological data, the model (i.e., the explicit realization of the theory) would be said to *account for* the experimental data.

Of course, the phrase ''account for'' must always be used with caution. Strictly speaking, it simply means that the model, when subjected to certain types of stimuli, responds in the same manner as does the physiological system. It does not necessarily *prove* that the model accurately reflects the basic mechanisms involved, though of course it may. In fact, there are often several quite different models that can account equally well for any limited set of responses. Naturally, if one particular model comes to account successfully for more and more of a system's behavior, it tends to dominate our thinking; and we begin to think that this model does indeed capture, to some extent at least, the mechanisms involved. It is this type of captivating model we utilize herein. In general, the simplest models that seem faithful to the basic processes involved are presented here, with ample references to models of more sophistication and complexity.

To help visualize some of the complicated mechanical motions and electrical processes that take place in the ear, yet another type of model can be used, computer *animation*. Sets of these pictorial movies have been developed by several research groups. Those developed here at the Department of Neurophysiology at the University of Wisconsin—Madison are available to the reader through the World Wide Web. These simulations, listed pictorially in Figure 1.1, are referred to at appropriate places in the book. Other animations and much other information regarding hearing are available in the ''virtual library'' maintained by the Association for Research in Otolaryngology on its web site (address: http://www.aro.org).

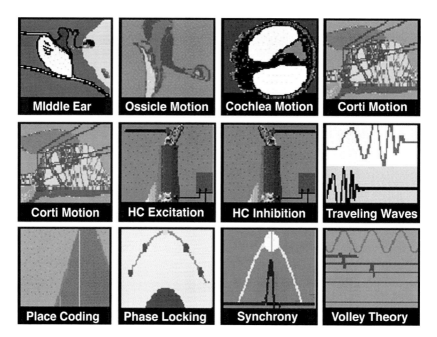

Figure 1.1. World Wide Web page that contains the icons of available animations. Click on the appropriate icon for desired animation. The web address is http://www.neurophys.wisc.edu/animations.

ENTRÉE

The tasks of the mammalian ear are accomplished by some astonishing and elegant mechanisms. As you read, I hope that you will come to share my great sense of awe for this beautiful system.

I

MECHANISMS OF THE EAR

2

SOUND WAVES

We live at the bottom of an ocean—an ocean of air molecules. Free to move independently, each molecule is in constant motion, colliding incessantly with its neighbors. Because the bouncing air molecules move randomly in every possible direction, they collide with any objects that happen to be around. It is the collective effect of all of these tiny molecular collisions on an object that produces "air pressure," as each collision produces a force (just as the collision of billiard balls does so). At sea level this air pressure is equivalent to that of a column of mercury 30 inches high.

It is *changes* in air pressure that we experience as sounds. Such changes may be minuscule or enormous, slow or rapid, localized or diffuse. The task of the ear is to detect them, translate them into the long-distance code of the nervous system (nerve pulses), and send the resulting signal to the brain. The very nature of air pressure imposes both the dimensions and the limitations of this task. For example, the randomness with which air molecules move ("Brownian motion") means that there is a randomness to the collision rate of air molecules with an object such as the eardrum. These unavoidable variations in collision rate produce small but continuous variations in pressure. These naturally occurring but meaningless pressure variations obscure smaller pressure signals, thereby setting a lower limit to the magnitude of the sounds the ear can detect. There are practical upper limits as well (see Frequency–Pressure Range of Human Perception, below).

Because of their obvious importance to our understanding of the ear's operation, this chapter is devoted to an exploration of some of the important attributes of air pressure and sound.

PROPAGATION OF SOUND WAVES

Air pressure variations do not remain where they are produced but propagate outward from the source at different velocities in different types of elastic media. At sea level, for example, the velocity of sound propagation in air is 344 m/sec, or about one-fifth of a mile per second (hence the ''5-second rule'' for determining approximate distance from a bolt of lightning). Such propagation occurs because of the dense packing of the air molecules. To understand this concept let us follow the events caused by the lateral movements of a thin, stiff plate at one end of a tube (Fig. 2.1). Assume that the plate is stationary in a vertical position until a certain time, denoted as $t = 0$, when it is given a small instantaneous displacement to the right of magnitude d (greatly exaggerated in Fig. 2.1). The air molecules located directly in front of the plate are of course pushed along in front of it and jammed

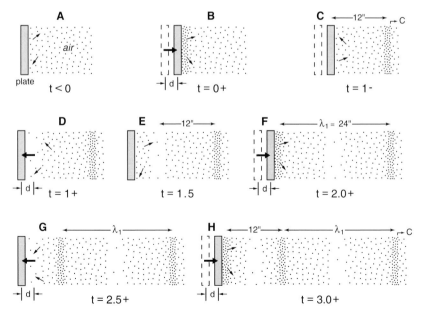

Figure 2.1. ''Snapshots'' obtained during the development of a sound wave generated by a pulsating flat plate at one end of a long tube. Wavelength (λ) is indicated. All features of the wave travel with the same velocity c. Exaggerated movements of two air molecules are indicated with thin arrows.

into the resident molecules in the next adjacent thin sheet of air (Fig. 2.1B). Thus immediately after the plate's movement (at $t = 0+$), a sheet of air bordering the plate has increased density (called *condensation*) because there has not been time enough for the molecules in that sheet to redistribute. They are therefore undergoing a higher collision rate than normal (as we would experience if walking in a suddenly more crowded shopping mall). Because collisions produce pressure, this increased collision rate means that an increased pressure now exists directly in front of the plate. This close correlation between density and pressure is an important aspect of sound propagation.

Consider now the evolution that occurs. The molecules originally pushed by the plate were given added velocity towards the right (hence extra energy and momentum). Through multiple collisions, this extra energy and momentum are quickly transferred to other molecules, literally bumping them to the right (see Fig. 3.2B). By that process the region of increased density also moves: It now appears in the second air sheet, just to the right of the first one. A similar sequence of events bumps molecules from the second sheet into the third, and so on. When we freeze this process just before $t = 1$ *msec* (Fig. 2.1C), we find that the thin sheet of condensation has moved far to the right (about 1 foot). It is important to realize that this traveling condensation (and traveling increased pressure) does *not* involve the long-distance travel of individual air molecules. Because of the close packing, the latter cannot move far in 1 msec (e.g., follow the two identified air molecules through the panels). The only things that move steadily away from the plate are the momentum and the energy generated by the plate's original movement. The properties of air are such that this sheet of condensation travels through the tube with relatively little change in its shape, although it gradually loses its sharp edges with distance.

Assume now that the plate is suddenly snapped back to its original position at $t = 1$ *msec*. Immediately after this movement the suddenly recreated volume of air space lying immediately in front of the plate contains a partial vacuum (called *rarefaction*) because molecules have not yet had a chance to flow into it (Fig. 2.1D). Thus molecules bordering that rarefaction undergo fewer bumps from right-moving molecules than from left-moving (there are fewer molecules to their left), and so they receive a *net* bump to the left. Accordingly, some border molecules flow leftward, eliminating thereby the rarefaction immediately in front of the plate, and creating an area of rarefaction in the space left behind. In other words, the sheet of rarefaction also travels, just as fast and just as securely as the sheet of condensation in front of it (Fig. 2.1E).

Finally, let us assume that the plate again moves instantaneously to the right at $t = 2$ *msec*. The same condensation process described above again occurs immediately in front of the plate, and so now two propagating sheets of condensation exist (Fig. 2.1F). Several important concepts can be clarified by examining this panel. First, note that the distance between the two regions of compression is 2 feet. This distance is appropriately called the *wavelength* of the pressure wave, assumed for the moment to repeat regularly (i.e., be "periodic"). This wavelength (usually indicated by the Greek letter lambda, λ) stays the same with time, as each segment of the wave is propagating at the same velocity. Second, because one full cycle of the wave took 2 msec to generate, 2 msec is the interval that separates the arrivals of the two condensations at any fixed location down the tube. This interval is called the *period* of the wave (often written as T). The wave's period and the wavelength are intimately related: the shorter the period, the shorter the wavelength. This relation can be written formally as

$$\lambda = cT \text{ or } c = f\lambda, \tag{2.1}$$

where c is the velocity of sound, and f is the frequency of the assumed periodic repetitions ($f = 1/T$).[1] This equation is well known, applicable to a wide variety of wave phenomena. Its validity is demonstrated in the last two panels of Figure 2.1, for which the assumption of periodicity was relaxed. Here only 1 msec separates the creation of the second and third compression sheets. Because sound propagation velocity remains constant throughout (ca. 1 foot/msec), the third sheet of condensation is now traveling only 1 foot behind the second. Thus as the first form of the equation states, halving the period of a wave segment halves its wavelength as well.

AMPLITUDES

Variations with Distance

Continuing the examination of Figure 2.1, note that the density of the compression segments is about twice that of the undisturbed air. This amount of compression, which could be created only by an explosion, is *far* beyond that encountered in everyday sounds. It is clear that much smaller compressions could have been created in our example simply by moving the plate shorter distances (displacing smaller volumes of air). The density variation in the wave therefore is another of its important parameters. Density is difficult to measure, so instead we measure pressure, the inevitably occurring consequence of the density variations. For the tube configuration of Figure 2.1 the pressure pattern produced by the traveling wave is one-dimensional and does not change appreciably with time or distance traveled. Thus the pressure pattern produced directly in front of the plate is virtually the same as that which eventually arrives far down the tube.

This conservation is not true for a sound wave propagating in free space. Consider, for example, the three-dimensional sound wave depicted in Figure 2.2. Imagine the sound source, which lies at the center of the figure, to be a sphere whose surface alternately expands and contracts at 1 msec intervals (i.e., in the same temporal pattern as the plate movements of Fig. 2.1A–F). Each expansion of the sphere's volume produces a thin shell of air compression (condensation) that propagates away from the source at the speed of sound. The wavelength of the resulting wave is then 2 feet, the same as it was in Figure 2.1F.

In this spherical case the pressure variations in the sound wave decrease as the wave propagates outward. The reason for this decrease can be heuristically couched in terms of energy. For the instant of the "snapshot" in Figure 2.2 there is a certain amount of acoustic energy contained within the thin shell of compressed air centered at radius R_1. That same amount of acoustic energy must be found within the shell when it has expanded to radius R_2, assuming that negligible amounts of energy are absorbed by the air in between. The volume of the expanding compressed-air shell (ca. $4\pi R^2$ * *thickness*) increases with the square of its distance from the center of the sphere, yet the total amount of acoustic energy contained within the shell must remain unchanged. Hence the *density* of acoustic energy (e.g., energy/ cm^3) within the shell must vary inversely with R^2 (the shell's thickness does not vary appreciably). Finally, because the acoustic pressure in a spherically expanding pressure wave is approximately proportional to the square root of its energy density (for large R), the acoustic pressure inside the expanding

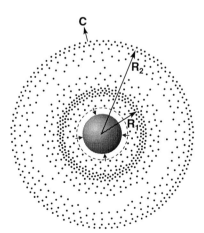

Figure 2.2. "Snapshot" showing the spherically expanding sound wave generated by a sphere periodically pulsating in its radius (arrows). The radii of two successive compression shells, each moving with velocity c, are given (R_1 and R_2).

shell of Figure 2.2 must be decreasing in proportion to its radius (because $\sqrt{R^2} = R$). That is, once away from the source, the pressure in the spherical sound wave is inversely proportional to the distance traveled (Beranek, 1993). Because sound sources in nature typically radiate sound energy in an approximately spherical fashion, at least until the wavefront is reflected from surrounding objects or the ground, this inverse relation between sound pressure and distance traveled accounts for the perception that sounds grow steadily weaker as one moves away from a source located out in the open.

Logarithmic (Decibel) Pressure Scale

Speaking of acoustic pressure, this is a good point at which to introduce the scales by which acoustic pressure is measured. For comparison purposes, note that sea-level atmospheric pressure is, in the metric-mks system, 10^5 Pascals (1 Pascal = 1 Newton/meter^2). Pressures of the weakest tones that average young human adults can hear (in our most favorable frequency range) have been measured at about $20*10^{-6}$ Pascals (20 μPa). This hearing "threshold" corresponds to an amazingly small fractional change of 2 parts in 10 billion ($2*10^{-10}$) in existing air pressure. We hear without difficulty sounds of increasing pressure until levels are reached that are more than a million times more intense than the threshold pressure (see Fig. 2.4).

This wide range of pressures presents two problems. The first is a minor display problem. How do we graph pressure? If we use a linear scale with, for example, 1,000,000 * threshold as the maximum value, all pressures less than about 10,000 * threshold (e.g., maximum/100) become indistinguishable on the graph. Yet those lower values form our most important acoustic region, the one where we spend most of our lives. One answer is to use a logarithmic scale, as we often do for systems that have large ranges of possible values ("dynamic ranges").

The logarithmic scale used with acoustic pressure is somewhat unusual in that it does not give absolute sound pressures but, rather, pressures relative to a "reference" pressure arbitrarily chosen to be the same 20 μPa threshold level mentioned above. Specifically, the logarithmic amplitude of any sound can be determined simply by taking the logarithm (base 10) of the *ratio* of that sound's pressure compared to 20 μPa. For historical reasons, the resulting number is multiplied by 20 and given the units of "*decibels sound pressure level*" (dB SPL). Thus the reference pressure itself has an amplitude of 0 dB SPL (its relative magnitude is unity, and the log of unity is zero), and a pressure of 2000 μPa has a value of 40 dB SPL (its relative magnitude is 100, and the log of 100 is 2). The useful range of sound pressures for human listeners extends over seven orders of magnitude: from

0 dB SPL (our most sensitive thresholds) to 140 dB SPL (painfully and dangerously loud).

The decibel scale has proved to be a natural and useful one for both physiological and perceptual investigations of hearing. This fit exists because, roughly speaking, both the neural encoding of sound magnitude (see Chapter 12) and its perception tend to be logarithmic in nature. Analogies are instructive for getting the ''feel'' for this measuring system. If we limit ourselves to the usually encountered 0- to 100-dB range, the monetary or fahrenheit-temperature scales are suggested. Such well known metrics, in addition to having the convenient span of 100, imply a more or less equal weighting of differences that occur anywhere within that span. For example, the difference between 25 and 30 cents is the same nickel difference as that between 70 and 75 cents. Subjective loudness judgments made by human subjects, in fact, do tend to behave in the same way. For example, the difference in loudness between tones of 70 and 80 dB SPL is judged to be similar to the difference between 40 and 50 dB tones.

A second, much more serious problem generated by the large dynamic range of acoustic signals was mentioned in Chapter 1: The range of incoming sound pressures with which the ear must deal covers more than seven orders of magnitude, whereas its output signals (the nerve pulses of auditory neurons) are functionally limited in rate to approximately two orders of magnitude (see Chapter 12). This large difference between input and output dynamic ranges means that the acoustic signals must somehow be ''compressed'' in amplitude as they proceed through the ear. This unavoidable compression, and the elegant way in which it is achieved, comprises one of the basic themes of this book.

An acoustic wave also possesses *intensity*, which is a measure of the acoustic *power* (energy per second) the wave transmits through a cross-sectional area of unit dimensions (i.e., 1 m^2) (Beranek, 1954). Although frequently used (incorrectly) to designate sound pressure, sound intensity is in fact proportional to the square of sound pressure.

WAVEFORMS

Fourier Analysis and Synthesis

If we were now to measure the pressure wave generated in Figure 2.1 as it passes some point down the tube, we would obtain a waveform with an alternating series of brief condensation and rarefaction pulses (idealized in Fig. 2.3A). Considering how arbitrary was its manufacture, it is clear that a literally infinite number of other waveforms could have been created. How

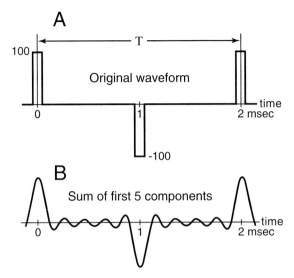

Figure 2.3. Example of Fourier series analysis and synthesis. *A*. Signal waveform. *B*. Sum of the first five components in the Fourier series representing the signal waveform *A*.

are we to organize our work in the face of such vast numbers? Perhaps a catalogue of all of the waveforms (e.g., pulses, smooth wiggles, jagged wiggles) should be created and the ear's processing of each type of waveform determined.

For reasons that become clearer as we progress, Fourier analyses are much more elegant and natural approaches to many acoustic problems (for review see Appendix A). With periodic pressure waves, for instance, we could utilize the following Fourier series method. First we would represent the acoustic waveform, regardless of its shape, as a sum of cosines and sines. This protocol amounts to decomposition of the waveform into sinusoidal elements and is allowable because Fourier's particular way of summing sinusoids is known to match exactly such a waveform. Next we would measure how the ear responds to each of the individual sinusoids making up the waveform. Finally, we would add all of the responses to these individual sinusoids to synthesize a single output waveform, which according to the theory would be virtually identical to the response generated by the ear were the original waveform to be used as the stimulus.

In other words, the *sum of the responses* produced separately by each of the individual sinusoids into which the waveform was decomposed is theoretically identical to the single response produced by presentation of the *sum of the input sinusoids* (i.e., the original waveform). As an example of this basic summation principle, consider the simple system whose function is to multiply its input by the constant A. Let x and y be two sinusoids; then $(Ax + Ay)$, the sum of the responses to x and y presented individually, is equal to $A(x + y)$, the response to x and y presented simultaneously.

The beauty of such a procedure (when it works) is that, regardless of the shape of the original waveform, we can accurately predict a system's response to it knowing only how the system processes a single type of signal, the sinusoid. Alas, this beautiful decomposition–recombination procedure has been tried on the ear and does not always give correct answers, particularly for inner ear processes. Why not? Because the ear is in general a "nonlinear" system, and Fourier processing works (perfectly) only for "linear" systems.[2]

Why then should we persist in using Fourier techniques if they do not work well? In fact, they work nearly perfectly for normal acoustic pressures and external ear processes (which are essentially linear), they give good first approximations for middle ear processes (which are nearly linear), and they even give ballpark estimates for many inner ear processes (some of which are strongly nonlinear). The latter estimates are possible because the inner ear, even though nonlinear, has an anatomical organization that, roughly speaking, does decompose each incoming waveform into many sinusoids (more precisely, bands of sinusoids—see Chapter 5). In fact, this separation into frequency bands accomplished by the inner ear is maintained throughout much of the brain's auditory nervous system. Just how these bands are recombined to provide the unitary nature of auditory perception (the "binding problem") is presently unknown.

To summarize, Fourier analysis has proved to be a useful tool for studying the ear. Like all tools, though, it must be used with care.

Example

Figure 2.3 illustrates the power of Fourier decomposition. Shown in Figure 2.3A is a pulse waveform of the type generated in Figure 2.1A–F. Let us suppose that this waveform, which has maximum pressures of 100 μPa and a duration of 2 msec, is repeated ad infinitum, creating a periodic acoustic wave whose period is 2 msec. Upon calculation, the first term of its Fourier series decomposition (the "fundamental" component) is found to be a cosine wave of 500 Hertz (Hz) with an amplitude of 19.5 μPa. The second and third terms in the Fourier decomposition are also cosine waves, having frequencies of 1500 and 2500 Hz, respectively, the third and fifth multiples (harmonics) of the fundamental component's frequency (the "fundamental frequency").

The sum of the first five Fourier components of the original waveform is shown in Figure 2.3B. Even though its major pulses are wider than those of the original and there are unwanted minor pulses between the major pulses, this sum has the same general shape as the original (alternating condensation and rarefaction pulses). Thus the claim made in Appendix A that an arbitrarily close fit to the original waveform (except at the discontinuities) could be achieved by adding more and more sinusoids becomes plausible. Examination of the waveform in Figure 2.3B gives a hint of how this increasingly accurate replica is manufactured by the "sum of sinusoids." For those moments during which the original waveform has large values the sinusoids add their values together (as the five cosines do at $t = 0$, and again at 1 and 2 msec), whereas for those moments when the original has small values the sinusoids tend to cancel each other out.

The question might be raised as to how we know that the Fourier decomposition of the original waveform is unique. Perhaps other combinations of sinusoids would give equally good approximations. Happily, there are none. It can be shown that *any* deviation from Fourier decomposition degrades the resulting approximation, creating mismatches that cannot be corrected, no matter how many terms are used in the sum.

FREQUENCY–PRESSURE RANGE OF HUMAN PERCEPTION

The propagation of sound in air is an essentially linear process for all the sound pressures we normally encounter. Thus application of Fourier analysis to virtually all of our acoustic problems is permissible, allowing us to regard any air-conducted sound as the sum of its sinusoidal components. Measurements made with individual acoustic sinusoids (tones) show that mammalian ears operate over rather large frequency ranges. For example, humans are sensitive to pure tones with frequencies ranging from about 10 Hz to 20 kilohertz (kHz), a range of more than three orders of magnitude (or "decades"), as shown in Figure 2.4 (note the logarithmic frequency axis). Also shown is the range of frequencies heard by the cat, the species from which much of our physiological data have been obtained. Note its extended high frequency hearing, up to 60 kHz. Bats are sensitive to higher frequencies still—as much as an octave (factor of 2) higher in some species (Fay, 1988; Popper and Fay, 1995).

Several other features of relevance to human hearing are shown in Figure 2.4, such as the borderline for pain near 140 dB SPL (von Békésy, 1960) and that for "high risk" of damage to the ear (Melnick, 1991). From 140 dB SPL to about 90 dB SPL is the range of sound pressures capable of producing permanent hearing loss (von Gierke and Ward, 1991). As a general rule for that high pressure region, the more intense the sound, the shorter the time to which a listener can be safely exposed. Note that both firearms

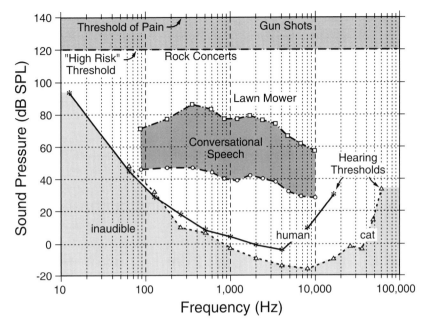

Figure 2.4. Plane showing the sound pressure levels and frequencies of tones (and tonal components of complex sounds) relevant to the hearing of most mammals, particularly humans and cats. Only those tones whose parameters fall above the "Hearing Threshold" curves are audible. The band of parameters that encompass normal English-language speech (Dunn and White, 1940) lies within the shaded area.

and rock concerts produce sound pressures that are well into the danger zone. Also shown is the classically determined range of normal English conversation (Dunn and White, 1940).

With the physical dimensions of perceptually important sound waves thus delineated, we can begin our consideration of the physiological mechanisms involved in their perception. The first step in this process is, of course, detection of the sound wave. As the detector cells are located deep within the head (see Chapter 4), the first job of the ear is to transmit a portion of the impinging sound wave to those cells with as little distortion of the waveform as possible. This transmission begins with the capture of the sound wave by the external ear.

NOTES

1. If the "period" of a periodic wave is (1/*N*)th of a second in duration, then N periods occur in 1 second: that is, the "frequency" (of repetition) of the wave is N per second (now designated as N Hertz)

2. By definition, a "linear system" can be described by a system of linear equations, either algebraic or integrodifferential in our field. Roughly speaking, linearity occurs when *each* variable in the equations appears in the first power only (neither higher nor lower), is never multiplied by itself (including its derivatives and integrals) or by any other variable, and is never subjected to a nonlinear operation (e.g., one, such as "squaring," that forces it into a higher power).

Various attributes of linear systems are mentioned at appropriate points in the text and are illustrated in footnotes. In this section the *distributive* property of linear systems is introduced: that is, any linear operation on the *sum of multiple inputs* produces an output equal to the *sum of the outputs* produced by each of the inputs acting separately. This property was demonstrated in the text for the linear operation of multiplication by a constant.

3

EXTERNAL EAR

The basic role of the external ear is to collect impinging sound waves and channel them toward the inner ear's sensory cells. If that were the whole story, why do we have two ears when one would suffice? An obvious answer is that two ears provide us with the means for capturing two samples of incoming sounds, allowing comparison between them. In fact, the differences between the sound waves arriving at the two ears *do* provide vertebrates with a great deal of information about the location of sound sources. This information is so complete and so accurate that the best auditory localizers, barn owls and some species of bats, can home in on prey with accuracies on the order of 1°. In this chapter we consider not only the mechanisms by which the external ear captures sound, but the resulting cues to the locations of sound sources that result.

ACOUSTIC CONSIDERATIONS

Interaction of Sound Waves and the Head

When propagating sound waves strike the head, they engulf it in a manner analogous to the way ocean waves wash around a small island. Shown in Figure 3.1, this engulfing produces a number of behaviorally important events. Most important of course is the direct exertion of the sound wave pressure on the head. Second is that the sound wave changes as it moves around the head, producing significantly different sound pressures at the two ears. In Figure 3.1, for example, the sound waves are produced by a source located to the right of the subject's head and because of their finite velocity they reach the subject's right ear first. As a consequence, there is a *time* difference in the arrival of the sound waves at the two ears.

In addition, the left ear lies out of sight, within the head's "sound shadow." Thus sound waves must diffuse around the head to reach the far ear, losing amplitude in the process. As a result, there is an *amplitude* difference in the sound pressures striking the two ears. Because this sound-diffusing process is a function of tonal frequency, there are also differences in the frequency compositions of a complex signal received by the two ears. These differences in the amplitude versus frequency profiles (or "spectra") of the two waveform samples thus produce a *spectral* contrast as well.

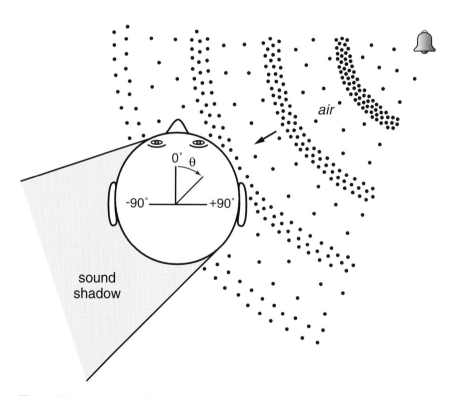

Figure 3.1. Acoustical effects of a source in the horizontal plane at a position ("azimuth") to the right of the midline on sound waves striking each ear. Wave fronts arrive at the near ear sooner and are generally more intense than at the far ear.

Because different locations in space obviously produce different inter-ear ("interaural") time, amplitude, and spectral profile differences, a catalogue of these differences would enable a listener to determine something about the location of the sound source. It should come as no surprise therefore to learn that some of the auditory centers of the vertebrate brain perform exacting temporal and magnitude comparisons between the neural signals coming from the two ears (see Irvine, 1992; Ehret and Romand, 1997).

Wave Transmission Across Boundaries

To detect sound pressures, a sensor of some sort is needed. Perhaps it should be located flush with the scalp, as depicted in Figure 3.2A. From a functional point of view, that is not a good idea, as there is a large mismatch between the physical properties of the air and the sensor, assuming that the sensor is filled with fluid (as in all vertebrate ears). The significance of these physical differences regarding the transmission of sound waves from one medium to the other can be appreciated by considering the greatly simplified situations illustrated in the rest of Figure 3.2.

When one idealized molecule collides dead center with a stationary molecule of equal mass, it can be shown by elementary dynamics that all of the first molecule's energy and momentum are transferred to the second. This transfer results in the abrupt halt of the first molecule and the departure of the second at the same speed (V_0) with which the incoming molecule arrived (Fig. 3.2B). This reaction is almost precisely what happens when two billiard balls collide head on and pictorially depicts collisions that occur between air molecules as sound waves propagate through space.

Consider what happens, however, when a lighter molecule (e.g., of mass m) hits a much heavier molecule (of mass $N*m$, where N is a large number). Upon collision the lighter molecule is bounced backward, with its speed

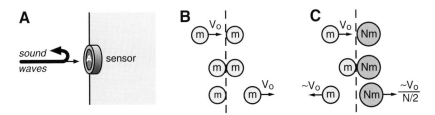

Figure 3.2. *A.* Large reflections of air-borne sound from a fluid-filled sensor. *A* is the area of sensor's input port. *B.* "Snapshots" of a particle with velocity V_0 hitting an identical twin; there is no rebound. *C.* "Snapshots" of one particle hitting a much heavier particle; almost total rebound of the smaller particle occurs, and the heavy particle absorbs little of the incoming energy.

(and therefore its energy) almost undiminished; and the heavier molecule, receiving only a small fraction of the energy originally carried by the lighter molecule, barely moves (Fig. 3.2C). When this example is multiplied many times over to include the myriad air molecules that contribute to air pressure, it can be appreciated that when a sound wave in air hits the surface of a much denser fluid almost all of its energy is reflected from the surface. Little sound is then transmitted into the fluid. In fact, more than 99.9% of the incoming acoustic energy would be reflected away were sound waves to be applied directly to our inner-ear sensors (Killion and Dallos, 1979).

Figure 3.2C suggests that the situation could be improved by somehow combining the energy of many light molecules to move the heavier one. One way to accomplish this (Fig. 3.3A) would be to provide a large movable plate (an "eardrum") as the receiver. When a compression wave now reaches the eardrum, a large number of air molecules strike it, each providing a tiny push inward. If the eardrum has an area that is, for example, 10 times the area of the sensor's input port (A), the total acoustic *force* exerted on the eardrum is 10 times that exerted on the surface-mounted sensor of Figure 3.2A. If this stronger force is transmitted without loss to a deeply sited sensor via a thin, rigid column (Fig. 3.3B), a tenfold increase occurs in the input force exerted on the sensor and thus in its input pressure (recall that pressure = force/area). This calculation of course depends on the assumed perfect transfer of force by the rigid column. The actual transmission efficiency of the middle ear is described in Chapter 4.

Review of Impedance

At the point we must pause to review the concept of impedance (see Appendix C). In every day usage "impedance" means resistance to movement.

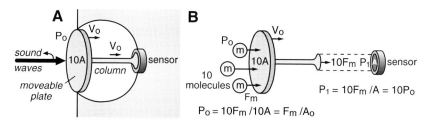

Figure 3.3. A. Large connected plate (i.e., an "eardrum") increases the sound pressure (P_1) exerted on a fluid-filled sensor. B. Pressures involved. The tenfold greater collecting area of the eardrum (10A) increases tenfold the pressure (P_1) exerted on the sensor. V_0, velocity; m, molecules; F_m, The acoustic force exerted by a token air molecule on the eardrum; P_0, pressure on eardrum; A, area.

"Acoustic impedance" is consistent with this usage, being the quantitative relation that exists between an acoustic drive (the pressure over some specified cross-sectional area) and the ensuing physical response (roughly the summed velocities of all the sectors in that cross section). More specifically, *acoustic impedance* is defined as the ratio of acoustic pressure to the "volume velocity" (velocity times cross-sectional area) (Beranek, 1954):

$$\text{Acoustic impedance} = \text{pressure}/(\text{velocity} * \text{area}) \qquad (3.1)$$

Let us assume that the pressure wave hits the eardrum with the magnitude P_0 (Fig. 3.3B). Because of that pressure, the eardrum is moving with velocity V_0. The acoustic impedance presented by the eardrum is therefore

$$P_0/(V_0 * 10A) = 0.1 P_0/(V_0 * A)$$

Focusing now on the sensor input port, we see that its velocity is the same as that at the eardrum (as each end of the rigid column must move at the same speed). Furthermore, the *forces* acting on the eardrum and on the sensor port are equal. However, because the sensor port is 10 times smaller than the eardrum, the *pressure* exerted on the sensor is 10 times greater than that exerted on the eardrum. Thus the acoustic impedance of the sensor is $10 P_0/(V_0 * A)$, or 100 times that of the eardrum.

This difference is of significance because it can be shown mathematically that only when the acoustic impedances of two conducting media are identical can a sound wave be passed from one to the other without some reflection. Thus because there is a ratio of 3880:1 between the measured acoustic impedances of water and air, an initial calculation suggests that the eardrum in our example should actually have had size $62A$ ($62 = \sqrt{3880}$) in order that all of the energy of the air-borne sound wave be transferred to the sensor (i.e., no sound energy reflected). More sophisticated impedance calculations show that this ratio is a function of tonal frequency but has indeed about this magnitude at frequencies above 2 kHz (Killion and Dallos, 1979).

Note that the scheme shown in Figure 3.3A implies that the thin column connecting the ear's outer surface and the acoustic sensor organ must be located in an air-filled chamber (if it were fluid-filled, we return to the original air–fluid mismatch of Figure 3.2C). Such an air chamber, called the "middle ear," is in fact a general characteristic of vertebrate ears. Somewhat startling is the close resemblance of some vertebrate middle ears to the sketch in Figure 3.3A (see Chapter 4).

The results just obtained put an upper limit on how large we can make a useful eardrum: Because acoustic impedances must be matched for efficient

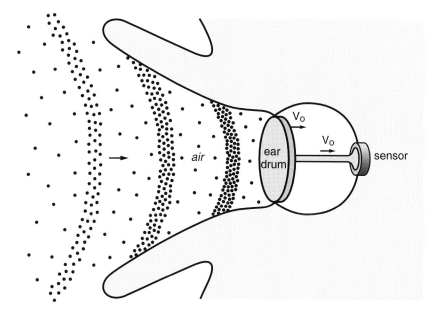

Figure 3.4. "Collecting horn" increases the sound pressure exerted on the eardrum. V_0, velocity.

sound transmission, too large an eardrum would be just as wasteful of incoming acoustic energy as one too small. There are, fortunately, still other ways to improve sound reception. One is simply to channel more sound energy to the eardrum. It can be shown that horns of certain types accomplish this task (Beranek, 1954). Roughly speaking, if the horn is hard and smooth and the taper is gradual enough, negligible sound reflection or absorption occurs at the walls of the horn. Because the *total* sound energy contained in an acoustic wave must be conserved and negligible energy is absorbed or reflected by the horn, the energy *density* of the incoming sound wave must be getting steadily larger as it progresses farther into the steadily narrowing horn (Fig. 3.4). An increase in energy density means an increase in pressure (see Chapter 2), so we indeed have another kind of pressure multiplier. The old-fashioned ear trumpet used by hearing-impaired people before the advent of electronic hearing aids is just such a device.

PHYSICAL MECHANISMS OF INTERAURAL SOUND DIFFERENCES

Amplitude Transformations

The mammalian ear is organized in a fashion similar to that depicted in Figure 3.4. As sketched for humans in Figure 3.5, there is a collecting horn,

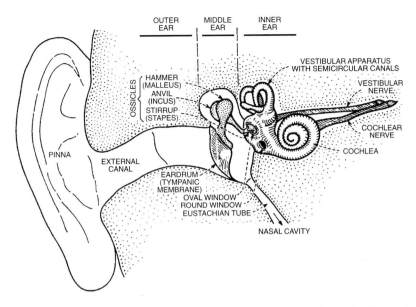

Figure 3.5. Human ear showing the outer, middle, and inner regions. For illustrative purposes, the sizes of the inner and middle ear structures have been exaggerated. (From Flanagan, 1972, with permission.*)

the fleshy shell extending from the side of the head (the *pinna*). It intercepts sound waves and channels them via the external ear canal to the eardrum. The resulting eardrum vibrations are transmitted through an air-filled middle ear by a three-bone structure (*ossicles*) to the inner ear's acoustic sensor (*cochlea*). Because the pinna is larger than the eardrum and the eardrum is larger than the input port of the cochlea (see Chapter 4), both of the pressure multiplications just discussed take place.

The pinnas of different species take on a fascinating array of shapes. Some are large and some small; many are pointed, but some are round; most point upward, but a few flop over (Fig. 3.6). Placement of the pinnas seems intimately related to the animal's behavior. In the moose, for instance, large upright pinnas are located far back on the head. Thus when the animal is grazing on aquatic plants in shallow water, its pinnas stay above the water, delivering acoustic information about its surroundings to the underwater head. Pinnas can also serve other functions, such as radiating heat or signaling mood.

How these pinnas operate acoustically has been quantitatively determined in several species. By inserting small sensing tubes into the external canal, pressures that exist at the eardrum have been measured in both humans (Shaw, 1974; Wightman and Kistler, 1993) and cats (Musicant et al., 1990).

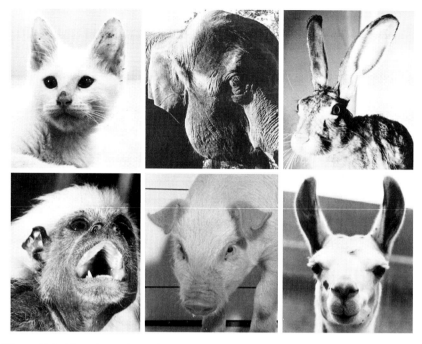

Figure 3.6. Note the variety of mammalian external ears. Clockwise, from top left: cat, elephant, rabbit, llama, pig, marmoset. (Courtesy of Welker, University of Wisconsin—Madison.)

The results are usually presented as a ratio: the pressure that exists at the eardrum compared to the pressure in the incoming wave (i.e., before it hits the head). Because sound propagation in air is basically linear[1] at normally encountered intensities, this ratio (usually expressed in decibels) holds for virtually all sounds of interest.

The amplitudes of the pressures produced at the human eardrum, relative to those of the incoming sound, are shown in Figure 3.7, for tones of different frequency. The different lines correspond to different horizontal angles (''azimuths'') between the midline of the head and the sound source (Fig. 3.1). There are a number of important features of these pressure ''transformations.'' First, pressure amplification does indeed occur. At the source's most favorable location, directly in line with the ear (top curve), pressure multiplication occurs at all frequencies, becoming greater than 5.6 (15 dB) over almost a two-octave frequency range (2–6 kHz). Second, and perhaps even more important from a behavioral point of view, the pressure at the eardrum becomes steadily smaller as the source moves around from the near side (top curve, +60°) to the front (0°) and then to the far side (bottom curve, −75°), casting a sound shadow. Third, all of the transformations share

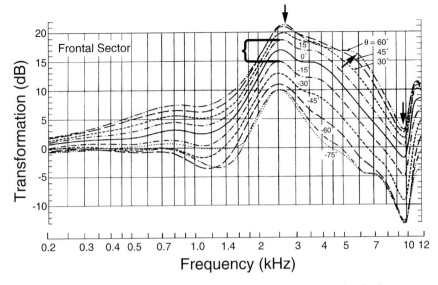

Figure 3.7. Curves showing the boost ("transformation") given by the human external ear to a tone's sound pressure level (in decibels), as the source azimuth in the horizontal plane was varied in 15° increments, as functions of frequency. Zero degrees corresponds to the midline. Arrows and brace indicate important features. (From Shaw, 1974, with permission.*)

some common features, such as the rounded peak at about 2.5 kHz and the sharper dip near 10 kHz (marked by vertical arrows).

The causes of these various features are well understood theoretically. For example, the common peak at 2.5 kHz is due to the "quarter-wave-length resonance" of the ear canal (see Appendix B), which affects equally sounds coming from all directions (because they all must pass through the canal). The other peaks in the transformations are caused by the pinna itself, which with its various cavities and edges supports a number of other resonances (Shaw, 1982a). Resonances depend on the match between cavity dimensions and wavelength, so the relatively small dimensions of the pinna's cavities mean that its resonance frequencies are higher than those of the ear canal. For instance, the small peak in the 5- to 7-kHz region (marked by a slanted arrow) is caused by resonances in the central depression (or *concha*) of the pinna. As shown in Figure 3.7, the magnitude of this concha resonance varies, depending on the horizontal position of the sound source.

The relative height of a sound source above or below the observer also affects the external ear transformations. The pressure-versus-frequency data in Figure 3.8A, from one human subject, show that source elevation determines the frequency of the dip ("notch") in the 6- to 12-kHz region (shown

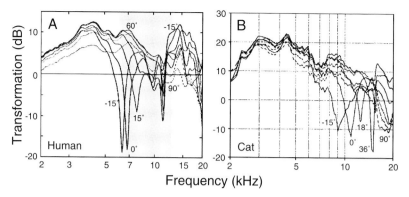

Figure 3.8. Curves showing the boost (''transformation'') given by the external ear to a tone's sound pressure (in decibels), as the source *elevation* in the midplane was varied, as functions of frequency. Zero degrees corresponds to the horizontal plane. *A.* Human subjects. The frequency of the large dip in the 6- to 12-kHz region (shaded) varies systematically with elevation. *B.* For the cat. (*A*: From Shaw, 1982b, with his permission. *B* From Musicant et al., 1990, with permission.*)

shaded). As seen in Figure 3.8B, a similar dependence of the major dip on source elevation occurs in the cat ear, although the frequencies are somewhat higher (Musicant et al., 1990). As expected theoretically, removal of the cat pinna results in large reductions in the magnitudes of these transformations and in the elimination of their major peaks and dips. In bats also—both those species that pursue prey using sonar echoes (Wotton et al., 1995) and those that hunt using prey-generated sounds (Fuzessery, 1996)—prominent notches exist at high frequency that change systematically with source elevation.

To summarize, the external ear transformations that occur at low frequencies (e.g., < 3 kHz in humans) are smoothly varying, with peaks and dips whose frequencies do not vary appreciably with source azimuth. However, these transformations do differ systematically in *magnitude* depending on source azimuth. At somewhat higher frequencies (5–12 kHz in humans), the location of the source in space, both its azimuth and elevation, affect the *shape* of the transformations. In particular, the elevation of a source determines the frequency of the major notch in the transformations. At still higher frequencies (> 12 kHz in humans), the transformations vary markedly with source location but in no simple pattern.

These external ear transformations are the basis for the newly developed ''virtual sound'' sources. For these perceptions of phantom sources, sounds are filtered according to the binaural transformations characteristic of a particular source direction in space. When presented through headphones, those filtered sounds give the impression of originating outside the head, coming from the direction corresponding to those particular transformations.

Complicating the picture for many mammalian species are highly mobile pinnas, which may be individually controlled. As indicated by direct experiments on the cat (Musicant et al., 1990), this type of pinna produces the largest responses when the sound source is broadcasting directly into the pinna (i.e., along the ''acoustic axis'' of the pinna). When the pinna rotates, this acoustic axis also rotates, directing the solid angle of maximum sensitivity toward the spatial region of the animal's concern. Such pinna movements are no doubt beneficial behaviorally, but by introducing another variable into the external ear transformations they complicate the source-localizing tasks of the brain.

Interaural Temporal Differences

Reference back to Figure 3.1 reminds us that the differences in the *arrival times* of a sound wave at the two ears also vary systematically with source direction: The farther the source is to one side (i.e., the greater its azimuth), the greater is the difference in the arrival times. Because the speed of sound propagation is the same at all auditory frequencies (see Chapter 2), this interaural time difference is the same for all sounds emitted by a single source, regardless of their frequency content.

FUNCTIONAL USAGE OF INTERAURAL DIFFERENCES

A great variety of animals use differences in the sounds received by the two ears to estimate the directions of sound sources, just as some use the differences in the images received by the two eyes to estimate the distance of objects. The primary acoustic localization cues known for mammals are the interaural differences we have just considered: amplitude, spectral profile, and time of arrival. In addition, monaural cues exist, such as the frequency of the notch in the 5- to 12-kHz region of the human transformation curve (Fig. 3.8A). At least some mammals appear to use all of these cues when localizing sounds (Blauert, 1983; Middlebrooks and Green, 1991; Wightman and Kistler, 1993).

To test the frequency ranges over which these various cues are utilized by human subjects, the temporal and amplitude differences normally produced at the two ears by different source placements were deliberately scrambled in one set of earphone experiments. The results obtained with bursts of ''broad-band'' noise (roughly, sounds composed of broad frequency bands) indicated that interaural time differences were the dominant localization cue so long as the noise bursts contained energy at frequencies below about 2.5 kHz (Wightman and Kistler, 1992). However, for noise bursts containing only higher frequencies (> 5 kHz), interaural amplitude differences were the dominant localization cue. There are both acoustic constraints[2] and physiological reasons (see Chapter 12) for this division of labor.

Also of interest is the finding that the subjects in this study located sources of broad-band noise more accurately than they located pure-tone sources (Wightman and Kistler, 1992). Perhaps comparisons between the differing spectral profiles of the sounds entering each ear (e.g. Fig. 3.7) were utilized in locating the noise sources, or perhaps interaural comparisons between the noise signals' unambiguous ''marker events'' were made (or both). We can also make monaural estimates of source elevation (Butler and Belendiuk, 1977).

Cats appear to utilize these same sound localization cues (Huang and May, 1996). In behavioral experiments, for instance, they executed accurate ''orienting responses'' (turning their heads toward the direction of a new sound) when presented with bursts of noise with a frequency content limited to their ''mid-frequency'' region (5–18 kHz). Examination of Figure 3.8B shows that this frequency region is precisely the one in which that species' external ear pressure transformations produce strong interaural azimuth and elevation differences. However, when the perception of these mid-frequency peaks and notches in eardrum pressures was denied to these animals by using bursts of a *single* mid-frequency tone, those head orientations became poorly directed, as they did when only high-frequency (>18 kHz) noise bursts were used. It thus appears that mid-frequency spectral cues play important roles in the cat's ability to localize sound sources.

An interesting difference appears to exist between the source localization mechanisms of humans and cats on the one hand and those of pigs on the other. The latter were able to localize low-frequency pure-tone pips well, but they failed absolutely to localize pips of tones having frequencies of 4 kHz or higher, despite hearing them very well (Heffner and Heffner, 1989). Extrapolating from human performance, where temporal localization cues seem to dominate at low frequencies, it appears that pigs utilize only interaural time-of-arrival differences for their sound-source localizations. Perhaps the pressure transformations created by their floppy pinnas are not as dependent on source direction as those observed in species with upright pinnas, such as the cat.

A marvelous variation on the manufacture of interaural amplitude differences occurs in the barn owl. This bird has no obvious external ears, yet the tightly packed feathers of its facial ruffs on each side provide effective acoustic channels for high-frequency sounds (Fig. 3.9). Particularly striking is the asymmetrical placement of the owl's ear openings. The left one is

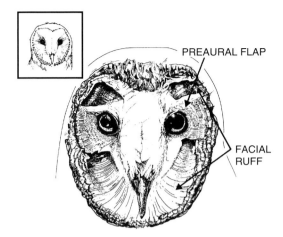

Figure 3.9. Facial ruff and asymmetrical ears of the barn owl. This sketch shows the face of the owl as it would appear if the facial ''disc'' feathers were removed (normal appearance shown in insert). The ear openings lie behind the preaural flaps. Note the asymmetry of the sound channels formed by the facial ruff. (From Knudsen and Konishi, 1979, with permission.*)

located higher in its channel than is the right. For frequencies above 4 kHz, this asymmetry causes the left ear to become more sensitive to sounds originating below the bird's horizontal plane and the right ear to sounds from elevated sources. As a result, this bird's external auditory apparatus plays a dual role. For tones with frequencies below 4 kHz, the ''plane of equal intensity'' (the imaginary surface composed of all locations from which a sound source would produce equal pressures at the two ears) is located vertically at the midline, as it is in humans. As sound frequency is increased above 4 kHz, this bird's plane of equal intensity gradually rotates from vertical to horizontal (Knudsen and Konishi, 1979). Thus a broad-band sound source obligingly provides interaural amplitude cues of both its horizontal and vertical coordinates. Utilizing such acoustic cues, these owls localize sound sources with such exquisite accuracy that they are able to hunt successfully in total darkness (Konishi, 1993).

IMPLICATIONS REGARDING PERFORMANCE OF THE AUDITORY SYSTEM

The acoustic cues used by an animal to estimate sound source direction provide us with useful gauges of the properties its auditory system must possess to utilize such cues. For example, the data in Figure 3.7 show that a source located 15° off the midline would produce in humans an interaural pressure difference of 3–5 dB in the mid-frequency range (the difference between the +15° and −15° curves in Figure 3.7, marked by a bracket). The accuracy with which we localize such sources is about 1.5° (Durlach and Colburn, 1978). Extrapolation from those numbers suggests that our cochleas encode stimulus amplitude with a precision no worse than about 0.5 dB (15°/1.5° = 5 dB/0.5 dB).

Interaural timing cues are dominant in low-frequency localizations, where human observers display accuracies of approximately 1° near the midline (Durlach and Colburn, 1978). A source that far off our midline produces an interaural time delay of only 10 microseconds (μsec) (assuming a 8-inch head diameter). Similar accuracy for a cat, with a much smaller head, would involve interaural delays of only a few microseconds. To achieve such judgments, it appears that mammalian cochleas must preserve interaural time differences with at least that same microsecond precision. Even greater temporal precision is suggested, at least for some species, by experiments that tested the range-finding abilities of big brown bats (Simmons et al., 1990). These animals demonstrated discriminations between two reflected signals that differed in their delays by less than 0.1 μsec.

In later chapters we consider some of the mechanisms by which the inner ear is able to perform such marvels. For the sake of continuity, however, we first must consider the manner in which the acoustic signals make their way from the ear canal into the cochlea. The route lies through the middle ear.

NOTES

1. A linear system has the property that the relation between the system's input and output is the same at *all* intensities. That is, the output "scales" with the input. For example, if $y(t)$ is the response generated in a linear system by an input $x(t)$, an input of $10*x(t)$ produces an output of exactly $10*y(t)$.

2. For *pure tones* having "high" frequencies, the interaural time-of-arrival differences give ambiguous localization cues. This ambiguity occurs whenever the interaural time delay is more than half the tonal period ($T/2$). For example, if a 10 kHz tone ($T = 100$ μsec) causes an interaural time delay of 50 μsec, does the sound wave at the left ear lead that at the right ear by half a cycle or lag by that amount? This ambiguity is eliminated in a broad-band signal containing those same high frequencies, as unambiguous marker *events* occur (e.g., aperiodic peaks in the waveform).

4

MIDDLE EAR

Transmission of sound through the mammalian middle ear is provided by a chain of the tiniest bones in the body. The physical properties of these bones and their supporting structures determine how efficiently this transmission is. In the absence of feedback from the central nervous system, middle ear mechanisms are essentially linear, allowing the highly developed techniques for analyzing passive mechanical systems to be employed. The fruits of those analyses give us a firm understanding of the general attributes of middle ear transmissions.

In the alert mammal, however, the middle ear is not a passive structure but one that is under continuous central control. We will review that control, highlighting its important protective features and its role in enhancing the usefulness of intense acoustic signals.

Because of their similar functions but simpler geometries, the middle ears of reptiles are a good place to start our considerations.

REPTILIAN MIDDLE EAR

A generalized sketch of the reptilian middle ear is shown in Figure 4.1. It is similar enough in structure to that of Figure 3.3A that we can deduce its

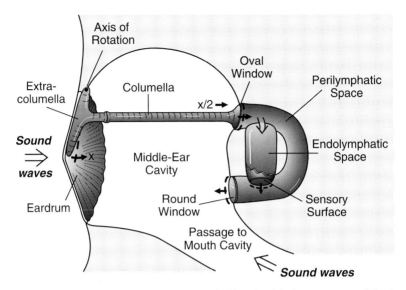

Figure 4.1. Cross section through the ear of a lizard, with the geometry of the inner ear greatly stylized. Because of the offset of the columella's shaft, the oval window vibrates with half the amplitude of the eardrum center. (Adapted from Manley, 1990.)

basic function readily. Sound waves strike the eardrum, located flush with the skin in this case, and cause it to vibrate. These vibrations are then transmitted by a two-element rod to the *oval window*, the input port of the sound-sensing organ (inner ear). There are many variations on this general theme, depending on the species, but this basic layout is common to the middle ears of reptiles, amphibians, and birds (for extensive coverage see books by Wever, 1978; Manley, 1990).

No ear canal is shown in Figure 4.1 because many reptiles do not possess one. In some lizards (e.g., the geckos), and in Crocodylia and birds, the eardrum lies well below the level of the skin, connected to the outside world by an ear canal. In many burrowing lizards this ear canal has only a tiny external opening. In some species even this tiny opening is lost, and the eardrum is covered by scaly skin that can become quite thick.

The eardrum shown in Figure 4.1 is not flat but slightly convex (pointing outward). Connected to the eardrum is the cartilaginous *extracolumella*, which comes in various shapes. In typical lizards it possesses a slender shaft and three or four finger-like processes that contact the eardrum. The shaft of the extracolumella is connected to one end of a thin rod, the *columella*, with a more or less flexible joint. The other end of the columella rests on the oval window.

Of relevance to sound detection is the position of the axis formed by this pair of *ossicles* (literally, "little bones"). Instead of extending from the center of the eardrum, as in Figure 3.3A, it lies closer to the edge of the drum. Thus when the center of the eardrum is deflected laterally by some amount (e.g., x, as in Fig. 3.3), the columella's shaft is deflected laterally by a lesser amount ($x/2$). This loss of deflection magnitude at first glance seems counterproductive. On the contrary, this arrangement acts as a lever system and provides yet another method of increasing pressure at the oval window.[1]

The sound-sensing organ depicted in Figure 4.1 represents no particular species but is presented in its simplest possible form to illustrate the universal organization of vertebrate inner ears. The sensing organ is composed of two abutting fluid-filled systems: perilymphatic and endolymphatic (with different chemical compositions—see Chapter 6). Sound waves, when introduced into the oval window by vibrations of the columella's footplate, propagate through the perilymphatic system and reappear in the middle ear at a membranous port, the *round window*. At first sight this arrangement seems curious. It appears that the sound makes a useless detour through the skull to finally end up back in the middle ear, which lacks acoustic sensors.

In fact, that is what happens, but it is not useless. During the process of traversing the perilymphatic system, the sound wave also enters and propagates through the endolymphatic system. During its travel through the endolymphatic system the sound wave encounters cells that sense sound pressure (actually displacement) and expends most of its energy in exciting these cells and their supporting elements. Thus the sound waves that leave the inner ear at the round window are weak echoes (energy-wise and thus pressure-wise) of the waves that entered the oval window.

Note that because of the virtual incompressibility of the fluids involved this reentry of the sound wave into the middle ear cavity has critical acoustic consequences. If the inner ear had but one port (the oval window) and so formed a closed fluid sack within the skull, the near incompressibility of both lymph and the surrounding bone means that the oval window could not move appreciably (and thus almost all of the incoming acoustic energy would be reflected away and lost). With the existing arrangement, the essentially incompressible fluids within the perilymphatic and endolymphatic systems are free to slosh back and forth. Thus as the oval window is pushed in, the round window is forced out an equal amount (Kringlebotn, 1995). In short, the incoming sound wave *vibrates* a small movable volume of fluids, rather than *pressurizing* the fluids within a rigid container. Nevertheless, even that small movable volume of fluid has a much higher acoustic impedance than an equal volume of air.

There is a seemingly endless variety of shapes in which this basic perilymph–endolymph arrangement is configured in various species, but it is the underlying structural plan of all vertebrate ears studied to date. Why two fluid systems? The sound-sensing cells need the special chemical composition of the endolymph, and the neurons connected to those sensory cells need the differing chemical composition of the perilymph. (see Chapter 7).

MAMMALIAN MIDDLE EAR

Basic Anatomy

The basic layout of the mammalian middle ear is similar to that of the reptilian ear. As shown in Figure 4.2, sound waves propagating in the ear canal strike the eardrum and cause it to vibrate. These vibrations are then

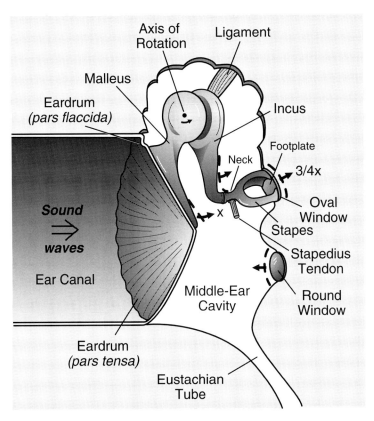

Figure 4.2. Cross section through the human middle ear. The oval window vibrates with three-fourths the amplitude of the eardrum center. Note that the axis of rotation passes through the main concentration of ossicular mass. The *pars flaccida* is a small, limp section of the eardrum that is unconnected to the ossicles. It appears to have several functions, including the release of static pressure within the middle ear (Teoh et al., 1997). (Adapted from Goodhill, 1979.)

transmitted through a three-element ossicular chain to the *oval window*, the input port of the *cochlea* (inner ear). The *round window*, acting here in the same basic manner as in reptilian ears, forms the cochlea's second port (see Chapter 5). Several animations of these middle ear vibrations are available for viewing on the World Wide Web (see Fig. 1.1).

The three ossicles are tiny, the smallest bones in the body. The last two in the guinea pig's chain, the *incus* and *stapes*, and part of the first, the *malleus*, are shown in Figure 4.3. At low frequencies, the ossicles appear to operate as a single rigid unit, principally executing rotary motion about an axis (marked in Fig. 4.2) that passes through the "heads" of the malleus and the incus (von Békésy, 1960). At higher frequencies the ossicular motions become complex, as do those of the eardrum (Decraemer et al., 1989, 1991). Nevertheless, as shown by the exquisite auditory sensitivities of some bats in the 100 kHz region, mammalian middle ears can still function superbly up to high frequencies. At all frequencies ossicular vibrations appear to be basically linear up to intensities of 130 dB SPL of more, so long as contractions of the middle ear muscles do not occur (Guinan and Peake, 1967).

The geometry of Figure 4.2 shows that both of the pressure-amplifying mechanisms of the reptilian middle ear are present in the mammalian middle ear as well. In humans and cats the area of the eardrum is about 20 times

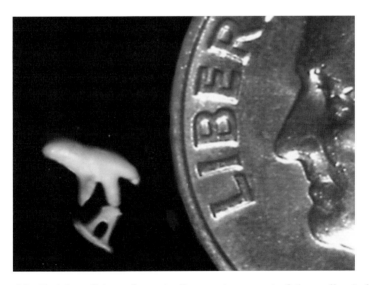

Figure 4.3. Ossicles of the guinea pig (incus, stapes, part of the malleus) shown with a dime for size comparison. (Courtesy of Cooper and Rhode, University of Wisconsin — Madison.)

larger than that of the oval window, and the "lever ratio" (eardrum displacement/stapes displacement) is more than unity: about 1.3 in humans and 2.0 in cats (Guinan and Peake, 1967). The combination of these two geometrical effects should result, theoretically, in a maximum middle ear pressure amplification of about 22 in humans and 43 in cats (but see Chapter 5).

Responses of the Middle Ear to Tones

Amplitudes of the stapes' movements produced in five vertebrate species by various pure tones presented to the ear at a fixed level of 100 dB SPL are shown in Figure 4.4. The curve for the cat is composed of two major segments, with 1 kHz being the dividing ("corner") frequency. Below this corner frequency the curve is approximately horizontal, and above the corner frequency the curve decreases at a more or less constant rate, diminishing by a factor of about 20 (26 dB) for every tenfold increase in frequency (i.e., −26 dB per decade). The stapedial responses measured in a number of other

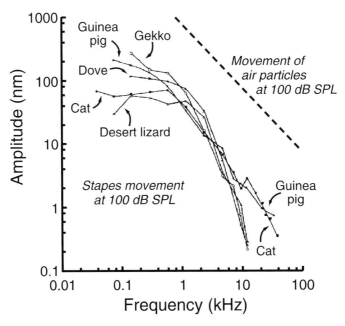

Figure 4.4. Amplitudes of the stapes vibrations elicited in several vertebrate species by tones of 100 dB SPL, plotted as functions of frequency. Note the much greater high-frequency responses of the mammals. Corresponding air particle amplitudes are shown for comparison (dashed line). (From Johnstone and Taylor, 1971, with permission*.)

mammalian species conform to this same overall pattern, differing mainly in the value of the corner frequency (Ruggero et al., 1990).

The relative invariance of the low-frequency segments of the curves in Figure 4.4 is reminiscent of the behavior of springs, which vibrate in response to a sinusoidal force with displacement amplitudes independent of stimulus frequency (see Appendix C). Accordingly, these low-frequency responses seem to be determined by the elasticity (springiness) of various middle ear structures, such as the joints and supporting ligaments of the ossicles, as well as the air in the middle ear cavity (see below).

Above the corner frequency, the response curves for the two mammals in Figure 4.4 have slopes nearly the same as that exhibited by air molecules in free space, which is also shown (dashed line). The constant slope of the latter curve (-20 dB per decade) is a consequence of the fact that a sound wave travels through air without appreciable amounts of its acoustic energy being either stored or reflected. Formally speaking, this property causes the acoustic impedance of a long column of air to be resistive,[2] meaning (among other things) that a pure tone propagating along that column is accompanied by air molecule displacements that are inversely proportional to the tone's frequency (see Eq. C.15). The descending slopes of the cat and guinea pig curves are only slightly steeper, suggesting that mammalian middle ears also pass on, albeit imperfectly, the high-frequency acoustic energy that impinges on them.

The vibrations of the mammalian ossicles elicited by sounds are *tiny*, only about $1/30$ those of the air molecule movements. At high frequencies the magnitudes of these vibrations become unbelievably small. For example, the data in Figure 4.4 show that a 20 kHz tone presented at 100 dB SPL causes stapes displacements of about 1 nanometer (nm) (10^{-9} meter). At the much smaller sound pressure level of 20 dB (still above the behavioral thresholds of many cats), stapes displacements would be 10^{-4} times smaller than that, or 0.0001 nm in magnitude. By comparison, the 0.1 nm diameter of a hydrogen atom is huge.

The stapes responses of several nonmammalian vertebrates, including a gecko lizard, are also shown in Figure 4.4. Note that the latter's sensitivity at low frequencies is even greater than that of the cat. Evidently, the columella type of middle ear can operate as efficiently at low frequencies as does the three-bone mammalian type. With increasing frequency, however, the sensitivity of the lizard middle ear deteriorates sharply; the slope of its high-frequency limb is steep, about -50 dB per decade. This sharp drop is attributed to flexing of the extracolumella process connected to the center of the eardrum (Fig. 4.1). That is, although the tip of this process might move a distance x, the process itself would be flexing like a fly-rod, reducing movements of the extracolumella's transmission shaft to much less than the $x/2$ shown in Figure 4.1.

Physical Factors Affecting Sound Transmission

Were the middle ear to do the job of sound transmission perfectly, it would transmit *all* of the acoustic energy impinging on the eardrum to the inner ear. Yet, no matter how well the middle ear is constructed, it *must* possess some finite amounts of mass, stiffness, and damping. Each of these fundamental properties exacts its toll from the sound wave, as summarized briefly below. In-depth mathematical analyses and models of the middle ear are available elsewhere (for review see Rosowski, 1996).

Stiffness

Because the acoustic impedance provided by stiffnesses increases as frequency decreases (see Appendix C), *below* some frequency the middle ear stiffness comes to dominate the composite acoustic impedance presented by the eardrum, and much of the incoming sound energy is reflected away. Greatly curtailed vibration amplitudes and energy transmission to the inner ear results.

The air contained within its cavity contributes to this middle ear stiffness (see Fig. C.1B). Relevant to this point, behavioral audiograms (threshold-of-hearing curves) for four small mammals are shown in Figure 4.5. The two desert rodents, gerbil, and kangaroo rat have much better low-frequency hearing than the other two. Major anatomical differences separating the two

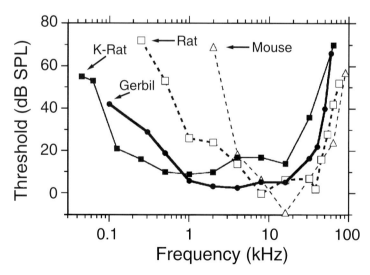

Figure 4.5. Auditory behavioral thresholds (''audiograms'') for the gerbil, house mouse, albino rat, and kangaroo rat (K-Rat). The desert rodents (gerbil and kangaroo rat), with huge middle ear cavities, have much better hearing at low frequencies. (From Ravicz et al., 1992, with permission*.)

groups are the larger eardrums and middle ears of the gerbil and kangaroo rat. Air trapped within the middle ear has a stiffness that varies inversely with its volume (Beranek, 1954), so the larger the size of the middle ear, the smaller is the stiffness presented by its trapped air. On theoretical grounds, it has been estimated that reducing the volume of the gerbil's middle ear by 75% would approximately triple the effective stiffness of the middle ear's input impedance (Ravicz et al., 1992) thereby elevating the animal's perceptual threshold below 2 kHz by as much as 12 dB (Ravicz and Rosowski, 1997).

Consistent with this estimate is the approximately fivefold (14 dB) loss of behavioral sensitivity to low-frequency stimuli suffered by kangaroo rats whose middle ear cavities had been three-fourths filled with clay (Webster and Webster, 1972). As the sound pressure emanating from a localized source drops off inversely with distance (see Chapter 2), this loss of sensitivity means that a predator generating low-frequency sounds could get much closer to these animals before being heard. In this case, that was too close: The kangaroo rats with partially plugged middle ear air volumes were much easier targets for snakes, which produce sounds having significant components at 1 kHz and below (Webster and Webster, 1971). The huge middle ear cavities of these desert animals, comparable in size to their brain cases, appear to be good investments.

Mass

In contrast to stiffness, the masses of the ossicles impede sound transmission at high frequencies. Because the impedance presented by a mass increases with increasing frequency (see Appendix C), *above* some frequency the impedances of the ossicular masses come to dominate the acoustic impedance presented by the eardrum, and so much of the incoming sound energy is reflected away. Consequently, as large animals are expected to have large ossicles, we would expect the upper frequency limit of an animal's hearing to be reciprocally related to its size.

The relations between the main ossicular masses (malleus and incus) and the mass of the skull are shown in Figure 4.6 for a large number of mammals (Nummela, 1995). Most of the ossicular masses fall within a three-decade range (0.1–100 mg), and the skull masses vary by some six orders of magnitude. Surprising is the demonstration that the theoretical pressure transformations of all of these middle ears are roughly comparable, varying between 30 and 80 (Hemilä et al., 1995).

Comparison between an animal's ossicular masses and the upper frequency limits of hearing yields approximately the expected inverse relation (Hemilä et al., 1995). In accordance with the theory, it was found that the behaviorally determined high-frequency hearing limits of a representative

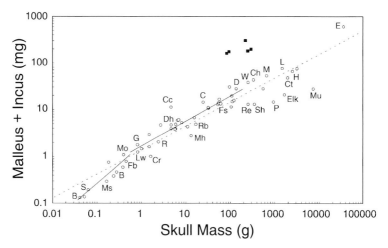

Figure 4.6. Combined mass of the main ossicles (malleus and incus) plotted against the skull mass (on log–log coordinates). Open circles, main group; filled squares, true seals. Regression lines are shown separately for the whole main group (dashed line) and for two selected sections. B, bat (*Myotis sp.*); C, Cat; Cc, chinchilla; Ch, chimpanzee; Cr. cotton rat; Ct, cattle; D, dog; Dh, desert hedgehog; E, Indian elephant; Fb, fish-catching bat; Fs, fur seal; G, Gerbil, Gp, guinea pig; H, horse; L, lion; Lw, least weasel; M, human; Mh, mountain hare; Mo, common mole; Ms, mouse; Mu, musk ox; P, pig; R, rat; Rb, rabbit; Re, reindeer; S, common shrew; Sh, sheep; W, wolf. (From Nummela, 1995, with permission*.)

group of mammalian species varied by approximately the inverse cube root of their ossicular masses. The usefulness of having small ossicular masses is apparent.

Damping (Energy Absorption)

As just demonstrated, efficient sound transmission through the middle ear is limited to some central frequency region, unavoidably degraded at either end of the frequency scale. In this mid-region the middle ear's resistive processes (e.g., friction), which we have so far ignored, become important. Their effects are summarized in Figure 4.7, which estimates the fraction of the energy entering the cat's middle ear that is delivered to the inner ear. As shown, transmission efficiency is roughly independent of frequency, averaging about 0.2.

Overall Efficiency

How well does the entire mammalian sound-capturing apparatus work? Channeled into the ear canal, reflected from the eardrum by middle ear stiffnesses and mass, absorbed by resistive elements all along the way, how

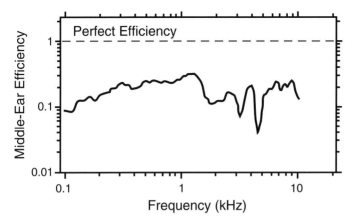

Figure 4.7. Middle ear efficiency (i.e., the fraction of sound power entering the middle ear that is delivered to the cochlea) in the cat, plotted as a function of tonal frequency. (From Rosowski, 1991, with permisison*.)

much of the incoming sound energy finally makes it through the gauntlet into the inner ear? Relevant data for the cat are shown in Figure 4.8 in the form of the ear's "effective" sound-collecting area for tones of different frequencies. To put it simply, each point shows the size of the input port needed by an ideal sound-collection system to deliver to the cochlea an amount of sound energy equal to that which it actually receives in nature.

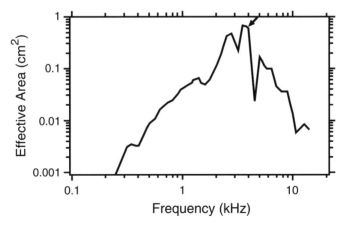

Figure 4.8. *Effective* area of the cat's sound-collecting apparatus (i.e., the cross-sectional area that a theoretically "perfect" external ear/middle ear system would need in order to deliver to the inner ear the same amount of sound energy transmitted to it in the living animal), plotted as a function of tonal frequency. Plane-wave sound source at 0° azimuth and elevation. (From Rosowski, 1991, with permission*.)

For instance, the data point at 4 kHz (Fig. 4.8, arrow) tells us that when tones of that frequency strike the cat pinna the external and middle ears transmit to the cochlea as much acoustic energy as would be captured from that same sound wave by an ideal sound catcher whose collecting surface had an area of about 0.6 cm^2.

The poor sound reception below 1 kHz can be attributed to the stiffnesses of the middle ear: Their high impedances at low frequencies reflect away most of the impinging sound energy. The peak at 4 kHz is due to ear canal resonance (see Fig. 3.7), and the plateau starting at about 10 kHz probably extends to much higher frequencies (Musicant et al., 1990). As these data were determined for a sound source located at 0° azimuth and elevation, considerable increases would occur were the source to be moved to the ''acoustic axis'' of the external ear (see Fig. 3.7).

These ''effective'' collecting areas may seem disappointingly small when compared with 13 cm^2, the typical collecting area of the cat pinna (Rosowski et al., 1988). Yet these numbers loom large when they are compared with the area of the cat oval window (ca. 0.01 cm^2), particularly when it is re-called that only a tiny fraction of *air-borne* sound energy striking the small oval window would actually make its way into the fluid-filled cochlea (see Fig. 3.2). It is thus clear from Figure 4.8 that the cat middle and external ears delivery far more sound energy to the inner ear than the latter could possibly capture by itself (Peake et al., 1992).

Other Interesting Features

To fulfill its functions, many important subtleties are involved in the con-struction of the mammalian middle ear. One concerns the influence of head motion on the middle ear ossicles. Important in this regard is the fact that the ''center of mass'' of the ossicles appears to lie close to the principal axis of their rotation (Bárány, 1938), just as it does for a wheel. For the wheel this conjunction means that when it is moved through the air (i.e., without touching the ground) the wheel does not rotate about its axle. Un-balance it, by putting an extra weight somewhere on the rim, and the wheel rotates when it is waved in the air. Fortunately for us, the mammalian middle ear appears to be well balanced, and so motions of the head theoretically cause minimal rotations of the middle ear ossicles (and consequent cochlear stimulation). Thus the construction of the ear reduces any self-stimulation of the cochlea that might occur during head movements, whether due to vocalizing and chewing or to changes of body position.

One final comparative note: The middle ear of mammals is basically a sealed chamber, with the Eustachian tube providing only sporadic access to the outside world (via the mouth cavity). Thus incoming sounds strike only the external surface of the mammalian eardrum. In other vertebrates the analogous connecting channel can be large and permanently open, creating a single acoustic volume that includes the mouth cavity and both middle ear spaces (and in the coqui frog the lungs as well) (Narins, 1995). As acoustic energy easily enters this volume, particularly if the mouth is open, some fraction of the sound energy striking the animal is conducted to the internal surface of the eardrum (Fig. 4.1). Consequently, with one sound wave pushing inward on the eardrum and another pushing outward, it is the *difference* between the two opposing sound pressure waves that drives the eardrum in this kind of ear. Such "pressure gradient" reception is thought to account for the sound-localizing abilities of small animals, such as the coqui frogs (about 1.5 inches in body length), whose heads are so tiny interaural time and pressure differences are minuscule (Narins, 1995).

MIDDLE EAR MUSCLES

The general scheme of this book is to follow, step by step, the progress of an acoustic signal on its journey into the mammalian brain. We must interrupt that progression here, and at a number of following stages, to consider the effects of feedback from more central locations. For the mammalian middle ear this feedback comes in the form of muscular forces delivered by the two smallest muscles in the body. One, the tensor tympani, is attached to the malleus. The other, the stapedius muscle, is connected to the neck of the stapes (see Fig. 4.2). These muscles, whose motoneurons are located close to auditory centers in the brain stem, modulate the acoustic properties of the middle ear and its response behavior (for comprehensive reviews, see Borg et al., 1984; Møller, 1984).

Acoustic Reflex

Conspicuous among the functions of middle ear muscles is the *acoustic reflex*, the attenuation of the vibratory input delivered to the cochlea during exposure to intense sounds. Best understood is the behavior of the stapedius muscle. From direct visualization, it is known that contraction of that muscle pulls the neck of the stapes slightly sideways, perpendicular to the axis of acoustic vibration (Fig. 4.2). Because the neck of the stapes is moved sideways, but its footplate cannot move in that direction (it is held snugly within the oval window), the stapes rotates or tilts about its footplate (Pang and Peake, 1986). This tilting (counterclockwise in Fig. 4.2) has the effect of stretching sections of the annular ligament which holds the footplate within the oval window, thereby increasing the stiffness the stapes–ligament complex presents to the incoming acoustic signal. Such an increase in stiffness, like that produced by reducing the air volume of the middle ear, increases the reflection of low-frequency sound from the eardrum and so reduces the magnitude of acoustic energy that reaches the cochlea.

The attenuations of input vibrations achieved with graded contractions of the stapedius muscle are shown in Figure 4.9A. As expected from our previous analysis, tones with frequencies below 1 kHz (where stiffness dominates middle ear impedance) were uniformly attenuated at all contractions. Unexpected and theoretically unaccounted for are the relatively large high-frequency attenuations produced by strong contractions of the muscle. As the acoustic reflex is a binaural phenomenon, the attenuation curve obtained with the smallest electrically produced contraction of the stapedius muscle (36 μm) is of particular interest. Its shape and magnitude are similar to those achieved by a strong tone delivered to the cat's opposite ear (Møller, 1965).

Recordings made from individual motoneurons of the stapedius muscle show that they respond directly to tones with a sensitivity that depends on tonal frequency. The minimum sound levels needed by tones of various frequencies to activate several such motoneurons are shown in Figure 4.9B. The pressure levels of these curves are high: Only tones with magnitudes of more than 90 dB SPL activate them. Not surprisingly, this level coincides approximately with the activation threshold of the acoustic reflex. Intriguing is the similarity between the differential sensitivity of these motoneurons to

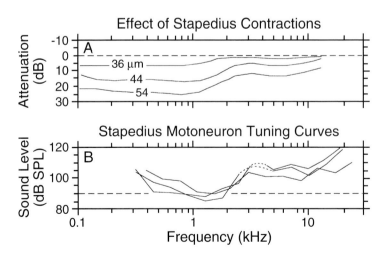

Figure 4.9. Comparisons between (A) the attenuation of middle ear sound transmission produced by stapedius muscle contractions of three amounts and (B) typical threshold level ''frequency tuning curves'' (see Fig. 5.8) for stapedius muscle motoneurons, all plotted as functions of tonal frequency. (A from Rosowski, 1991, with permission*; B from Kobler et al., 1992, with permission*.)

tones of various frequencies (Fig. 4.9B) and the relative effectiveness of the stapedius muscle in attenuating those very tones (Fig. 4.9A).

The other middle ear muscle, the tensor tympani, is known to participate in the middle ear reflex in some mammals, such as cats, but apparently not in humans (but see below). Experiments have shown that contraction of this muscle pulls the eardrum inward, toward the middle ear; but why this movement causes attenuation of sound transmission is not clear. Perhaps in a manner analogous to the action of the stapedius muscle, the forces exerted by the tensor tympani increase the stiffness of the eardrum or of its suspension.

To summarize, contraction of the middle ear muscles in the mammalian ear reduces the transmission of intense sounds to the inner ear. This graded feedback, only the first of many amplitude–compression mechanisms employed by the auditory periphery to handle the huge dynamic range of incoming sounds (see Chapter 2), has proved to be important in preserving the intelligibility of speech presented at high volume (Borg and Counter, 1989).

The middle ear muscles are far more than just adaptive signal processors. They are the principal line of defense against intense sounds, which can wreak havoc within the inner ear. Not only are the large vibrations produced by such sounds capable of causing appreciable impairment of behavioral sensitivity that can last for hours, they can cause long-term damage, including destruction of the cochlea's sensing cells. In one dramatic case, a chinchilla taken out for a single evening of rock music was found to have suffered significant degeneration of the sensory cells within localized sections of the cochlea (see Chapter 16).

Activation During Vocalizations

Bat cries, indeed the loud vocalizations of humans, routinely develop sound pressures in the immediate vicinity of the head that exceed 100 dB SPL. These intense sounds are of course attenuated by the middle ear muscles. Rather than awaiting the arrival of self-vocalizations and then taking action, the mammalian brain utilizes its information regarding planned actions and activates the middle ear muscles *prior* to the vocalizations. Thus the protective mechanisms are in place when the sounds arrive. The precision of this process has been raised to an incredible degree in species of bats that emit rapid sequences of short cries (O. W. Henson, 1965; Suga and Jen, 1975). Just before each cry is emitted, the middle ear muscles quickly contract, reaching their maximum contraction as the cry is emitted. The conduction of the cry through the middle ear is thereby attenuated. Immediately following that cry, the muscles partially relax, allowing the faint returning echoes to be transmitted with less attenuation. Conducted on a millisecond time scale, this sequence of muscular contraction and relaxation continues tirelessly, sometimes at rates exceeding 100 cries per second. Not surprisingly, the middle ear muscles in these bats are huge and loaded with mitochondria and sarcoplasmic reticula (cellular organelles needed for intense muscular activity).

The extensive frequency range over which attenuation is produced by middle ear feedback in these bats is particularly interesting. In the little brown bat, it extends up to 100 kHz (Suga and Jen, 1975). This extensive range, which cannot be accounted for theoretically, means that the bat's middle ear "automatic volume control" system[3] operates effectively over the entire frequency range of its cries.

Human middle ear muscles (both of them) are also activated prior to self-vocalizations. Unlike the high-intensity thresholds that operate with externally generated sounds (e.g., 90 dB SPL), muscle activation thresholds for self-vocalizations are an order of magnitude lower, at about 70 dB SPL (Borg and Zakrisson, 1975). As a result, the middle ear muscles are activated prior to all but the softest speech. Muscular contractions above that threshold increase approximately monotonically with speech intensity, with the half-strength contraction point occurring at the level of loud speech (ca. 80 dB SPL). Accordingly, it has been recommended that a person should hum while shooting a gun, so as to activate the middle ear muscles before, rather than after, the arrival of destructively large gunshot pressures (Borg and Counter, 1989).

The middle ears of many species of reptiles, amphibians, and birds also receive central feedback. In contrast to the mammalian ear, the feedback to the middle ears of these animals is usually exerted by a single muscle, which may have several points of connection along the ossicular chain. In contrast to mammalian ears, presentations of intense sounds fail to elicit acoustic reflexes in many species of birds (Borg and Counter, 1989). It appears therefore that protection of the inner ear from self-vocalizations (which reach the 100 dB SPL level in some species) may be the *only* role of the middle ear muscle in birds.

DIAGNOSTIC TESTS INVOLVING THE MIDDLE EAR

Changes in the input impedance of the eardrum provide the basis for several diagnostic tests (Wiley and Block, 1984). Consider, for example, the increase in the effective stiffness of the eardrum caused by contraction of the middle ear muscles. This increased stiffness causes increased sound reflections from the eardrum, the analysis of which can be used to cast light on the integrity of the acoustic reflex. Because this reflex involves a complete collector–sensor–brain–muscle loop, lesions and abnormalities anywhere along the line can produce irregularities. As these irregularities differ, depending on the sites and causes of the problem, a differential diagnosis is possible. For example, certain types of brain stem tumors produce rapid tiring of the acoustic reflex. Fluid in the middle ear, on the other hand, simply causes large eardrum reflections.

RECAPITULATION

The middle ear, via the vibrations of its ossicles, transmits sound signals from one acoustic medium to another: Air-borne sound waves are turned into mechanical vibrations, which in turn launch new sound waves within the fluids of the cochlea. This transmission is done efficiently and, in the absence of central control, virtually linearly.

Fortunately, the central nervous system is continually on guard, reducing the middle ear transmission of intense sounds, whether generated externally or self-vocalized. This signal compression has an important protective effect, limiting the amplitudes of the pressure waves launched within the cochlea. The fate of these fluid-borne waves is our next concern.

NOTES

1. To assure ourselves that pressure amplification occurs, assume that there are no reflections of energy from the eardrum or from the oval window. Under this assumption, energy delivered to the inner ear is simply the product of force times distance. Call the force that the columella normally exerts on the oval window F_0. The energy transmitted to the oval window by one eardrum deflection of magnitude x is therefore $F_0 x/2$. With no reflections allowed, that must be the energy in the incoming sound wave as well. If, on the other hand, the columella were to be centered on the eardrum, its displacement would be x. With the incoming energy fixed at $F_0 x/2$, the force exerted on the oval window would be reduced to $F_0/2$, half that of the normal case. Thus the offset of the columella amplifies the acoustic forces delivered to the oval window by a factor of 2, in this case (ignoring subtleties).

2. The passing of a sound wave down an infinitely long tube of air is endless, and so the acoustic energy never returns. Therefore so far as any one particular cross section of the tube is concerned, the energy passing through it is lost. Mathematically, this type of energy loss means that the acoustic impedance seen looking into the tube is purely resistive. Reference to Appendix C shows that the *velocity* of the response excited in a resistive impedance is independent of frequency; hence the response *displacement* (obtained by integrating the response velocity) is inversely proportional to frequency. When expressed in decibels, this inverse relation means

that one order of displacement magnitude (20 dB) is lost for every tenfold increase in frequency (expressed as −20 dB per decade). At −26 dB per decade, the slopes of the mammalian middle ear amplitude–frequency curves are not much different.

3. "Automatic volume control" is similar to the adaptive volume control of microphone systems used at sporting events. When the announcer is speaking (close to the microphone), the volume is set low to provide a comfortable listening level. When the speaking is over, the volume is automatically turned up, so the distant and (usually) much quieter crowd noises become audible.

5

SOUND-INDUCED VIBRATIONS IN THE INNER EAR

According to present knowledge, the sound-sensing cells in vertebrate inner ears respond only indirectly to sound. They are stimulated by sound-induced mechanical vibrations of their surrounding structures, rather than by the sound pressures that exist within the inner ears per se. That being so, our next step must be to consider the processes whereby fluid-borne sound waves within the inner ear produce such structural vibrations. In the mammalian ear this transformation is complicated. Three of the next five chapters are devoted to examining its mechanisms, one step at a time. We start by considering the sound-induced mechanical motions of the membrane-like structures that support the sensory cells.

BASIC ANATOMY

Although the shape of the mammalian inner ear is much more complicated than that of reptiles (see Fig. 4.1), the two have the same basic organization. In both cases there is a continuous perilymphatic duct system that has two openings into the middle ear, one of which is vibrated by an ossicle, as well as an endolymphatic volume connected acoustically to the perilymphatic system through two flexible membranes, one of which houses sensory cells.

55

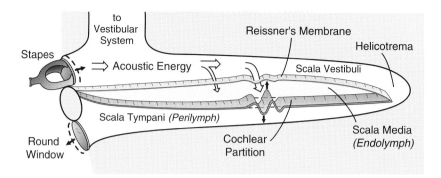

Figure 5.1. Stylized mammalian cochlea, shown as if the cochlear partition were straight. The acoustic energy produced by a *loud* tone of mid-frequency (e.g., 2 kHz) flows along the cochlear partition (open arrows) toward the one particular segment tuned to 2 kHz. Most of the sound energy is absorbed by the cochlear partition in the vicinity of the 2 kHz section, where broadly tuned oscillations are produced. Because of fluid incompressibility, volume displacement of the round window equals that of the oval window.

A schematic sketch of the mammalian cochlea is shown in Figure 5.1. The perilymphatic space has the shape of an elongated U, the top arm of which is called *scala vestibuli* (reflecting proximity to the vestibular system) and the bottom arm the *scala tympani* (reflecting proximity to the round window). For the purpose of illustration, the relative dimensions of these scalae have been deliberately distorted. They are actually very narrow and long, not unlike the arms of a hairpin. The head of that hairpin is the *helicotrema*, a short duct connecting the two perilymphatic scalae. Thus when the stapes pushes inward, the U-shaped column of perilymph is free to slide through its casing, as an arm through a sleeve, and push the round window outward (Kringlebotn, 1995).

Inserted between the two arms of the mammalian perilymphatic space is the endolymphatic space, appropriately labeled *scala media*. An extremely thin *Reissner's membrane* separates scala media from scala vestibuli; and the *cochlear partition*, a flexible structure that contains the sensory cells, separates scala media and scala tympani.

SOUND PROPAGATION IN THE INNER EAR

Because of its much simpler geometry, let us first consider sound propagation within the reptilian inner ear (see Fig. 4.1). When the oval window is pushed inward by the columella, the increased sound pressure that results in the endolymphatic space pushes uniformly on the flexible sensory surface, bulging it slightly toward the return arm of the perilymphatic space. The perilymph so displaced pushes out the round window. The reverse process occurs when the columella is pulled outward, creating reduced pressures inside the oval window.

The process in more complicated in the mammalian inner ear, as the greatly elongated perilymphatic scalae force the sound waves to travel a long distance to reach the round window: all the way out to the helicotrema around and back. Along the way, the sound waves must traverse the entire surface of the cochlear partition, each part of which absorbs some of the passing acoustic energy. Although this interaction between sound wave and membrane is complex (Patuzzi, 1996; de Boer, 1996), its basic consequences are illustrated in Figure 5.1.

As the acoustic wave formed by stapes vibrations propagates through scala vestibuli[1] it causes the flexible cochlear partition to vibrate. These vibrations are not uniform along the cochlear partition as they are in the reptile (see Fig. 7.6A). Rather, as we see in the next section, the vibrations of the cochlear partition in mammals vary in position depending on the nature of the acoustic stimuli being used.

MECHANICAL MEASUREMENTS IN DEAD COCHLEAS

The first descriptions of cochlear partition vibrations, measured mostly in dead cochleas, were reported by von Békésy during the 1940s (collected and published as a book on 1960). At that time they were an extraordinary achievement, earning him a Nobel Prize. One of his illustrations, showing cochlear partition displacements produced along a section of a dead human cochlea by a 200 Hz tone, is reproduced in Figure 5.2. To aid in appreciating the nature of these displacements, he plotted them at two instants during one period of the 200 Hz stimulus, the dot-dashed curve occurring one-fourth of a cycle after the solid curve. Also shown is the displacement wave's "envelope," the points of maximum upward and downward displacement (dashed lines).

These measurements show that a *traveling wave* of displacements existed on the cochlear partition. That is, each of the displacement peaks (and valleys) traveled farther from its starting point at the stapes during the 1.25 msec that elapsed between the two "snapshots." Note that each point on the cochlear partition just moved up and down. What traveled laterally, away from the stapes, were sound pressure waves in the scalae (unseen) and the pattern of cochlear partition displacements they produced. (Animations of the traveling displacement waves produced by tones of different frequency are available for viewing on our World Wide Web site.)

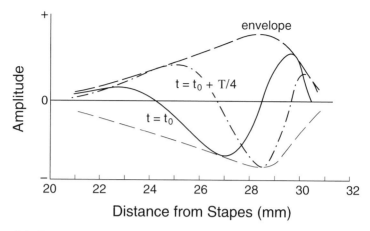

Figure 5.2. Two "snapshots" of cochlear partition oscillations produced in a dead human cochlea by a tone of 200 Hz. The dot–dashed curve was measured 1.25 msec (one-fourth period) after the solid curve, showing that all features of the displacement (e.g., the peaks) were moving away from the stapes. The "envelope" of the displacement wave (e.g., the set of maximum displacements) is marked with dashed lines. (From von Békésy, 1947, with permission.*)

Of fundamental importance is the relation that exists between stimulus frequency and the cochlear partition's displacement pattern. Shown in the top panel of Figure 5.3 are von Békésy's recordings of the displacement "envelopes" produced by tones of several frequencies. As can be seen, each tone produced a localized response in a distinct place: The lower the frequency of the tone, the farther from the stapes was the whole vibration pattern located.

The phases of the cochlear partition displacements, relative to those of the stapes, produced by those same four tones are shown in the bottom panel of Figure 5.3. For any one frequency, the phase curve is the classic signature of a traveling wave. It shows that any particular feature of the displacement wave (e.g., one peak) occurred later and later in time as the distance of the location away from the stapes increased. For example, with 200 Hz excitation, a phase lag of about π radians existed in the response which occurred at a location 27 mm from the stapes (top arrow). In other words, the cochlear partition at the 27 mm point responded to a 200 Hz tone with sinusoidal vibrations that lagged behind those of the stapes by about 2.5 msec (half a period). Slowing down, the 200 Hz displacement wave took more than another 2.5 msec to travel only 3 mm farther, down to the 30 mm point (bottom arrow).

Von Békésy used stroboscopic flashes of ordinary visible light for his measurements. With then-extant techniques, the smallest response ampli-

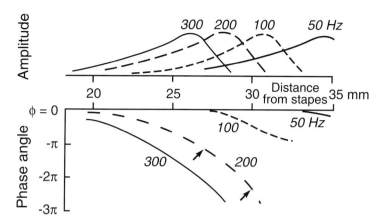

Figure 5.3. *A.* Envelopes of the sinusoidal displacements produced in a dead human cochlea by tones of four low frequencies. The higher the frequency, the closer is the peak to the stapes. *B.* Phase angles (re: stapes) for the displacements in *A.* For each tone, progressively greater phase *lags* (negative values) occurred with increasing distance from the stapes, indicative of a wave of displacement traveling away from the stapes. The two upward-pointing arrows on the 200-Hz curve indicate phase shifts at 27 and 30 mm, respectively. (From von Békésy, 1947, with permission.*)

tudes he could measure were of the same order of magnitude as the wavelengths of that light (ca. 500 nm). During the decades since, cochlear vibrations have been measured much more precisely using more modern techniques. Despite the dramatically improved measuring instruments, however, the basic pattern observed by von Békésy characterizes virtually all existing cochlear partition measurements. That is, a tonal stimulus sets up a displacement wave on the cochlear partition that travels away from the stapes and peaks in a restricted region whose location is determined by the stimulus frequency.

The intracochlear pressures responsible for these displacement waves have been measured in several species. Those recorded from inside the cat cochlea, near the stapes, are shown in Figure 5.4. In the scala vestibuli, just inside the oval window, the pressure rises steadily with the frequency to about 1 kHz and then plateaus. This pattern is expected from our middle ear considerations. Above 1 kHz, sound energy is transmitted efficiently to the inner ear, producing pressures in the scala vestibuli that can reach values more than 20 times those recorded at the eardrum (compare with the theoretical value of 43) (see Chapter 4). As frequency is reduced below that corner frequency, stiffness increasingly dominates the middle ear's acoustic impedance and reflects away increasing fractions of the incoming acoustic energy. Note that the sound pressures in the scala tympani were much

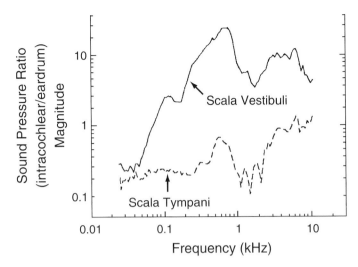

Figure 5.4. Ratio of intracochlear sound pressures to pressure at the eardrum, plotted as a function of tonal frequency. Solid line shows pressure in scala vestibuli (near the stapes); dashed line shows pressure in scala tympani (near the round window). Note the large pressure *differences* that developed across the cochlear partition at frequencies above 500 Hz. (From Nedzelnitsky, 1980, with permission.*)

smaller than those in the scala vestibuli at virtually all audible frequencies. For any one tone, the difference in those two pressures forms the effective sound stimulus for the inner ear (Voss et al., 1996). Similar pressure transformations take place in the human inner ear (Puria et al., 1997).

MODEL OF COCHLEAR PARTITION VIBRATIONS

The displacement responses described in the dead cochlea can be readily accounted for with a simple model. To form the model, the cochlea is first sliced perpendicular to its main axis, like a loaf of bread. Then, as shown in Figure 5.5, the cochlear partition in each slice is represented as a thin, rigid plate, connected to lateral supports by springs. The plate has mass, and its movements are subject to friction. Because of the negligible acoustic impedance of Reissner's membrane, the pressure in scala media is assumed to be identical to that in scala vestibuli (P_v). That pressure pushes down on the partition slice (or "section"), and the pressure in scala tympani (P_t) pushes up on it. The difference between the opposing pressures ($P_v - P_t$), the *net* pressure acting on the mass, is used as the driving term in a differential equation describing the movements of the spring-tethered mass. One equation is written for each section, and then equations are written to de-

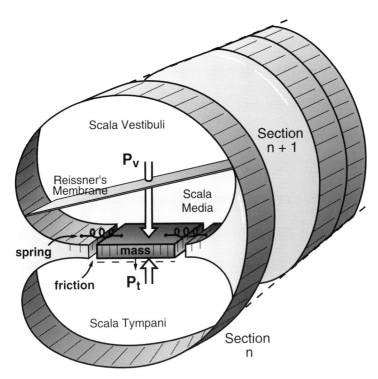

Figure 5.5. Mechanical model of a section of the cochlear partition (n). A flat plate possessing mass is suspended between scala vestibuli and scala tympani by springs, with motion impeded by friction. The plate is driven by the net pressure across it ($P_v - P_t$). Plate motions of successive sections are coupled through displaced fluids.

scribe the physical motions of the fluids within each scala. Finally, the entire set of equations, describing all of the mass and fluid motions, are simultaneously solved by computational techniques.

Such models do indeed produce traveling pressure and displacement waves that propagate to specific places along the (simulated) cochlear partition. The output of one such model, constructed to mimic the 25 mm long cat cochlea, is shown in Figure 5.6. When 300 Hz stimulation was used, the response was a traveling wave (as indicated by the steadily increasing phase lags) that peaked far from the stapes, almost at the helicotrema. Qualitatively, it is similar to the 300 Hz response observed by von Békésy in cadaver ears (Fig. 5.3). For 9 kHz stimulation, the peak of the traveling wave response occurred much closer to the stapes, as in the real cochlea (see Fig. 5.8).

Key to this successful mimicking of responses to different frequencies is the assignment of different values of stiffness to the supporting springs of the different cochlear slices. This variation in stiffness values is based largely

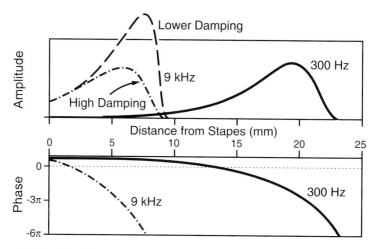

Figure 5.6. *A.* Envelopes of the sinusoidal cochlear partition displacements produced in a hydromechanical model of the cat cochlea with tones of 300 Hz and 9 kHz, the latter used with two different values of section friction: the lower the damping, the larger the peak. *B.* Phase angles of the displacements in *A*, indicative of traveling waves. (From the Geisler-Sang model (1995), with no "amplification").

on other experimental measurements of von Békésy (1960), who showed that cochlear partition elasticity decreases dramatically with the distance from the stapes. Based largely on extrapolations of his data, this model was constructed with spring stiffnesses that decreased in an approximately exponential manner with distance from the stapes (but see Chapter 9). Each section was assumed to have the same mass.

The consequences of this stiffness variation are illustrated in Figure 5.7, a broadside sketch of the cochlear-partition model, with three representative sections drawn. The stimulus is assumed to be sinusoidal with a particular radian frequency of ω_0. Each cochlear partition section, made up as it is of a mass (M) constrained by both stiffness (K) and damping (D), has an acoustic impedance to movement whose magnitude $|Z|$ is given as

$$|Z| = (1/A^2)\sqrt{[(M\omega_0 - K/\omega_0)^2 + D^2]} \tag{5.1}$$

(see also Eq. C.20). Assume that ω_0 has a value just equal to $\sqrt{(K_2/M)}$, where K_2 is the stiffness of the middle section in Figure 5.7. Substitution of this frequency into Eq. 5.1 shows that the "reactive" component of that section's acoustic impedance, $(M\omega_0 - K_2/\omega_0)/A^2$, goes to zero. "Resonance" for that particular section has occurred. That is, the motion-impeding influences of the spring and mass have canceled each other, and the acoustic impedance of that segment drops to its lowest possible value (D/A^2), deter-

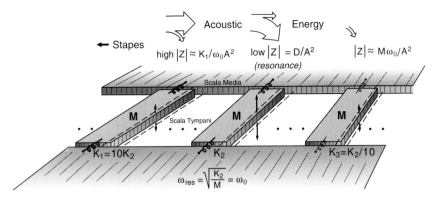

Figure 5.7. Interior lateral view of the hydrodynamic model, with only 3 of 350 plates shown. The middle plate is tuned to the frequency of the stimulating tone (f_0) and so has a low impedance (D/A^2). The left plate is tuned to a higher frequency and has a much higher impedance ($\approx K_1/\omega_0 A^2$). The right plate is tuned to a lower frequency and also has a higher impedance ($\approx M\omega_0/A^2$). The middle plate therefore moves most readily.

mined entirely by section damping. Thus the lower the damping, the lower is the total impedance.

For any partition section with much larger values of stiffness (e.g., the left-hand section with $K_1 = 10K_2$), the stiffness term in Eq. 5.1 is much larger than the mass term at frequency ω_0 and so comes to dominate that section's acoustic impedance (e.g., $|Z_1| \approx K_1/\omega_0 A^2$, assuming a relatively small damping value). That section also resonates with sinusoidal excitation but at a resonant frequency ($\omega_{res} = \sqrt{K_1/M}$) about three times *higher* than ω_0.

For sections with much smaller values of stiffness (e.g., the right-hand section, where $K_3 = K_2/10$), the contribution of the mass to the section's acoustic impedance is much larger at radian frequency ω_0 than that of the spring. Accordingly, the acoustic impedances of those sections at that frequency are largely determined by their masses (i.e., $|Z_3| \approx M\omega_0/A^2$), again assuming relatively little damping. These sections also resonate but at frequencies *lower* than ω_0.

To summarize, the acoustic impedance of each mass–spring–damper section has its minimum value at one particular (resonant) frequency, which is determined by the stiffness/mass ratio. Tones with frequencies higher or lower than that encounter increased impedance. Moreover, because the stiffness of a section decreases exponentially with its distance from the stapes, the resonant frequencies of successive sections also decrease exponentially.

Armed with this information, let us follow the progress of a sinusoidal sound wave with radian frequency ω_0 as it propagates along the surface of this simulated cochlear partition. Initially, the wave moves past sections of the cochlear partition that are much stiffer than K_2 and thus far from resonance. Their acoustic impedances are accordingly large; consequently little displacement of the cochlear partition is produced, and little acoustic energy is absorbed. With little energy lost to the partition and negligible reflections (Zweig et al., 1976), the wave must travel on.

As it progresses along the cochlear partition, the wave encounters progressively lower acoustic impedances (since membrane stiffness decreases monotonically with distance from the stapes). Thus increasingly large section deflections and more energy absorption results, but still much energy (and therefore pressure) remains in the acoustic wave. Eventually, the pressure wave encounters the resonant section and, faced with its small impedance, produces relatively large displacements,[2] which absorb most of the remaining energy. What little energy is left in the wave is quickly dissipated in the mass-dominated sections lying beyond. The lower the damping in the model, the larger is the response peak, as shown for the 9 kHz responses seen in Figure 5.6.

There is overwhelming evidence that the same basic phenomena depicted in the model occur in dead or badly damaged mammalian cochleas.

MECHANICAL MEASUREMENTS IN LIVING COCHLEAS

The modern era of measuring cochlear vibrations began with the initial employment of the Mössbauer effect (Johnstone and Boyle, 1967). To utilize this quantum mechanical phenomenon in which the velocity of a radioactive source modulates the frequency (energy) of the γ-photons it emits, a tiny radioactive source is placed on the cochlear partition; and the frequency of its γ-ray emissions is determined. This Doppler shift effect, used in conjunction with the then newly invented laboratory computer (Clark and Molnar, 1965), made it possible to measure instantaneous cochlear partition displacements at the nanometer level—more than a 100-fold improvement in resolution over von Békésy's measurements.

Responses of the Region Tuned to High Frequencies

The results obtained were astonishing. Only at high sound levels were cochlear vibrations highly damped and poorly localized, as in the dead cochlea. In striking contrast, a lightly damped and well localized deflection peak occurred at low sound levels (Rhode, 1971). Although initially met with widespread skepticism, these results have now been repeated many times over; and they have been extended, most recently with the more powerful laser interferometric techniques (for review see Ruggero, 1992). Representative data,[3] obtained with a *velocity*-sensitive interferometer, are shown in Figure 5.8A. Repeating the basic theme discovered by Rhode, the data show a narrow peak at the lowest sound level (3 dB SPL) that gradually grows and broadens as the level is raised. Note the strong compressions involved. For example, although a 9 kHz tone presented at its lowest level (3 dB SPL) evoked a velocity response of nearly 0.1 mm/sec (bottom curve), it could

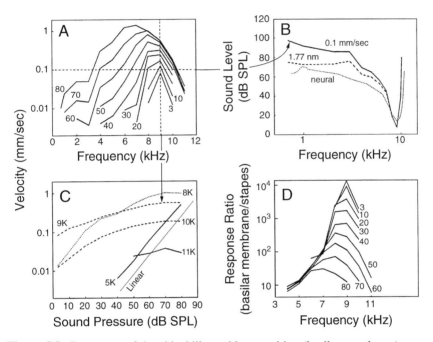

Figure 5.8. Responses of the chinchilla cochlear partition (basilar membrane), near the stapes, to various tones. *A*. peak velocities of responses elicited by tones of various frequencies. All responses obtained at one sound level (dB SPL) are joined with an appropriately labeled solid line. *B*. "Frequency tuning curves" (i.e., stimulus levels that just produced a criterion response) for the data in *A*, using either a velocity criterion of 0.1 mm/sec (along the horizontal dashed line in *A*) or a displacement criterion of 1.77 nm (dashed line). For comparison, the threshold-level frequency tuning curve of a typical primary afferent neuron innervating that location (see Chapter 12) is also shown (dotted line). *C*. "Level response" curves (i.e., response amplitudes plotted as functions of the sound level) derived from *A* for tones of selected frequencies, such as 9 kHz (along the vertical dashed line). Note the "compression" of responses to the highest frequencies. *D*. Ratio between the responses in *A* and the corresponding responses of the stapes. The high "gain" at low stimulus intensities collapses as the intensity is raised. (*A* and *B*: From Ruggero and Rich, 1991, with permission.* *C*: From Ruggero, 1992, with permission.* *D*: From Ruggero et al., 1992, with permission.*)

barely quadruple the size of that response when presented at a level of 80 dB SPL, almost 10,000 times more intense (top curve).

If the amplitudes of the responses to 9 kHz tones (along the vertical dashed line) are plotted as a function of stimulus level, we obtain the 9 kHz input–output curve of Figure 5.8C. Several more of these response-versus-level curves, obtained with tones of other frequencies, are also shown. Note that the 5 kHz curve has unity slope, and so would plot as a straight line of unity slope on linear coordinates as well. In other words, that point on the cochlear partition responded to 5 kHz stimulation in a *linear* fashion.[4]

Strongly compressive responses were obtained with all tones whose frequencies were near 9 kHz (slopes are much less than unity) (Fig. 5.8C). This compression has obvious functional importance. For example, were the system to respond linearly to 9 kHz tones the response at 83 dB SPL would be exactly 10,000 times greater than the response at 3 dB SPL. Such a velocity would amount to *displacements* of 18,000 nm (18 μm) in amplitude. Such huge displacements are known to have highly destructive effects. Fortunately for us, the living cochlear partition strongly compresses the responses to high-frequency tones. Thus in the case at hand, the response of the living cochlear partition evoked by *any* tone presented at less than 80 dB SPL was limited to velocities of less than 1 mm/sec (which corresponds to a 18-nm displacement at 9 kHz).

The *ratios* of the cochlear partition responses of Figure 5.8A relative to the corresponding linear responses of the stapes are plotted in Figure 5.8D. This form of display highlights the extraordinary nature of the responses to weak tones. For weak 9 kHz stimulation, the cochlear partition's response was 10,000 times larger than that of the stapes. With increasing intensity, this ratio drops precipitously. The large response peaks evoked at low stimulus levels have proved vulnerable to experimental damage, and they disappear rapidly (within minutes) upon the death of the animal (Rhode, 1973). Although the mechanisms involved are still a matter of debate, there is little doubt that these mountainous low-level peaks exist, and that they are caused by some sort of on-board ''amplifying'' system located within the cochlea itself (see Chapter 9).

Figure 5.8B shows a measurement display that appears often in later chapters, the *isoresponse level* curve (usually called the frequency tuning curve). Unlike the usual response displays, which plot output–amplitude versus frequency of stimulation for a *fixed* input level (as in Fig. 8.5A, D), an isoresponse curve plots the stimulus levels *needed* to produce a criterion level of output. Such displays are useful when the stimulus has a wide range of levels (as does sound), but the amplitude range of the responses is much more limited. Thus when the criterion response level of 0.1 mm/sec is applied to the data of Figure 5.8A, the sound levels that produced this strength of response (the intersections of those response curves with the dashed horizontal line) are plotted in Figure 5.8B as a function of frequency (solid curve).

At the recording site of these data, located fairly near the stapes, tones with frequencies below 3 kHz required high levels (> 80 dB SPL) to produce the criterion response. Evidently those low-frequency sound waves were just passing by, depositing little of their energy. By contrast, the 9 kHz tones must have dumped most of their energy in the immediate neighborhood of the recording spot to produce the criterion response at a level of only 10 dB SPL.

Note that the isoresponse level curve in Figure 5.8B is much sharper in character than most of the isoinput level curves of Figure 5.8A. Such shape disparities hold true for all compressive systems. Only for a linear system do these two curves have the same shape (when the two are plotted on log–log coordinates).

Perhaps it is membrane *displacement* rather than membrane velocity that is important physiologically. In that case, a constant displacement–amplitude criterion can be used to form an isoresponse curve. For example, a displacement criterion of 1.77 nm applied to the data of Figure 5.8A produced the dashed curve of Figure 5.8B. It is similar to the velocity tuning curve near 9 kHz but departs from it increasingly at lower frequencies. For comparison, the (threshold level) frequency tuning curve of a primary auditory neuron (see Chapter 12) is also shown (dotted curve). Note how well it matches both the displacement and velocity curves in the vicinity of the 9 kHz "tip." At lower frequencies the neural tuning curve falls somewhat below the two partition response curves.

A useful measure of the sharpness of a cochlear frequency tuning curve is the so-called Q_{10} factor, which is the ratio between the curve's tip frequency and its bandwidth (the width of the curve at a sound level 10 dB higher than that of the tip). For the 0.1 mm/sec curve of Figure 5.8D, for example, this 10 dB width is 1.2 kHz, so the Q_{10} of that tuning curve is 7.5 (9.0 kHz/1.2 kHz). For most mammals this degree of sharpness is typical for the mechanical tuning curves obtained in the cochlea's high-frequency region at low sound pressures; it is also typical for the associated neural tuning curves (see Chapter 12).

For mustache bats, however, which echolocate flying insects in the forest canopy, the cochlear partition is tuned so sharply that Q_{10} values sometimes reach the incredible value of 610. That is, for tones in their main sonar frequency region (ca. 60 kHz), these flyers have frequency tuning curves whose bandwidths are less than 100 Hz (Russell and Kössl, 1995).

Not shown here are examples of the phases of the responses obtained with modern techniques. They almost universally show large phase lags that increase monotonically with frequency (as in Figs. 5.3 and 5.6), indicative of traveling waves.

Responses of the Region Tuned to Low Frequencies

Because of the corkscrew geometry of the mammalian cochlea (see Chapter 6), it has been extremely difficult to measure cochlear partition vibrations in the low-frequency regions of the living cochlea. Fragmentary information about this region was obtained in the intact animal some time ago (Rhode, 1978), and more recent experiments using isolated temporal bone preparations have yielded useful data (Ulfendahl et al., 1989; Gummer et al., 1995). Systematic measurements of mechanical vibrations at the apical end of the cochlear partition in the living animal have only recently been accomplished (e.g., Rhode and Cooper, 1996).

A set of these new measurements, the displacement responses of the chinchilla cochlear partition obtained with fixed-amplitude tones of various frequencies, is shown in Figure 5.9A. In contrast to the basal-turn data of Figure 5.8A, the shapes of these curves do not change much with stimulus level. Response-versus-level curves derived from these data at various frequencies (e.g., along the vertical dashed line in Fig. 5.9A) show that the responses are linear for all tones presented at low intensities, and that higher level compression occurs at all frequencies as well (Fig. 5.9C and shaded portion of Fig. 5.9A).

These unique attributes are made even clearer when the responses are normalized to those of the middle ear (Fig. 5.9D). As the lowest intensity responses have the largest relative amplitudes, the cochlear amplifier must have been at work in the apex as well, amplifying low-intensity tones. In marked contrast with amplification in the basal turn, however, apical turn amplification is relatively small (< 20 dB) and is not confined to frequencies near the characteristic frequency. In short, the responses to *all* low-level tones are boosted a bit, with little change in frequency selectivity as intensity is increased. This dramatic difference in the mechanical behavior of the two cochlear regions has no theoretical explanation as yet. We shall see its neural counterpart in the different response behaviors of neurons innervating these different parts of the cochlea (see Chapter 12).

A frequency tuning curve for this animal's mechanical responses is shown in Figure 5.9B, along with that of another chinchilla (solid lines). Typical (threshold-level) frequency tuning curves of afferent neurons innervating this apical region are also shown (dashed lines). The two sets of curves are similar, with differences at the low frequencies attributable to the peculiar manner in which the principal sensory cells are stimulated at low frequencies (see Chapter 8).

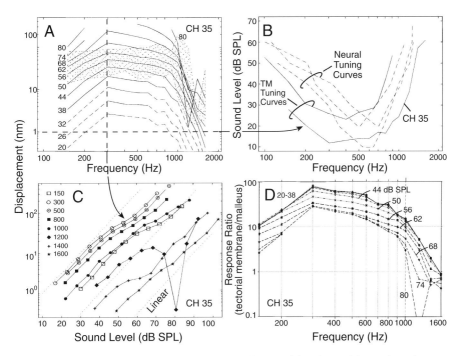

Figure 5.9. Responses of the chinchilla cochlear partition (tectorial membrane), near the apical end, to various tones. Format is the same as in Figure 5.8. *A*. Peak displacements of responses elicited by tones of various frequencies. Animal CH35. *B*. Frequency tuning curves for the tectorial membrane with a response criterion of 1 nm (along the horizontal dashed line) for two animals (solid curves). Typical frequency tuning curves for primary afferent neurons innervating that area are shown for comparison (dashed curves). *C*. Level response curves derived from *A* at selected frequencies (e.g., along the vertical dashed line for 300 Hz). *D*. Ratio between the responses of *A* and the corresponding responses of the malleus. (*A−C*: From Rhode and Cooper, 1996, with permission.* *D*: Courtesy of Rhode and Cooper).

RESPONSE PATTERNS TO COMPLEX SOUNDS

The fundamental behavior of cochlear partition responses is that originally observed by von Békésy: a pure tone forms a displacement wave on the cochlear partition that propagates away from the stapes until it peaks at a particular location unique to that frequency. It is somewhat like a piano being used as a receiver of sound rather than as its producer. With such role reversal, incoming air-borne tones of a particular frequency would enter at the treble end and pass over the various strings sequentially, causing the one particular string tuned to that frequency to resonate and vibrate more strongly than any other string. The lower the frequency, the farther from the treble end this resonant string would be located. The cochlea behaves in an analogous manner but has the handicap of being immersed in fluids that have considerable viscous friction (which limits response amplitudes at resonance).

From this piano-like organization of the cochlea, the basic response patterns of the cochlea excited by complex sounds can be predicted using the Fourier analysis. To satisfy the formal mathematical requirements for the use of such analysis, let us first consider the responses of the dead cochlea, as it is known to behave in an essentially linear fashion.

To start the process, Fourier analysis is used to decompose the incoming complex sound wave into a series (or continuum) of sinusoidal components. The responses of the linear inner ear are then determined for each of these sinusoidal components presented separately: The low-frequency components would propagate far down the cochlear partition, and high-frequency waves would peak near the stapes (Fig. 5.6). Finally, because the dead ear behaves linearly, we simply sum all of the responses evoked by each of the individual components to obtain the response to the initial complex wave.

The data we have reviewed show that the living cochlea does not behave in a linear fashion, so Fourier theory cannot be applied rigorously to its operation. Nevertheless, even here the propagation of acoustic waves *within* the cochlear fluids is basically linear: It is the cochlear partition that is behaving nonlinearly. Thus an incoming acoustic stimulus can still be decomposed legitimately into its sinusoidal components. The low-frequency components still propagate far down the partition, and the high-frequency components peak more basally. What does differ from linear behavior in the living cochlea among other things is that the different frequency components interact wherever they happen to coexist, producing novel effects. For instance, sound pressure components having completely new frequencies are created and broadcast in all directions, even out of the ear (see Chapter 10).

A LOOK AHEAD

Figure 5.6 showed the responses of a simple linear model to a pure 9 kHz tone presented at two levels of cochlear partition damping. The simulated response obtained with the high level of damping (dot-dashed curve) is qualitatively and quantitatively similar to the response patterns produced in the dead cochlea or in the living cochlea by intense tones (see the 80 dB curve in Fig. 5.8A). This fit suggests that the model is adequately representing the living cochlea's physiological mechanisms *only* under those high-level conditions.

The 9 kHz response in Figure 5.6 obtained with the lower level of damping (dashed curve) is larger and more peaked than that produced with high-level damping. This trend suggests that the cochlear mechanisms responsible for the sharper and relatively larger low-level responses observed in living animals (Fig. 5.8) may somehow be involved in reducing intrinsic damping. Identifying these mechanisms has proved difficult. They are subtle enough that theoreticians were unable to guess their modes of operation in the absence of detailed measurements and difficult enough to measure that, until recently, there has not been enough experimental data with which to work. Thus only now, nearly 50 years after the first mathematical models of the cochlea appeared (Zwislocki, 1948; Peterson and Bogert, 1950; Ranke, 1950), are accurate models incorporating physiologically reasonable mechanisms starting to appear (see Chapter 9).

The principal reason for this improved modeling of cochlear mechanisms has been improved understanding of how the sensory cells work. Before the physiology of the sensory cells can be examined, however, we must consider their locations within the cochlear partition and the ways in which they are stimulated by vibrations of the cochlear partition.

NOTES

1. Scala vestibuli is separated from scala media by Reissner's membrane, which is so thin and so flexible it is presumed to have virtually no influence on acoustic waves. Thus the entire fluid space above the cochlear partition appears as a single duct to sound waves.

2. It is the *ratio* of pressure to impedance that determines section velocity. Because the magnitudes of both pressure and section impedance drop steadily with distance from the stapes, the section that displays the largest displacement cannot be easily predicted. The larger the internal friction of the model, the more rapidly is energy (thus pressure) extracted from the progressing sound wave, and so the closer to the stapes lies the section displaying the maximum displacement. Only for minuscule damping is the maximally displaced section the resonant one.

3. The measurements in Figures 5.2 and 5.3 are of displacements produced by single *tones*, plotted as functions of distance. By contrast, the measurements in Figures 5.8 and 5.9 are of velocities and displacements produced at one *point*, plotted as functions of tonal frequency. Nevertheless, the two types of plot look similar and, with certain assumptions, can be transformed from one into the other (Geisler and Cai, 1996).

4. Recall that the output of a linear system scales with its input. Hence the input–output curves of any linear system *always* have slopes of unity (i.e., if we increase the amplitude of the input by any numerical factor, the amplitude of the output increases by exactly that same factor).

6

TRANSFER OF SOUND-INDUCED
VIBRATIONS TO SENSING CELLS

The sound-sensing cells of the mammalian cochlea are situated in a geo-metrically complex structure that transfers the sound-induced vibrations of the cochlear partition to its embedded sensory cells. Anatomical and phys-iological evidence indicates that this transfer is efficient, providing the sen-sory cells with a faithful, robust version of the partition's vibrations. Ex-amining the nature of that transfer is the main task of this chapter.

Also considered are attributes of the fluids that bathe the sensory cells. The strikingly different chemical properties and electrical potentials of en-dolymph and perilymph create for these cells a unique electrochemical environment.

FUNCTIONAL ANATOMY

The dimensions and geometry of the cochlear sketch in Chapter 5 (see Fig. 5.1) were deliberately distorted to make clear the path taken by incoming acoustic energy. One of the major distortions was a drastic shortening of the organ. In the cat cochlea, for example, the cochlear partition is nominally 25 mm (1 inch) long, whereas the areas of the scalae are less than 1 mm^2 over most of their lengths (Dallos, 1970). The first step toward appreciating the cochlea's true form therefore is to stretch the cochlea of Figure 5.1 out to its full length (about 10 times that shown in Fig. 5.1). Then take the stretched out cochlea by its tip and coil it back on itself several complete turns, like a corkscrew, except that each successive turn is smaller than the previous one. The result is a compact, cone-shaped helix about the size of a peppercorn in humans. The number of turns and overall shape is specific to each species. From an acoustic point of view, the curvature of the scalae is negligible; it is so slight compared to the cross sectional dimensions of the scalae that the sound waves propagate in them almost exactly as they would in a straight cochlea.

A photomicrograph of a partially dissected chinchilla cochlea is shown in Figure 6.1. The remnants of the cochlear partition are prominent in each

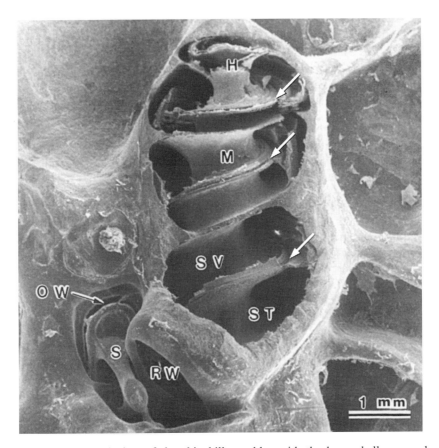

Figure 6.1. Lateral view of the chinchilla cochlea with the bony shell removed. Arrows point to remnants of the cochlear partition in the various turns. H, helicotrema; M, modiolus; OW, oval window; RW, round window; S, stapes; ST, scala tympani; SV, scala vestibuli. (From Harrison and Hunter-Duvar, 1988, with permission.*)

turn (marked by arrows), separating the two perilymphatic scalae. The conical nature of the overall structure allows us to introduce standard nomenclature. The region of the cochlea adjacent to the stapes, shown inserted into the oval window, is called the *base*. The cochlear turn that includes the base is referred to as the *basal* (or *first*) turn. The other turns are simply numbered sequentially upward from there. The region farthest away from the stapes, at the top of the cone, is appropriately named the *apex*. The center shaft of the cone, called the *modiolus*, is hollow and forms the passageway for the axons of the neurons which innervate all turns of the cochlea. Incidentally, note that the cochlea protrudes far into this animal's middle ear (the viewpoint of the photograph), as is common in rodents, making it accessible for experimental manipulation.

The basic structure of the cochlear partition is shown in Figure 6.2, a cross-sectional sketch of a radial[1] slice taken from the guinea pig's second turn. Forming the basic platform of the partition is the *basilar membrane*, which is not really a membrane. Rather, it is a composite acellular plate containing a thin sheet of fibers and unstructured matrix material. The fibers,

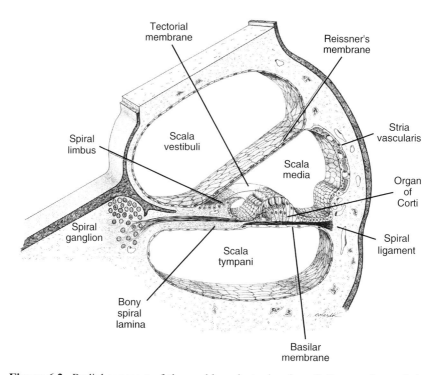

Figure 6.2. Radial segment of the cochlear duct, showing all three scalae and the basic divisions of the cochlear partition. The modiolus is to the left. (From Fawcett, 1994, with permission.*)

possibly containing collagen, are all oriented in radial directions. On the side closest to the modiolus, these basilar membrane fibers insert into the *bony spiral lamina*, and on the farthest side they are continuous with the *spiral ligament*. As suggested in Figure 5.1, the basilar membrane is narrower (and thicker) in the base than it is in the apex. These longitudinal[1] differences in the structure of the basilar membrane are presumed to account in large part for the different resonant frequencies measured at different points along the cochlear partition (see Fig. 5.3).

Delicate probing of the basilar membrane suggests that it is not under tension, at least in the dead cochlea (von Békésy, 1960, p. 465). However, tension fibroblasts (cells containing actin filaments) exist in the spiral ligaments of a wide variety of mammals (Henson and Henson, 1988; Kuhn and Vater, 1997), suggesting that the basilar membrane, particularly in basal regions, may be under radial tension (see Chapter 9).

Resting on the basilar membrane is a small but complicated superstructure, known as the *organ of Corti*, which contains the sound-sensing cells. Information is carried from these sensory cells into the central nervous system via the afferent axons of bipolar neurons whose cell bodies are located close by in the aptly named *spiral ganglion* (see Chapter 11). Efferent axons also exist, originating in neurons of the brain stem, which carry information from the brain into the organ of Corti (see Chapter 15). Note also the *stria vascularis*, located on the outside wall of scala media above the spiral ligament.

Of great functional importance is the *tectorial membrane*, shown here as being transparent: it extends from the lip of the *spiral limbus* to overlie the apical surface of the organ of Corti. Here is another misnomer, as the tectorial membrane is not a membrane but an acellular gelatinous structure containing several classes of proteins (Steel, 1983). More than one type of collagen has been identified in its composition.

An expanded view of the organ of Corti, with nearly a score of its various cell types identified, is shown in Figure 6.3 (for a comprehensive review see Slepecky, 1996). Its chief structural members appear to be the column-like *pillar* cells, which exist in two forms: the inner[2] pillar cells and the outer pillar cells. These pillar cells, whose trunks are composed of dense matrices of interlaced microfibrils and microtubules (Angelborg and Engström, 1972), are paired off, one of each forming a pair. The apical[3] surfaces (the ''heads'') of these two pillar cells are locked together, and their bases (or ''feet'') contact the basilar membrane at widely separated points, creating a cell-free space between them. The joined pairs of pillar cells stand head to head in a longitudinal row, creating a sidewalk-like surface on top and the *tunnel of Corti* underneath. Gentle mechanical probing of the cochlear partition from the basilar membrane side suggests that the pillar cell complex

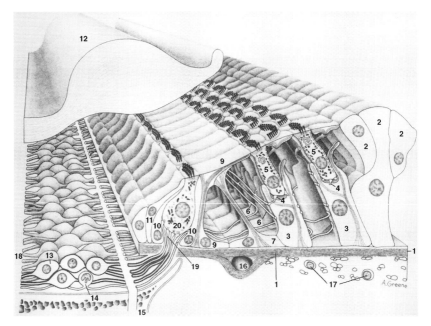

Figure 6.3. Typical organ of Corti in the basal turn, showing its many cell types. 1, basilar membrane; 2, Hensen's cells; 3, Deiters' cells; 4, nerve endings; 5, outer hair cells; 6, outer spiral axons; 7, outer pillar cells; 8, tunnel of Corti; 9, inner pillar cells; 10, inner phalangeal cells; 11, border cell; 12, tectorial membrane; 13, type I spiral ganglion cell; 14, type II spiral ganglion cell; 15, bony spiral lamina; 16, spiral blood vessel; 17, spindle cells; 18, axons of spiral gangion cells (auditory nerve axons); 19, peripheral axon; 20, inner hair cells. (From Kiang, 1984, with permission.*)

is relatively rigid compared to surrounding structures (Olson and Mountain, 1994). It appears that the pillar cells form the struts of a relatively stiff three-dimensional structure with a triangular cross section, reminiscent of the trusses used for bridge building.

On the modiolar side of a pair of the joined pillar cell heads lies a single sound-sensing cell, an *inner hair cell*, one of a row of such cells that runs uninterrupted from base to apex. This flask-shaped cell has a flat top that is exposed directly to endolymph (or some close relative). Conspicuous on this cell top are a number of protruding *stereocilia* (see Chapter 7). These "cilia" (an often used contraction) can be considered the mechanical focus of the entire inner ear—indeed of the entire peripheral ear. As shown in the following chapters, the angular deflection of these cilia is the final *mechanical* step in the ear's transduction of acoustic signals into neural pulses. Supporting cells, whose functions have not been closely investigated, invest all sides of the inner hair cell.

On the far side of a pillar-cell pair lie a related group of sound sensors, three *outer hair cells*, arranged in a more or less radial line. Each of these cylindrically shaped cells is also one of a row that runs longitudinally from base to apex. Like the inner hair cells, the outer hair cells have flat apical surfaces that bear cilia. In addition to differences in their shapes, there are a number of other distinctions between the two forms of hair cell (see Chapter 8). For instance, the outer hair cells are supported only at their bases and apexes by specialized *Deiters' cells*. This end-only support leaves the sides of the outer hair cells mostly free of cellular contact, an arrangement believed important to their functioning (see Chapter 9). Beyond the outer hair cells are several types of supporting cells, with only the *Hensen's cells* shown. Their functions are largely unknown.

Overlying this whole superstructure is the tectorial membrane. Usually dislodged from the organ of Corti during histological processing, this gelatinous structure is nevertheless known to be firmly attached to the Hensen's cells and the cilia of the outer hair cells in the living cochlea.

A micrographic view of a partially dissected organ of Corti is provided in Figure 6.4, obtained from an elevated "outside" position, looking down

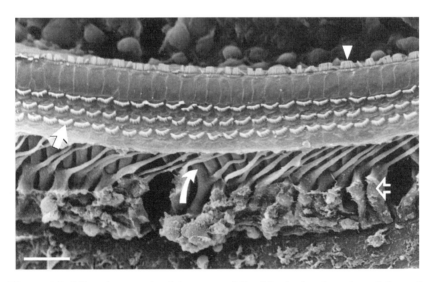

Figure 6.4. Microphotograph of the organ of Corti in the basal portion of the mole rat cochlea; the stapes is toward the left. Inner hair cells form a single row (triangle points to cilia); outer hair cells form three rows (solid arrow points to cilia). The latter are cylindrically shaped and tilted toward the stapes (curved arrow). From the Deiters' cells (open arrow) extend oppositely tilted phalangeal processes to the reticular lamina. Bar, 25 μm. (From Raphael et al., 1991, with permission.*)

and inward toward the modiolus. Prominent are the three rows of outer hair cells separated from the single row of inner hair cells (top of Fig. 6.4) by the smooth tops of the inner pillar heads. Because the cilia of each inner hair cell are formed into straight rows oriented in the same longitudinal direction as the hair cell row itself, an almost unbroken "fence" of inner hair cell cilia is formed. The cilia of each outer hair cell, by contrast, have a more complicated pattern, resembling the letters V and W.

Also noteworthy are the long, slender processes that arise at the bottom of Figure 6.4 and run upward toward the right. Each process is the single *phalangeal process* of a Deiters' cell, originating near the "cup" with which that cell cradles the base of a single outer hair cell and extending obliquely upward to the reticular lamina. The outer hair cells also have a longitudinal tilt, but in the opposite direction.

The connection between an outer hair cell and its companion Deiters' cell is shown more clearly in Figure 6.5. Note the closely packed microtubular arrays of the Deiters' cell main trunk and phalangeal process. Similar to pillar-cell structure, these arrays suggest columnar rigidity. Proteins identified in various parts of these two abutting cells are also shown in Figure 6.5.

As can be seen in Figures 6.4 and 6.5, the flat tops of the phalangeal processes end at the same level above the basilar membrane as do the flat tops of the outer hair cells. In fact, the interlacing flat tops of these two types of cell are connected tightly together to form the lateral section of the *reticular lamina*, the upper surface of the organ of Corti.

A close-up view of this luminal surface is provided in Figure 6.6. Interspersed between several rows of outer hair cells are the dumbbell-shaped tops of the Deiters' cell phalangeal processes (one is marked). Also striking on close examination is the precision with which the cilia are arranged on the apical surface of each outer hair cell. Five or six curved rows are formed, each row composed of cilia having approximately the same height. The shortest row on each hair cell faces the modiolus (to the left), and each successive row behind it stands slightly taller.

It is to this apical surface of the organ of Corti that the tectorial membrane adheres, partly to the cilia of the outer hair cells and partly to the Hensen's cells (Tonndorf et al., 1962). It has been suggested that their connections with the tectorial membrane account for the V shape taken by the ciliary rows of an outer hair cell. This peculiar shape not only provides each outer hair cell with more cilia than could be packed into the same number of straight rows, but the orientation of the rows, concave toward the modiolus, appears to provide the whole ciliary complex with some structural stiffness in the radial direction. Such stiffness seems useful for tethering the tectorial membrane.

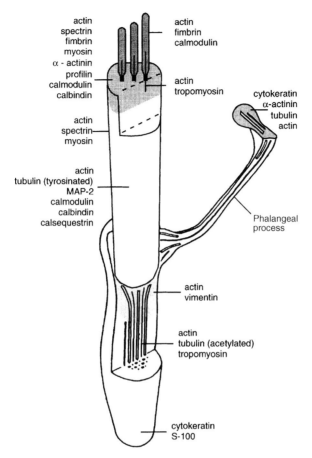

actin
spectrin
fimbrin
myosin
α - actinin
profilin
calmodulin
calbindin

actin
fimbrin
calmodulin

actin
tropomyosin

cytokeratin
α-actinin
tubulin
actin

actin
spectrin
myosin

actin
tubulin (tyrosinated)
MAP-2
calmodulin
calbindin
calsequestrin

Phalangeal
process

actin
vimentin

actin
tubulin (acetylated)
tropomyosin

cytokeratin
S-100

Figure 6.5. Outer hair cell and the (partially dissected) Deiters' cell supporting its base, with known protein constituents. The parallel arrays of structural proteins in the trunk and phalangeal process of the Deiters' cell suggest structural strength. The opposing longitudinal tilts of the outer hair cell and the phalangeal process of the Deiters' cell (see Fig. 6.4) place the tip of the phalangeal process among the apical surfaces of other outer hair cells. (From Slepecky, 1995, with permission.*)

By contrast, anatomical and physiological evidence strongly indicates that the tectorial membrane does not touch the cilia of the inner hair cells, at least in adult animals (Slepecky, 1996). If dissected away from the organ of Corti, the tectorial membrane displays a narrow longitudinal ridge (*Hensen's stripe*) on its undersurface that appears, from geometrical analysis, to lie directly over the single row of inner hair cells in the intact cochlea. Just how the tectorial membrane is connected to the organ of Corti in this vicinity is not clear, but the presence of wispy spindles (''trabeculae'') often seen protruding at regular spacings from Hensen's stripe in extracted specimens

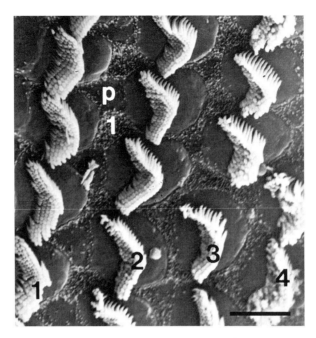

Figure 6.6. Microphotograph of the endolymphatic surface of the reticular lamina of the lower basal portion of the mole rat cochlea, showing three rows of outer hair cells (black numbers 1–3, from medial to lateral) and an occasionally present fourth row of outer hair cells (black 4). First-row outer hair cells are separated by outer pillar heads (p), and the second and third rows are separated by the apical tips of the phalangeal processes of Deiters' cells (white number 1 shows the first row phalangeal process tip). The modiolus is to the left. Bar, 5 μm. (From Raphael et al., 1991, with permission.*)

suggests that the tectorial membrane is normally moored just above the tips of the inner hair cell cilia by these trabeculae (Lim, 1980). To underline the importance of the tectorial membrane, note that some gelatinous structure, extending from the substrate to the ciliary tips of hair cells, exists in almost all vertebrate inner ears studied to date (but see below).

BASIC MECHANICAL MOTIONS

Deflection of the Cilia of Outer Hair Cells

Figure 6.7 shows our current understanding of how basilar membrane motion is transformed into the ciliary deflections of the *outer* hair cells during intense stimulation (i.e., when all ''amplifying'' mechanisms are negligible).

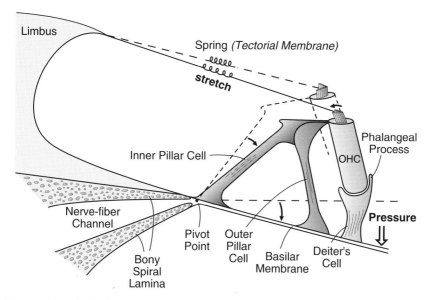

Figure 6.7. Mechanism thought to deflect the cilia of the outer hair cells. As the outer hair cell (OHC) is moved away from (toward) the spiral limbus by the vibrating basilar membrane, the tectorial membrane pulls (pushes) on the retreating (advancing) cilia.

For simplicity, a spring[4] represents the effect of the tectorial membrane on the cilia of this particular hair cell. As the basilar membrane is deflected downward by acoustic pressure, the relatively rigid triangular pillar cell complex keeps its shape and pivots clockwise about the foot of the inner pillar cell, which is situated near the edge of the relatively immobile bony spiral lamina. The outer hair cell, cradled by the Deiters' cell, is carried along with the basilar membrane, moving away from the spiral limbus. The tectorial membrane, attached to both the stationary limbus and the cilia of the receding outer hair cell, is stretched.

For their part, the hair cell cilia are known to be stiff (like rods) but readily rotatable about their insertions into the tops of the hair cells (see Chapter 7). Hence the force with which the stretched tectorial membrane pulls on the cilia causes them to rotate in a counterclockwise direction. The exact angle of ciliary deflection depends on the magnitude of their rotational stiffness relative to the stretching stiffness of the tectorial membrane.

Several estimates suggest that the maximum deflection possible for the ciliary tips of an outer hair cell is nearly equal to the deflection of the point on the basilar membrane that is located directly underneath that particular hair cell (e.g., Geisler, 1993). Thus the organ of Corti does an efficient job of transferring the vibrations of the basilar membrane to the cilia of the outer hair cells.

Deflection of the Cilia of Inner Hair Cells

The production of deflections in the cilia of the inner hair cells is somewhat less direct because, as mentioned, these cilia apparently do not contact the tectorial membrane in the adult. Therefore instead of the pulling action of the tectorial membrane, which moves the cilia of outer hair cells, it appears to be the movement of the fluid trapped in the subtectorial space (i.e., that sandwiched between the reticular lamina and the undersurface of the tectorial membrane) that deflects the cilia of the inner hair cells.

This process is outlined in Figure 6.8. The counterclockwise rotation of the outer hair cell cilia pictured in Figure 6.7 displaces some endolymph medially, toward the inner hair cells. Some of this displaced fluid presumably flows through the narrow gap separating the tectorial membrane (Hensen's stripe) from the tips of the inner hair cell cilia, pulling the latter radially inward toward the modiolus by viscous friction. The remainder of the moving fluid pushes directly against those cilia. These two forces, frictional and inertial, combine to cause a counterclockwise rotation of the inner hair cell cilia. Exactly the reverse process occurs when the basilar membrane is displaced upward. Experiments monitoring the output of the inner hair cells (see Chapter 8) indicate that for tonal stimulation at frequencies below about

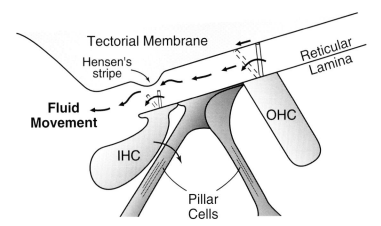

Figure 6.8. Mechanism thought to deflect the cilia of the inner hair cells (IHC). As the outer hair cell (OHC) cilia are deflected, the fluid thereby displaced flows over the tips of the IHC cilia, deflecting them as well. The width of the gap between the cilia and the tectorial membrane is unknown, as is the role of Hensen's stripe.

1 kHz the friction forces are the major rotating agent, whereas for higher frequencies the direct inertial push is dominant (Patuzzi and Yates, 1987). Theoretical analyses support this conclusion (Freeman and Weiss, 1990a,b). However, since the motions depicted here have never been observed directly, other mechanisms may also be involved, as indeed is indicated by the complexities of the primary neural responses to pure tones (see Chapter 12).

Returning to Figures 6.3 and 6.4 for a moment, we can appreciate now that the inner hair cell cilia are arranged in a manner ideally suited to sense this radial flow of fluid. Lined up in long, straight rows perpendicular to that flow, these cilia present to it an almost uninterrupted barrier. With the tectorial membrane presumably moored just above those cilia, the fluid displaced by the outer hair cell cilia has only the thin gap between the tectorial membrane and the tips of the inner hair cell cilia through which to flow. The result is relatively high fluid velocities and the high viscous friction forces that result (recall that friction force is proportional to velocity).

Animations of the idealized ciliary deflections produced by cochlear-partition vibrations are available on our World Wide Web site (see Fig. 1.1).

Comparison with a Reptile Ear

An instructive comparison can be made with the workings of the alligator lizard's basilar papilla (the reptilian analogue of the organ of Corti). Situated between the endolymph and perilymph, as depicted in Figure 4.1, this small sensing organ is in the form of an elongated rectangle, approximately 400 μm long and 50 μm wide (Fig. 6.9). The papilla carries approximately 200 hair cells, arranged in five or six parallel rows running the full length of its endolymphatic side (the vantage point of Figure 6.9). Especially interesting about this papilla is the division of its hair cells into two groups: those that contact an overlying tectorial membrane and those that do not (the "free-standing" ones).

A cross section through the portion of this papilla containing the tectorial membrane is shown in the bottom inset of Figure 6.9. The cilia of the five hair cells are relatively short and contact the tectorial membrane directly. A fascinating stop-action video recording of the ciliary motions that occur in this portion of the papilla has been made in an excised preparation, looking down on it through the virtually transparent tectorial membrane (Davis and Freeman, 1995). This recording shows that the tectorial membrane, with the tips of the hair cell cilia embedded in it, undergoes relatively little lateral motion, whereas the apical surfaces of the hair cells, containing the rootlets of those same cilia, are carried laterally back and forth by the acoustically induced movements of the whole papilla. It appears that the mass (inertia) of the tectorial membrane makes it difficult to move rapidly. Thus with their

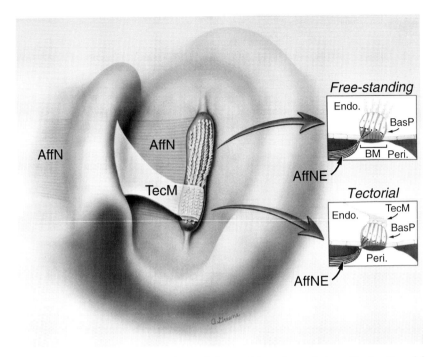

Figure 6.9. Endolymphatic surface of the cochlear duct of the alligator lizard in vitro. The papilla measures approximately 400 × 50 μm and contains about 200 hair cells innervated by about 900 nerve endings (AffNE), the terminals of the innervating axons, most assumed to be afferent (AffN). In one region a tectorial membrane (TecM) contacts the hair cell cilia, whereas in the other region the cilia are free-standing. The auditory receptor organ (basilar papilla, BasP) is attached to the basilar membrane (BM), which separates the endolymphatic space (Endo.) from the perilymphatic space (Peri.). Depending on the location, the cilia are either free-standing (top inset) or embedded in the tectorial membrane (bottom inset). (From Freeman et al., 1993, with permission.*)

tips fixed but their rootlets moving to and fro, the hair cell cilia are forced to rotate. These ciliary rotations are the only ones to have been directly observed so far in an intact auditory organ, although it is presumed that something similar happens in the mammalian cochlea because relative motions between the tectorial membrane and the reticular lamina must also exist there (Figs. 6.7 and 6.8).

A similar cross section through the uncovered section of the alligator lizard papilla is shown in the top inset of Figure 6.9. As discussed in more detail later (see Chapter 7), it appears that it is the mass (inertia) of the endolymph itself that forces a similar type of rotation on these free-standing cilia as their hair cells are carried along with the acoustically induced vibrations of the underlying basilar membrane.

Finally, note the nerve fibers that arrive at the left side of the papilla in a thin sheet. These fibers innervate the hair cells along the entire length of the papilla. In a similar fashion, the nerve fibers serving the mammalian cochlea penetrate the organ of Corti in a thin sheet (Fig. 6.3), although it is much longer than that of the alligator lizard and is wound into a helix (see Fig. 11.1).

CHEMICAL AND ELECTRICAL MILIEU OF THE ORGAN OF CORTI

The sound-sensing behavior of the organ of Corti cannot be understood without an appreciation of the strong chemical and electrical gradients that exist there. Endolymph, the fluid of scala media that appears to bathe the cilia and apical surfaces of mammalian hair cells (Fig. 6.10), is unique among the body's extracellular fluids (for review see Wangemann and Schacht, 1996). Chemically, it has a high concentration of potassium ions (K^+), about 150 millimolar (mM) in the guinea pig, and a low concentration of sodium ions (Na^+), about 1 mM (Sellick and Johnstone, 1975). These extracellular concentrations are most unusual, resembling those found *within* most mammalian cells. Scala media also contains an electrical voltage, the *endocochlear potential*, which is +60 to +100 millivolts (mV) relative to that of the animal's vascular system (von Békésy, 1960).

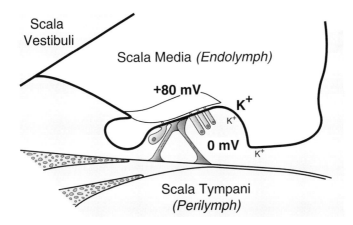

Figure 6.10. Electrochemical environment of the organ of Corti. The boundary between endolymph and perilymph is indicated by the heavy line. The apical surfaces of the hair cells face a high positive voltage (e.g., +80 mV) and a high concentration of K^+ ions, whereas the neural innervation and basolateral surfaces of the hair cells are bathed in an electrically neutral solution poor in K^+ ions (though rich in Na^+ ions).

Perilymph, on the other hand, has properties similar to those of the normal extracellular fluid that exists between most mammalian cells: high Na^+ and low K^+ concentrations and an electrical potential approximately the same as that of the vascular system.

Contrary to what might be expected from its gross structure, the boundary between endolymph and perilymph that exists in the organ of Corti does *not* occur at the basilar membrane but, rather, at the reticular lamina. Experiments with dyes have shown unequivocally that the former is permeable to small molecules, whereas the latter is not (e.g., Tonndorf et al., 1962). This separation of lymph is accomplished by tight junctions, which connect the tops of the various cell types that border scala media (Gulley and Reese, 1976). Because the fluid in the subtectorial space appears to have a composition much like that of endolymph (Flock, 1977), it is believed that the cilia and tops of the hair cells are bathed by a fluid of high positive voltage and high K^+ concentration.

By contrast, because the hair cells' basolateral surfaces and their neural innervation lie below the reticular lamina, they are in contact with perilymph (whose high Na^+ concentration is needed for nerve-pulse conduction). The result (Fig. 6.10) is that large electrical and ion concentration gradients are developed across the different surfaces of the hair cells, gradients that power the sound-sensing functions of these cells (see Chapter 8).

The important role of the *stria vascularis* in maintaining the organ of Corti's unusual chemical and electrical milieu should be mentioned. This prominent structure, which occupies almost the entire outer wall of scala media (Fig. 6.2), produces both the endolymph of scala media and its positive electrical potential (Kuijpers, 1972). As its name implies, the stria vascularis, composed of three cell layers, is richly supplied with blood. Immediately adjacent to the endolymph are the *marginal*, or *dark*, cells. These cells are strange, one of the few cell types in the mammal to have *positive* intracellular resting potentials (ca. $+80$ mV). Still debated, the molecular mechanisms responsible for the highly unusual properties of stria vascularis have been modeled in several ways (Wangemann, 1995; Wangemann and Schacht, 1996).

The ready oxygen supply provided by the stria's rich blood supply is vital to its functioning, as the endocochlear potential drops rapidly, even going negative, within a minute or so after breathing is arrested (Kuijpers, 1972). It is worth noting that hair cells per se do not require the large positive potentials of normal cochlear endolymph to function: The endolymph that fills the membranous labyrinth of the vestibular system, with its several types of hair cell, has electrical potentials of only a few millivolts (Goldberg and Fernández, 1972).

NOTES

1. The cochlear coordinate system, as described in this book, is as follows: *Radial* is the direction, in any cross-sectional view of the cochlear partition, that extends outward from the axis of the modiolus, parallel to the line of the basilar membrane (i.e., forms a spoke sprouting from the modiolar axis). *Vertical* is the direction in that same cross-sectional view of the cochlear partition that is perpendicular to the basilar membrane. *Longitudinal* is the direction in the plane of the local basilar membrane that is along the helix (i.e., parallel to the axes of the scalae), with the stapes serving as the starting point.

2. There are several types of cells within the organ of Corti which come in two distinct and geographically separated forms. The form located closest to the modiolus is identified as "inner"; the form located farther out radially is labeled "outer."

3. Standard nomenclature considers the basilar membrane as forming the "base" of an upright organ of Corti. Thus the "basal" segments of organ of Corti cells are those nearest the basilar membrane (scala tympani), and "apical" surfaces are those nearest scala media. These names are unfortunate, as they are also used to describe the longitudinal position within the cochlea. Nevertheless, it is usually clear from the context the structures or sections that are being referenced.

4. It is not known how to represent accurately the hydromechanical properties of the tectorial membrane. Extensively hydrated, its mass is assumed to be virtually that of an equal volume of endolymph; but only one in situ measurement of its static stiffness has been reported (Zwislocki and Cefaratti, 1989). Its viscoelastic properties are virtually unknown. For present purposes, an exact representation of the tectorial membrane is not important, provided it acts passively (i.e., not powered metabolically) and presents some sort of mechanical impediment to movement of the ciliary tips. The available experimental evidence indicates that these two conditions are satisfied, justifying the "spring" representation used here. Various other models have been proposed (e.g., Zwislocki and Kletsky, 1979; Allen, 1980).

II

Hair Cell Functions

7

TRANSDUCTION PROCESSES IN
HAIR CELLS

The hearing organs in vertebrates, their vestibular apparatus, and (in fish and some amphibians) the lateral line organs, share the need to transduce minute mechanical disturbances into receptor potentials. These organs, which together make up the *acousticolateralis* system, accomplish this task with specialized displacement-sensing cells. Although they come in various shapes and sizes, each of these *hair cells* is characterized by a group of cilia or "hairs" protruding from an approximately flat surface making up one end of the cell (Flock, 1971). The deflection of these cilia is the crucial mechanical step in the hair cell's transduction process (Hudspeth and Corey, 1977).

To produce these deflections, the various sensory systems harness forces through a variety of ingenious accessory structures. In the semicircular canals of the vestibular system the rotational inertia of a ring of fluid (one for each dimension) creates differences in motion between the fluids and their rotating sleeves; in the utriculus and sacculus the force of gravity (or its equivalent, acceleration in a straight line) pulls on heavy crystals; in the externally located lateral-line organs the momentum of water flowing over the skin of the animal is tapped; and in the hearing organs acoustic forces cause various substrate or tectorial structures to vibrate.

In this chapter we review attributes of hair cells in general. In Chapter 8 we examine their specializations for the cochlea.

STRUCTURAL ANATOMY

The basic structure of a generalized hair cell is shown in Figure 7.1. At the apical end of the cell, cilia protrude from a rigid, flat *circular plate*. All but one of these cilia are *microvilli*, tubular protrusions of the cell composed of parallel actin filaments tightly packed into hexagonal arrays and oriented along the long axis of the cilium. Cross-sectional views of these microvilli, known as *stereocilia*, are observable in the photomicrograph at the right in

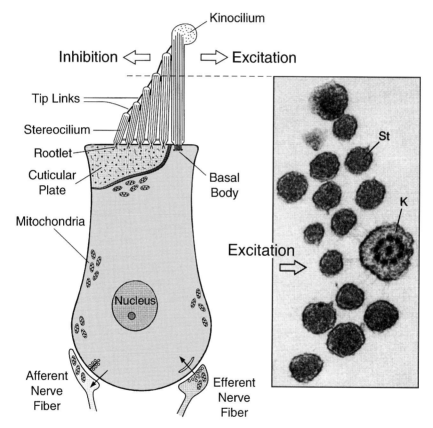

Figure 7.1. Stylized vertebrate hair cell. Deflection of the stereocilia toward (away from) the kinocilium results in excitation (inhibition) of the hair cell. *Inset.* Ciliary cross sections in an electron micrograph obtained from a turtle cochlea, in a plane parallel to the cuticular plate, at the height of the dashed line. Note the ''9+2'' organization of the microtubule doublets in the kinocilium (K) and the tightly packed actin rods of the stereocilia (St). (Photomicrograph: From Hackney et al., 1993, with permission*.)

Figure 7.1. Fimbrin appears to crosslink these actin strands together (Flock et al., 1981) into what proves to be a stiff rod, with a diameter of 0.1–0.3 μm. Note that the diameter of each stereocilium is considerably reduced at its insertion into the cuticular plate. This reduction in ankle diameter coupled with its stiffness ensures that a stereocilium remains rigid (like a tin soldier) when subjected to lateral forces, pivoting stiffly about the narrow *rootlet* that connects it with the cuticular plate. Although their functions are not clearly understood, a number of other proteins, such as myosin and tropomyosin, have been identified in the cuticular plate (see Fig. 6.5).

The stereocilia are arranged in rows or clusters (depending on the organ), whose orientation is determined by the single *kinocilium*. This cilium, which is always located at an edge of the ciliary cluster, has its own base, or *basal body*, located just outside the cuticular plate. The kinocilium is different from the stereocilia, having a cytoplasmic core containing the 9+2 arrangement of microtubular doublets characteristic of true cilia (cross section at right in Fig. 7.1).

The function of the kinocilium, which has different relative lengths in different types of hair cells, is not completely understood. It does not seem to be related to the transduction function in any basic way, as not all hair cells have them. Moreover, even in hair cells that do have them, their removal does not impair transduction (Hudspeth and Jacobs, 1979). The tip of the kinocilium is often connected to an overlying tectorial structure, and so in those cases at least it serves to transmit movements of that tectorium to its stereociliary neighbors through numerous interconnecting crosslinks (Thurm, 1981). In any case, the kinocilium, or its basal body (which *does* appear in all hair cells), forms the functional axis of the hair cell. Roughly speaking, rotations of the stereocilia toward the kinocilium (basal body) result in electrical depolarization of the cell, whereas tip movements in the opposite direction produce hyperpolarization (see animations). Movements at right angles to these cardinal directions produce little or no response (Flock, 1971).

The stereocilia are arranged in different configurations on the cuticular plate, depending on the identity of the hair cell. A common pattern, seen for example in the bullfrog sacculus, is for the stereocilia to be tightly packed within a circle, at the edge of which is found the single kinocilium. By contrast, as shown earlier (Figs. 6.3, 6.4), the stereocilia of each cochlear hair cell in the mammal are arranged in rows, much like ranks of soldiers. Despite this diversity, common to *all* of these deployments is a stair-step arrangement of the stereocilia. If a kinocilium is present, the stereocilia that stand closest to it are the tallest, with the ones behind becoming progressively shorter. If only a basal body is present, as in cochlear hair cells, the

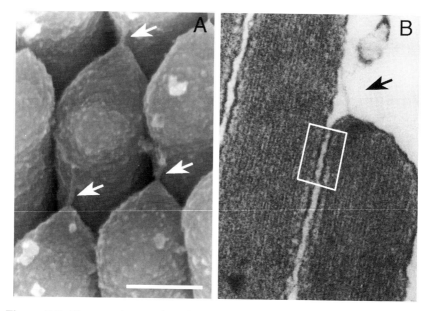

Figure 7.2. Electronmicrographs of tip links between hair cell stereocilia in the turtle cochlea. *A*. Scanning electron micrograph. Tip links are indicated by arrows. Bar, 0.2 μm. *B*. Transmission electron micrograph. Tip link is indicated by the arrow. Rectangle encloses an area of close ciliary apposition. (*A*: Courtesy of Hackney and Furness, University of Keele, UK. *B*: From Hackney et al., 1993, with permission*.)

row of stereocilia closest to it is tallest, with the rows behind successively shorter.

The necessary consequence of this ordered ranking of heights is that, except for the tallest, each stereocilium stands behind a taller one. Such staggering of heights permits the existence of *tip links*, fine strands (possibly of elastin) that connect the top of the shorter stereocilium with the lateral wall of its taller neighbor (Fig. 7.2). These universally occurring tip links, discovered by Pickles et al. (1984), are in addition to lateral links, which run in all directions between neighboring stereocilia. Each end of a tip link forms an electron-dense plaque (Hackney et al., 1993).

TRANSDUCTION OF CILIARY ROTATIONS INTO CELL POTENTIALS

Location of Transduction Sites

There is much evidence that these tip links are essential parts of the motion transducers. For example, when tip links are destroyed, either by treatment with the proteolytic enzyme elastase (Preyer et al., 1995) or by removal of

Ca^{2+} ions from the external medium (Assad et al., 1991), the transduction processes of the hair cells are irreversibly lost as well. A possible mechanism for this transduction is depicted in the "trapdoor" model shown in Figure 7.3. At rest (Fig. 7.3B), the tip link is slightly stretched, allowing an attached stretch-sensitive cationic channel to conduct only occasionally, perhaps 10% of the time. A small steady flux of K^+ ions, occurring in high concentration in the endolymph (see Fig. 6.10), is thus driven into the cell through these flickering channels by the strong electrical potential that exists between the positively charged endolymph and the negatively charged interior of the cell. A "resting" depolarization of the hair cell results (see Fig. 8.3).

Positive stimulation occurs when external forces push cilia in the direction of their taller neighbors, thereby rotating each stereocilium about its rootlet and further stretching the interconnecting tip link (Fig. 7.3C). The "trapdoor" is opened more frequently by the increased tension in the tip link, K^+ ions flow inward at a higher average rate, and the cell is further depolarized. *Negative* stimulation occurs when stimulating forces push the ciliary tips in the opposite direction, toward their shorter neighbors (Fig. 7.3A). In that case, the tension in the tip link is reduced below its resting value. With

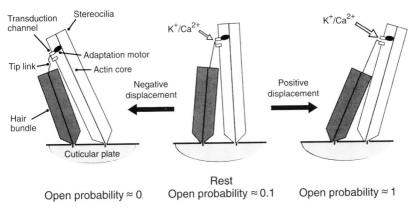

Figure 7.3. "Trapdoor" theory of hair cell excitation. Changing tension in the tip link is hypothesized to change the conduction probabilities of a related nonspecific cation-conducting channel. For displacements toward the kinocilium (*C*), the tip link is stretched, increasing the opening probability of the trapdoor. For displacements away from the kinocilium (*A*), tip link tension is relaxed, and the trapdoor is less readily opened. "Adaptation" of the hair cell's responses (Fig. 7.4) is attributed to adjustment of tip-link tension by an "adaptation motor" located at the upper end of the tip link (*A*), so as to reestablish at the new "resting" position the initial value of tip link tension and hence of channel conductance (*B*). (From Gillespie, 1995, with permission*.)

less pull on the ionic trapdoor, the probability of channel opening is accordingly reduced, the flow of K^+ ions is stifled, and the cell potential sinks below its unstimulated value.

This "trapdoor" model has considerable support, including the finding that the whole-bundle stiffness of a frog saccular hair cell is indeed a function of the open probabilities of its transduction channels and thus presumably of the average tension in its tip links (Hudspeth, 1989). Moved by forces not much bigger than those required to activate its presumed sensors, it appears that the ciliary tufts in such hair cells are about as pliable as they could possibly be.

Theoretical analyses show that tip links are beautifully positioned to act as sensors of ciliary deflection. Not only is the stretch on the tip links calculated to be directly *proportional* to the angle of stereociliary deflection, but the height of the cilia appears to have little influence on this stretch (Geisler, 1993; Pickles, 1993). Thus tip links between neighboring stereocilia of any length appear to be almost equally effective and accurate sensors.

Another possibility for the hair cell transduction mechanism has been suggested by attempts to label the transduction channels immunocytochemically (Furness et al., 1996). Successful labeling did occur but not at the upper end of the tip link as expected. Instead the labeled particles congregated in the *tip junction* region, just below the lower end of the tip link, where the tip of the shorter cilium comes into close proximity (perhaps even contact) with the taller cilium (region indicated in Figure 7.2B). Theoretical analysis indicates that the stretching of such a ciliary contact point during small deflections would be similar to the stretching of the neighboring tip link (Furness et al., 1997).

With either scenario the transduction channels are located in the tip-link region, where several independent lines of experimental evidence site the hair cell's transduction channels. Earlier, a sampling of voltages at points all around the ciliary tuft of a saccular hair cell showed that mechanical deflection of the tuft produced transduction currents that were strongest in the vicinity of the ciliary tips (Hudspeth, 1982).

More recently, calcium imaging techniques have shown that, upon positive deflection of the ciliary tuft, free calcium ion concentrations rose sharply in the stereocilia with a concentration gradient that decreased from tip to rootlet (Denk et al., 1995). Moreover, the number of stereocilia responding was proportional to the transduction current. Evidently, calcium ions flowed into the stereocilia through transduction channels located somewhere in the ciliary tips. An unexpected finding was that some of the shortest stereocilia sometimes sustained calcium ion influxes. Are there "trapdoors" on both sides of the gating structure?

Effect of Ciliary Deflections on Ion Flows

A dramatic example of a transducer channel at work is shown in Figure 7.4A, the "whole cell" voltage-clamp[1] recording of a turtle hair cell having only one functional transduction channel. At rest (the condition at the beginning and end of the plot), the probability of channel opening was small. With an excitatory stepwise movement of 200 nm on the ciliary tuft (Fig. 7.4A, top tracing), the probability of opening was greatly increased, and the channel rapidly flickered open and closed, allowing a channel current of about 9 picoamperes (pA) (pico = 10^{-12}) to flow nearly half the time for an average value of about 5 pA (Fig. 7.4A, bottom tracing). It is the sum of all such randomly pulsating transduction currents that make up the responses of a hair cell.

The magnitudes of such responses recorded from a more nearly normal turtle hair cell are shown in Figure 7.4B as a function of ciliary bundle displacement. At rest, only a small transduction current existed, averaging about 9 pA (Fig. 7.4B, open circle at zero displacement). At the existing cell potential (-85 mV) it corresponded to a cell resistance of about 10^{10} ohms, or 100 picoSiemens (pS) conductance (conductance = 1/resistance).

Displacements of the stereociliary tips in the direction of the kinocilium caused increasing current flow: the larger the displacement, the larger the flow (Fig. 7.4B, open circles). For large positive displacements, an asymptote of about 250 pA was reached, corresponding in this case to about 3400 pS. Values as high as 5500 pS have been observed (Fettiplace et al., 1992). This maximum conductance is significant, as it is about 55 times that of a single channel. If we assume that the asymptotically large current flows shown in Figure 7.4B were achieved only when all transduction channels were conducting simultaneously, this ratio indicates that the hair cell possessed about 55 channels. Because 50–100 stereocilia comprise each ciliary bundle, the obvious conclusion is that a fully functional turtle hair cell has somewhat less than one channel for each of its stereocilia, consistent with both the tip link and tip contact models.

The resulting transduction mechanism has a number of stunning attributes. First, it is *extremely* sensitive. Estimates for several vertebrate species (guinea pig: Sellick et al., 1982; turtle: Fettiplace, 1992) indicate that the ciliary tip displacements of auditory hair cells at behavioral threshold are on the order of 0.3 nm (Hudspeth, 1989). For a 5 μm cilium this displacement causes angular rotations of less than 0.003°. This angle is so tiny it is even less (by an order of magnitude) than the random deflections of the ciliary tips caused by the Brownian motion of the surrounding fluid mole-

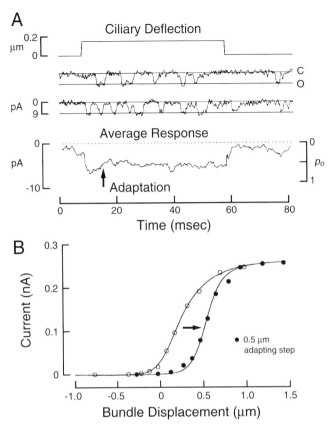

Figure 7.4. Excitation of hair cells isolated from turtle cochlea. *A.* Middle traces are two individual "whole cell" recordings taken from a hair cell having only a single operational ion channel. The conducting time of the channel, which was either fully open (O) or fully closed (C), was increased during positive stepwise ciliary deflection (top trace). The average of 55 individual recordings (bottom trace) shows that the ciliary deflections caused an average increase of about 5 pA in the ion channel's current. The right-hand ordinate is p_0, the channel's probability of being open. *B.* Peak amplitudes of average transducer current elicited in a more nearly normal hair cell by stepwise ciliary displacements of various magnitudes, some preceded by an adapting bias of +0.5 μm (closed circles) and some not (open circles). (*A:* From Crawford et al., 1991, with permission*. *B:* From Fettiplace, 1992, with permission*.)

cules (Denk et al., 1989). It is the angle moved by the minute hand of a clock during 30 msec.

The system is also very fast. Channel-opening times of less than 50 μsec have been measured in some hair cells, strongly indicating direct mechanical action on the channels rather than a second messenger system.

Adaptation

The second set of data in Figure 7.4B (closed dots) provide yet another remarkable characteristic of the transduction apparatus, *adaptation*. When the stereocilia are subjected to an abrupt stepwise displacement in the excitatory direction, the magnitude of transducer current slowly decreases, or "adapts," to a new lower level. An example of this adaptation can be seen in the average response in Figure 7.4A. If such a stair-step displacement is maintained long enough, the stereocilia gradually change their properties such that the cell's "transfer" characteristic (i.e., current-versus-displacement curve) recenters itself about the new position of static displacement. The great importance of this sort of self-centering is clear: Without it, the contact region between two stereocilia would have to be constructed and maintained in place with nanometer accuracy despite any static deflections that might occur in the ciliary tuft.

The molecular mechanisms of this adaptation are not clear at this time. One essential factor has been identified: an ample supply of Ca^{2+} ions. Specifically, when the Ca^{2+} concentration of the solution bathing these isolated turtle hair cells was reduced from its usual value near 3 mM to 1 mM, the rate of adaptation became slower, apparently vanishing completely when the concentration was reduced still further to 50 μM, near the in vivo level in the turtle ear (Crawford et al., 1991). Lowering the Ca^{2+} concentration also increased the asymptotic value of the transduction current and changed the "resting" point on the cell's transfer curve.

The adaptations exhibited by such isolated hair cells may not be characteristic of hair cells in situ. Work with an in vitro preparation of the whole turtle cochlea indicates that rapid hair cell adaptation can exist with low extracellular concentrations of Ca^{2+} ions (Ricci and Fettiplace, 1997). The essential factor seems to be the *internal* concentration of free Ca^{2+} ions, not their extracellular concentration.

It has been proposed that this adaptation is caused by the action of myosin molecules, which have been discovered near the upper end-plaque of the tip link (Hudspeth and Gillespie, 1994). With this scheme the myosin molecules would interact as a group with the cilium's actin filament matrix, which has its functional polarities oriented downward, toward the cuticular plate (Flock et al., 1981). Assuming the type of actin–myosin interaction that occurs in striated muscle cells, the myosin group would climb upward along the actin matrix toward the ciliary tip until a balancing amount of tension would be developed in its tip link tether (Fig. 7.3B). Were the cilia to be biased in the excitatory direction (Fig. 7.3C), increased tension in the tip-link would drag the myosin "adaptation motor" downward, gradually reducing that tip-link tension until a new balance point was reached. Reciprocally, were the cilia to be biased in the inhibitory direction (Fig. 7.3A), existing tension in the tip link would be reduced and the motor would be freed to climb farther upward, until balancing tension was again restored.

There is much indirect support for this motor hypothesis (Gillespie, 1995), but it cannot account for such adaptation phenomena as the previously mentioned change in the cell's "resting" point, which occurs with reduced Ca^{2+} concentrations.

An alternate hypothesis is that calcium ions themselves interact directly with a transducer channel to determine its state of adaptation: the higher the local Ca^{2+} concentration, the more highly adapted the channel (Fettiplace, 1992). A static excitatory deflection of the hair cell cilia would allow an increased flow of Ca^{2+} ions to enter the ciliary tip, thereby increasing the Ca^{2+} concentration near the channel, whereas a steady inhibitory deflection would diminish the inward flow of calcium ions and their concentration at the tip. The solid lines of Figure 7.4B were produced with an explicit version of this hypothesis under the assumption that each ion channel had one open state and two closed states, one of which bound Ca^{2+} ions.

Conversion of Ion Flows into Cell Potentials

From a simplified point of view, the conversion of ion flows into hair cell *transduction potentials* is straightforward. The nonspecific cation-selective transduction channels in its stereociliary tips admit into each hair cell a steady flow of positively charged particles, principally K^+ ions. With the increased flow of these cations, which results from excitatory deflections of the ciliary bundle, the concentration of positive ions within the cell rises, causing the cell's electrical transmembrane potential[2] to rise also. By the same token, inhibitory deflections of the ciliary bundle reduce the cation influx below resting level, the concentration of positive ions within the cell drops, and accordingly the cell potential drops.

An explicit electrical circuit model of this process, which also takes into account the ion channels that exist in the basolateral surface of a hair cell, is described in Chapter 8.

Amplification of Signal Power

During the process of transforming mechanical motions into electrical potentials, the hair cells may amplify the power[3] of a signal many times over. A simplified ballpark calculation bears this contention out. Consider first the power transferred to a hair cell by an incoming sinusoidal signal. The absorption of power by an ideal mechanical element can be shown[4] to equal the magnitude of its damping (D) multiplied by the square of its velocity

(v^2) (i.e., Power = $D * v^2$). The damping of a frog saccular hair cell tuft has been estimated at about $200 * 10^{-9}$ Nsec/m (Denk et al., 1989). Therefore a tone of 160 Hz, vibrating the ciliary tip at an amplitude of 10 nm (velocity $\approx$ 10 μm/sec), delivers to the hair cell (and its immediate fluid environment) approximately $2 * 10^{-17}$ watts of power.

So far as the hair cell itself is concerned, we know that a ciliary deflection of 1 μm produces a transmembrane potential of about 100 mV (Denk and Webb, 1992). Thus with a tip deflection of 10 nm, the corresponding hair cell receptor potential would have an amplitude of about 1 mV. As power dissipated by an electrical element is equal to the square of the voltage (E^2) across its terminals divided by its resistance (R) (i.e., power = E^2/R), and the resistance of these cells is estimated at 400 MΩ, the signal power dissipated electrically in the cell would be approximately $2.5 * 10^{-15}$ watt. Thus, at this frequency there is a 100-fold boost in the power of the signal as it changes media, a factor that decreases as the square of the stimulus frequency.

The added power is provided by the energy stored in the voltage and concentration differences created across the cell's plasma membrane by the long-term homeostatic mechanisms. By functioning as valves that control the flow of charged ions, the stereocilia can control the flow of more power than they themselves absorb. In this sense, they are behaving like electronic amplifying elements such as the transistor.

MECHANISMS OF HAIR CELL FREQUENCY SELECTIVITY

The magnitude with which a hair cell's stereocilia respond to externally applied sinusoidal forces is always related to the frequency involved. Some sinusoids vary too rapidly for the cilia to follow fully,[5] and some vary too slowly. Without exception, hair cells of every type display greater sensitivity to sinusoids of certain frequencies than of others. In fact, as far as we know, every auditory hair cell is tuned to a relatively narrow band of tonal frequencies. A surprising variety of mechanisms are used to achieve this sharp frequency tuning in the hearing organs of various vertebrate classes.

Substrate Vibrations

An obvious tuning mechanism is to site the hair cell on a movable support that is itself tuned. This situation pertains in the mammalian cochlea, where the frequency selectivity of the hair cells is largely determined by the motion of the hair cells' substrate, the basilar membrane. Intracellular data obtained

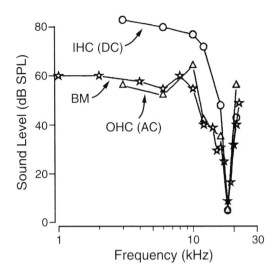

Figure 7.5. Frequency tuning curves for hair cells and basilar membrane at a basal location in the guinea pig cochlea. The tip of the curve for the basilar membrane (BM) compares favorably with those of both the outer hair cell (OHC) and the inner hair cell (IHC). Amplitude criteria used to create these isoresponse plots were 0.35 nm for BM, 0.5 mV AC receptor potential for OHC (corrected for equipment and cell wall filtering), and 0.8 mV DC receptor potential for IHC. (From Russell et al., 1995, with permission*.)

from cochlear hair cells located near the 18 kHz region of the guinea pig cochlea are a case in point. As shown in Figure 7.5, both the inner and outer hair cells displayed frequency tuning curves that had virtually the same frequency selectivity as the tuning curve of the underlying basilar membrane in the vicinity of their common ''characteristic frequency'' (i.e., that frequency of sinusoidal stimulation to which an element is most sensitive). Thus we may say that the frequency selectivity of cochlear hair cells is principally determined by the frequency selectivity of that section of the basilar membrane on which they ride.

Despite this close agreement between the sharp frequency tuning characteristics of cochlear hair cells and the basilar membrane in mammals, it would be wrong to assume that hair cells in the mammalian cochlea are simply passive recorders of basilar membrane vibrations. They are not. On the contrary, as is shown in Chapter 9, the outer hair cells play a crucial role in determining not only the amplitudes of those substrate vibrations but, in the cochlear base, their frequency selectivities as well.

Mechanical Tuning of Hair Cells

Other tuning mechanisms are brought into play in lizards, as the basilar membranes of at least two species do not appear to be as sharply or as differentially tuned as their output neurons (Peake and Ling, 1980; Manley et al., 1988). For example, displacement measurements obtained at various points along the bobtail lizard's basilar membrane (Fig. 7.6A) have much the same frequency selectivity: a poorly tuned "band-pass" curve with a peak somewhere between 1.0 and 1.5 kHz. Yet the frequency tuning curves recorded from the basilar papilla's primary sensory neurons in that species all displayed much sharper frequency selectivities, tuned to characteristic frequencies that varied over two full octaves, from 1 to 4 kHz (Fig. 7.6B). Each of these individual neural responses was successfully modeled using a spring-mass system sharply tuned to the neuron's particular characteristic

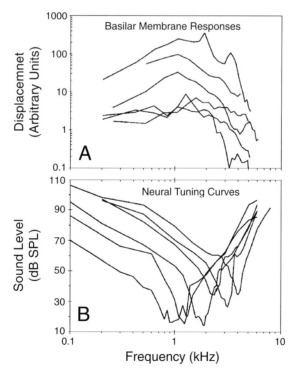

Figure 7.6. Frequency selectivity in the inner ear of a lizard, the Australian bobtail skink. *A.* Typical response curves of the basilar membrane (BM) at different points with tones of fixed amplitude and varying frequency. *B.* Family of (threshold level) frequency tuning curves for individual primary auditory neurons of the bobtail skink's ear. Contrast the broadly tuned BM peaks with the sharply tuned neural curves. (From Manley et al., 1988, with permission*.)

frequency (recall that $\omega_{res} = \sqrt{K/M}$), superimposed on the more broadly tuned basilar membrane vibrations.

A more recent modeling effort by that same group (Authier and Manley, 1995) suggested that the postulated secondary resonant system does indeed exist, constructed from the summed stiffnesses (*springs*) of all of the stereocilia in a small group of hair cells and the *mass* of the small, free-floating tectorial structure overlying that particular group of hair cells (many such groups exist side by side) (Manley, 1990). It thus appears that, at least in these lizard ears, the basilar membrane provides broad, similarly tuned substrate vibrations to all of its resident hair cells, each group of which then responds uniquely according to its own specific mechanical properties.

Yet a different arrangement occurs in the frog's basilar papilla, one of the two hearing papillae that exist within each of its inner ears. In this small high-frequency organ, a narrow crest of hair cells sits on an *immobile* cartilaginous substrate with their cilia embedded in the edges of a curtain-like tectorial membrane that partially occludes the endolymphatic duct (Geisler et al., 1964). Here the collective properties of all of the hair cell cilia (probably their stiffnesses) combine with those of the thin tectorial membrane (presumably its mass) to achieve a single, sharp hydromechanical resonance shared by all of the hair cells, as evidenced by the similar characteristic frequencies of their afferent neurons (Capranica, 1978).

The ultimate refinement of this individualized tuning is provided by a variety of lizard hair cells that contact *no* tectorial structure whatsoever (see Fig. 6.9). Measurements show that the ciliary tuft of each "free-standing" hair cell has an individualized resonance whose frequency depends on the length of its cilia, a feature that varies systematically along the papilla (Frishkopf and DeRosier, 1983). Theoretical analysis suggests that it is the springiness of each hair cell's ciliary tuft and the mass of the endolymph surrounding it that determine the specialized part of the sharp, individually tuned responses displayed by its afferent neurons (Freeman and Weiss, 1990). It appears that the surprisingly sharp tuning for these hair cells depends on the extraordinary lengths of their cilia, necessary in order for them to extend beyond the thin "boundary" layer of high friction forces (Freeman and Weiss, 1988).

Electrical Tuning of Hair Cells

Individualized frequency tuning of hair cells also exists in the turtle's basilar papilla, which like the lizard's papilla is broadly tuned throughout its length to a single frequency. Utilizing electrical rather than mechanical means, the individualized resonances of the turtle's hair cells are achieved by the interplay of incoming and outgoing cations (Fettiplace, 1987).

The process is perhaps best illustrated with an excitatory stepwise displacement of the ciliary tuft (Fig. 7.7). Commencing with the onset of ciliary displacement, a steady positive current of magnitude I_0 enters the cell through the suddenly opened transduction channels (Fig. 7.7, top trace). This current gradually charges up the cell's transmembrane voltage (bottom trace), which then opens voltage-controlled calcium pores (Ca_v), permitting Ca^{2+} ions to flow into the cell. In turn, these Ca^{2+} ions gradually activate the membrane's calcium-activated potassium pores ($K_{(Ca)}$), allowing a gradually increasing number of K^+ ions to escape the cell down their electrochemical gradient (Fig. 7.7, middle trace).

When this increasing efflux of K^+ ions just equals the influx of positive ions (time a), the membrane voltage momentarily stabilizes. However, the

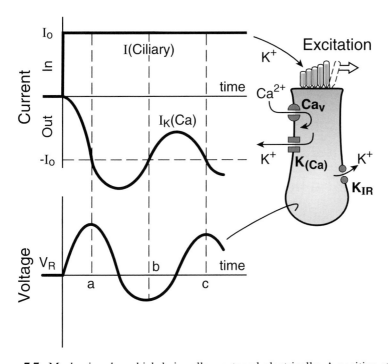

Figure 7.7. Mechanism by which hair cells are tuned electrically. A positive stepwise deflection of the ciliary bundle causes an incoming ciliary current I(Ciliary) (top trace). The depolarization (bottom trace) created by the incoming cations begins to open voltage-activated Ca^{2+} channels (Ca_v). The incoming Ca^{2+} ions, in turn, open Ca^{2+}-activated K^+ channels ($K_{(Ca)}$). The growing efflux of K^+ ions [I_K(Ca)] (middle trace) eventually exceeds the influx I(Ciliary), and the hair cell becomes hyperpolarized, choking the influx of Ca^{2+} ions and thus starting the shutdown of I_K(Ca). Delays in the activation processes allow voltage overshoots, and the cycle is repeated. Times a, b, and c mark moments of zero net current. (Adapted from Hudspeth and Lewis, 1988.)

slowly reacting K^+ pores further activate, allowing the cell's cation efflux to exceed its influx for a short time. This net loss of K^+ ions hyperpolarizes the cell, deactivating the voltage-controlled Ca^{2+} pores and slowing the influx of Ca^{2+} ions. The resulting reduction of Ca^{2+} ions internally begets deactivation of the calcium-activated K^+ pores, and a decline in the magnitude of $I_K(Ca)$ follows. Eventually, the now decreasing cation efflux again equals influx (time b), and the membrane voltage reaches stability once more. However, the sluggish K^+ pores continue deactivating, allowing the incoming cation current once more to dominate and begin to repolarize the cell. The next cycle has begun, though it will have a lower amplitude than the first, and so on. As in any resonant system, the closer the match between the period of a tonal stimulus (T) and the period of the hair cell's intrinsic oscillations ($t_c - t_a$), the larger is the magnitude of the transduction voltage.

Detailed modeling of the electrical tuning of turtle hair cells, which incorporated known types and numbers of membrane channels, gave excellent agreement with experimental results, accounting for resonant (characteristic) frequencies in the range of 16–600 Hz (Wu et al., 1995). Over most of that range the kinetics of the Ca^{2+}-activated K^+ channels (modeled with five closed states, three open states, and two blocked states) were the principal determinants of resonant frequency. Inwardly rectifying K^+ channels (K_{IR}), whose existence in the hair cells has been demonstrated experimentally, were also included in the model. The latter channels were necessary for the achievement of adequate frequency sensitivity at frequencies below 200 Hz.

Electrical tuning of acousticolateralis hair cells has been observed in a number of other species, including the cochleas of the chick and alligator (Fuchs and Evans, 1988; Fuchs et al., 1988) and the frog's low-frequency auditory organ (the amphibian papilla) and sacculus (Pitchford and Ashmore, 1987; Hudspeth and Lewis, 1988). Suggestive of common ionic mechanisms, the model for turtle hair cells was successfully extended to chick hair cells, producing resonant frequencies up to 4.3 kHz, near the upper limit of hearing for these birds (Wu et al., 1995).

The chick's ear is particularly interesting because the chicken's basilar membrane has also been shown to possess differential frequency tuning (von Békésy, 1960), although with poor selectivity (Gummer et al., 1987). Thus mechanical and electrical tuning coexist in the avian ear, prompting the suggestion that, as in the lizard ear, the self-tuning of the hair cells determines the sharp frequency selectivity displayed by the afferent neurons (Klinke and Smolders, 1991). A similar situation occurs in the crocodilian ear (Manley, 1990). Electrical tuning has been observed in the cochlear hair cells of lizards as well. However, the electrical resonances observed in those animals were at frequencies a full tenfold below the characteristic frequencies displayed by the afferent neurons when excited by tones (Eatock et al.,

1993). Although suggestive, this finding by itself does not disprove an important role of electrical resonance in vivo, as the hair cells involved in the measurements may have been damaged in preparation, thereby lowering their resonance frequencies (a known effect).

The essential role of calcium ions in the electrical tuning of vertebrate hair cells is but one of the many processes in which they play a key part. They also affect mechanoelectric adaptation, as discussed in the previous section, and trigger the exocytosis that delivers neurotransmitter to the afferent neurons (see Chapter 11). This many-faceted role of calcium ions requires exquisite control of its concentration throughout the cell, a process aided by strategic placement of the calcium pores.

Electrical recordings from resonant saccular hair cells of the grass frog indicated that almost all of a hair cell's Ca^{2+} channels and Ca^{2+}-activated K^+ channels, occurring in a 2.6:1.0 ratio, clustered together in a score of small patches on its basolateral surface (Roberts et al., 1990). As these "hot spots" coincided in number and distribution with the number of afferent synaptic contacts typically observed on these hair cells, it was concluded that the patches were the "active" zones of the synaptic contacts (see Chapter 11). It is difficult to imagine how the calcium pores could have been located any closer to their work sites.

Hot spots of clustered calcium channels have also been observed in the cochlear hair cells of turtles (Tucker and Fettiplace, 1995). In a three-dimensional model of calcium ion diffusion within these hair cells, the growth and dissipation of the domain of elevated Ca^{2+} concentration created by transient excitation of a hot spot agreed qualitatively with the experimentally measured Ca^{2+} transients (Wu et al., 1996). The role of diffusible calcium buffers was crucial to the model's success.

Summary

It appears that almost all vertebrate inner ears, despite their enormous structural differences, depend on hair cells to play the major role in providing refined frequency selectivity. Though the substrate may be rigid (auditory papillae of frogs), tuned to one frequency (lizard and turtle papillae), differentially but poorly tuned (avian and crocodilian ears), or differentially and sharply tuned (basal section of mammalian cochleas), the activity of hair cells is necessary to provide the sharp frequency tuning which the neural outputs of these organs all display. The only exception to this general pattern seems to be the low-frequency section of the mammalian cochlea (see Fig. 5.9). It seems therefore that the relatively large structures that support acoustically sensitive hair cells do not as a rule achieve sharp frequency selectivity by themselves.

NOTES

1. ''Voltage clamp'' recordings are made with a penetrating or ''patching'' micropipette connected to an electronic circuit that controls the transmembrane voltage of the cell during experimental manipulation. To maintain that voltage constant, the circuit must keep the net concentration of free ions near the plasma membrane virtually constant, supplying (or extracting) amounts of current *exactly* equal to the current that flows through the cell's plasma membrane. Thus by recording the current delivered by the electronic circuit to the micropipette transmembrane current is measured.

2. The electrical voltage that exists across a cell's plasma membrane is determined directly by the *net* concentration of unpaired electrical charges within the cell (i.e., the concentration of positive charges minus the concentration of negative charges). Thus any change in the internal concentration of *any* ion alters the cell's transmembrane potential.

3. The *power* of a signal is simply the rate with which energy flows: power = energy/time. Because by definition a sinusoid is infinitely long, it also possesses infinite energy. Hence the use of total energy to describe a sinusoidal process is meaningless, and power considerations are used instead.

4. An ideal frictional element is one whose force–velocity relation is linear, represented by the equation $F = D * v$, where D is the damping constant (see Appendix C). It can be shown that the power absorbed by such a frictional element is equal to the product of force times velocity (power = $F * v$). Substituting the first equation into the second, we find that the power absorbed by the element is equal to $D * v^2$.

5. Newton's second law ($F = ma$) states that the force needed to change the velocity of a mass (m) is proportional to the *rate* with which that velocity changes (the definition of acceleration, a). Because acceleration is thus the second time derivative of displacement, the acceleration of a sinusoidal displacement is equal (phase shifts ignored) to that displacement waveform multiplied by the square of the frequency (i.e., $a = \omega^2 x$). Thus as the frequency of the sinusoidal stimulation rises, the forces required to maintain a constant displacement amplitude must increase with the square of the frequency (i.e., $F = ma = m\omega^2 x$). As a consequence, *every* finite stimulating system, no matter how strong, eventually encounters a frequency above which the forces required to maintain constant displacement exceed its capacity, and diminishing response ability results.

8

HAIR CELLS OF THE
MAMMALIAN COCHLEA

Although hair cells of the mammalian cochlea share the general characteristics of all hair cells, they have some unique properties. Alone among hair
cells, their apical surfaces are subjected to large positive extracellular potentials. Moreover, neither type of hair cell has a kinocilium, but a basal
body is found in the usual location of the kinociliary insertion into the
cuticular plate. *Most* unusual is the ability of the outer hair cells to modulate
their shapes when stimulated electrically.

STRUCTURAL ANATOMY

The two types of cochlear hair cell have rather different anatomical characteristics. The inner hair cell is flask-shaped, with its tallest row of cilia
standing quite a bit taller than the other two rows (Fig. 8.1A). Synapsing
on its basolateral surface are a large number of afferent neuron terminals,
but it has little or no direct contact with axons originating in the central
nervous system. Efferent neurons do run near inner hair cells, but they synapse instead with the axons of the afferent neurons (see Chapter 15). Within
the organ of Corti the inner hair cells are completely surrounded by supporting cells.

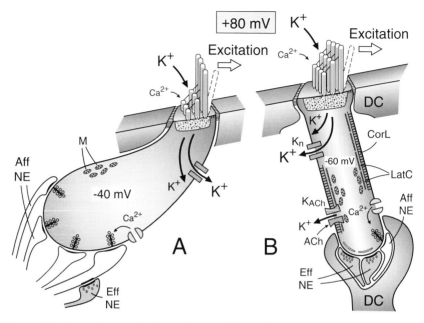

Figure 8.1. Inner hair cell (*A*) and outer hair cell (*B*). Modiolus is to the left. Excitation for both types of hair cell is ciliary deflection in the same radially outward direction (i.e., away from the modiolus). AffNE, afferent nerve ending; CorL, cortical lattice; DC, Deiters' cell; EffNE, efferent nerve ending; K_{ACh}, potassium channel activated by acetylcholine, an efferent neurotransmitter (see Chapter 15); K_n, potassium channel activated by large negative membrane potentials; LatC, lateral cistern; M, mitochondria.

By contrast, the outer hair cell is cylindrically shaped, and its several rows of cilia have uniformly staggered heights (Fig. 8.1B). The base of each outer hair cell is cradled by a single Deiters' cell, leaving its lateral wall largely free of cellular contact, directly exposed to the perilymph that fills the organ of Corti (see Fig. 6.4). Outer hair cells have both afferent and efferent innervation, with the latter predominating.

Unique to the outer hair cell are three concentric cylindrical components that occur near its outer shell (Holley, 1991). Outermost is the plasma membrane. Just inside that, linked to it, is a filamentous cytoskeleton called the *cortical lattice*. Just inside the lattice, also linked to it, is a multilayer system of membrane lamellae, the *lateral cisternae*. The latter structures appear to be involved in the electromotility of outer hair cells [see Motility of Outer Hair Cells (''Reverse Transcription''), below].

An outer hair cell is about 10 μm in diameter, no matter what its location within the cochlea; but its length can have a value anywhere between 10 and 90 μm, depending on the characteristic frequency of its cochlear location. In cochlear regions tuned to low frequencies, the outer hair cells are long; in high-frequency regions, they are short. This systematic relation between length and characteristic frequency holds within single mammalian species as well as across species (Pujol et al., 1992). In the guinea pig cochlea, for instance, the outer hair cells vary in length from 20 μm in the base to almost 90 μm in the apex (Preyer et al., 1996). Even smaller outer hair cells are found in the extreme base of some bat cochleas. The functional consequences of this length gradation are unclear, aside from the obvious reduction in mass that accompanies the shorter length. The lengths of inner hair cells also vary systematically with cochlear location, but not as markedly as those of the outer hair cells (Lim, 1980).

ION FLOWS THROUGH PLASMA MEMBRANES

With a large positive endocochlear potential on one side and a negative intracellular potential on the other, the apical surfaces of both inner and outer hair cells have large voltage differences across them (> 100 mV). These huge transmembrane potentials force cations, chiefly K^+ ions, into the apical section of each hair cell. In common with all hair cells, changes in the conduction of the transduction channels caused by rotation of the stereocilia modulate the magnitude of this K^+ current. Once inside the cell, the K^+ ions partially depolarize it, producing the transduction potentials. K^+ ions leave the hair cell through highly selective ion channels in the basolateral plasma membrane.

   Note that each hair cell has two completely different electrochemical gradients for K^+ ions, provided by the two entirely different media that bathe their various surfaces. Surrounded by perilymph, the basolateral membrane of the hair cell has the usual outward-directed gradient for K^+ ions, allowing them to leave the hair cell without requiring additional energy for the transit. By contrast, a strong inward-directed gradient for K^+ ions exists across the hair cell's apical surface. Unopposed by a significant Nernst potential,[1] the large transmembrane potential that exists there pushes K^+ ions into the hair cell, again requiring no energy from the hair cell itself. Thus the cochlear system has lifted the heavy energetic burden of powering the steady K^+ currents that flow through the hair cells from the hair cells themselves and shifted it onto the marginal cells of the stria vascularis (see Chapter 6). As a result, the extensive and therefore heavy blood supply needed for this and other ion-pumping tasks does not need be located on the otherwise lightly loaded and precisely tuned basilar membrane.

   When the outer hair cell's transmembrane voltage is in its normal operating range (-60 ± 10 mV), the main K^+ current flowing through its basolateral membrane is contributed by voltage-activated channels, represented in Figure 8.1B with the conductance K_n (n for "negative") (Housley and Ashmore, 1992). This channel, activated at large negative potentials (-90 to -50 mV), is highly selective for K^+ ions, which is advantageous in reducing the burden on the hair cell of extruding any other cations that might flow in through these channels. Also present are other ion channels, such as outwardly rectifying K^+ channels, which are activated at potentials more positive than -35 mV. The roles of these other channels are presently unknown.

The outward currents of the inner hair cell have also been investigated (Kros and Crawford, 1990). Pharmacological dissection of these currents indicated that these hair cells have two different potassium conductances, both of which are activated over the normal range of the cell's membrane potential.

Making up a small part of the currents that flow in through the transduction channels in the apical surface of the hair cells are other cations present in the endolymph (Ikeda et al., 1994). Important among these entering cations, which must be extruded from the cell, are Na^+ ions. Their low concentration in the endolymph (and the small Na^+ influx that results) is another boon bestowed by the strial cells on the hair cells, which must pump out any incoming Na^+ ions against the large electrochemical gradients that exist for these ions on all surfaces of the hair cells.

Some Ca^{2+} ions also flow in through the hair cell transduction channels. Of the two general mechanisms known for extruding these ions from neurons—a Na–Ca exchanger and a Ca^{2+} ATPase enzyme pump—it is the latter mechanism that seems operative in hair cells, at least those of the turtle cochlea (Tucker and Fettiplace, 1995).

BASIC ELECTROPHYSIOLOGY

The transducer voltages generated inside a cochlear hair cell by low-frequency tones can be estimated from the simple electrical circuit model of Figure 8.2. The conductance of the hair cell's apical membrane is composed of a resting value (G_{ap}: the reciprocal of its resistance R_{ap}) plus the changes $\Delta G \times \sin \omega t$, brought about by ciliary rotations (presumed sinusoidal in this case). The unchanging resistance of the hair cell's basolateral surface is represented by the fixed resistor R_{bas}; and the resistances of scala media and scala tympani are represented by the resistors R_{SM} and R_{ST}, respectively, both of which are much smaller than the two cell membrane resistances. The source of scala media voltage and the potassium Nernst potential for the basolateral surface are each represented by an appropriately

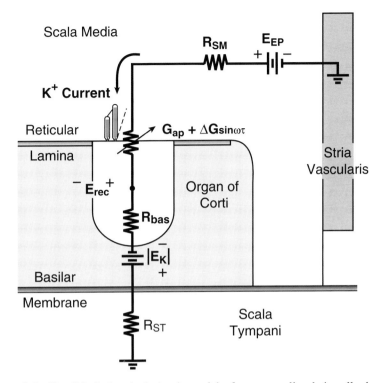

Figure 8.2. Simplified electrical circuit model of a mammalian hair cell, showing the generation of receptor potentials for weak tonal excitation at low frequencies. Potassium ions are forced into the apical surface by a large transmembrane voltage and out from the basolateral surface by the usual potassium electrochemical gradient. Sinusoidal deflections of the cilia cause sinusoidal changes $E_{rec}(t)$ in the hair cell's membrane potential. Adaptation effects (see Fig. 7.4), if any, have been ignored. At higher frequencies, the membrane capacitances become a factor; for strong excitation, modulation of the apical conductance becomes highly nonlinear.

labeled voltage source. The Nernst potential at the apical surface is set at zero.[1]

It can be shown, by straightforward use of Ohm's law ($E = iR$), that the current $i(t)$, which flows through the model's hair cell during small ciliary deflections ($\Delta G \ll G_{ap}$), is approximately

$$i(t) = I_0 + (\Delta G I_0 R_{ap}^2 / R_{tot}) \times \sin \omega t, \qquad (8.1)$$

where R_{tot} is a constant, the sum of all four resistances at rest conditions ($R_{SM} + R_{ap} + R_{bas} + R_{ST}$), and I_0 is also a constant, consisting of the sum of the two voltage sources, ($E_{EP} + |E_K|$), divided by R_{tot}. Note that sinusoidal modulation of the model's ciliary resistance has produced a sinusoidal modulation of the hair cell's K^+ current. This current flowing through the basolateral membrane (R_{bas}) creates a sinusoidal transmembrane "*rece*ptor" potential (E_{rec}), whose magnitude is directly proportional to ΔG.

Because a steady hair cell current of magnitude I_0 exists in the absence of sound stimulation, it has been termed the "silent current" (Zidanic and Brownell, 1990). Note that its existence is needed to register *decreases* in the cell's apical conductance ($\Delta G < 0$). That is, a resting level of current flow is needed before amplitude *deceases* in that current can occur. In that sense, the "silent current" is analogous to the well known "dark current" of retinal receptor cells. In both cases maintenance of this steady current is the price paid for providing the receptor mechanisms with something to modulate.

TRANSDUCTION POTENTIALS

Low-Frequency Stimulation

Through Herculean efforts, recordings have been made from both inner and outer hair cells in vivo, and their transduction potentials have been measured. Summaries of the relation obtained with low-frequency stimulation between sound pressure and receptor voltages (i.e., the "input–output" curves) for hair cells located in the basal region of the cochlea are shown in Figure 8.3. Both curves have the typical S-shape obtained from other hair cells (see Fig. 7.4B), two more in the sequence of compressive mechanisms possessed by the auditory periphery. A significant difference in the two curves is the location of the resting point. For the outer hair cell it is nearly at the midpoint, implying that approximately 50% of the transducer channels conducted, on average, in the absence of sound. By contrast, the resting condition for the inner hair cell is heavily biased toward its negative asymptote (all channels closed).

One consequence of this difference in resting points is illustrated in the output waveforms derived from the these curves using a moderately intense pure-tone input (Fig. 8.3, lowest curve). The response of the outer hair cell (Fig. 8.3, lower trace on right) is almost symmetrical, having a negligible average value; but it is not quite sinusoidal: Its peaks have been flattened. As can be seen (by following the arrows) this squashing is due to the compressive nature of the outer hair cell's input–output curve. For weaker stimuli, the relevant (central) part of this input–output curve is approximately a straight line. Thus the transducer potentials of outer hair cells in the cochlea's high-frequency region are predicted to be virtually linear at low intensities, as they seem to be at least for low frequencies (Russell et al., 1995).

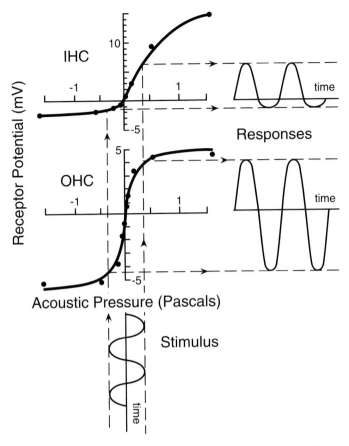

Figure 8.3. Generation of receptor potentials in an inner hair cell (IHC, top panel) and an outer hair cell (OHC, middle panel), with tonal excitation of about 84 dB SPL at low frequencies. The acoustic stimulus (bottom trace) changes the transmembrane potential according to each hair cell's input–output curve (left) resulting in the respective receptor potentials (right). (The input–output curves were obtained from Russell et al., 1986, with permission*.)

Before leaving the subject of outer hair cell transduction, note that the current flowing through the hair cell in Figure 8.2 also flows through the two scala resistances (R_{SM} and R_{ST}), producing transduction voltages in both scala media and scala tympani. As currents from *all* outer hair cells in the "vicinity" (electrically speaking) also have to flow through these same two resistances on their way to electrical "ground" (the vascular system), the total current flowing through them is the sum of all of these individual hair cell currents. Thus the voltages developed in the scalae are composed of contributions from many hair cells. The time-varying (or "AC") portions of those voltages are known as the *cochlear microphonic potentials*, and they can be recorded even at locations exterior to the cochlea (Dallos, 1973). These extracellular potentials provide information about the overall state of hair cells within specific cochlear regions but virtually nothing about individual hair cells.

Returning to Figure 8.3, we see that the input–output curve of the inner hair cell (upper trace on the right) is highly asymmetrical; accordingly, its output shows a large average value (sometimes called the "DC" component). Even for weak stimuli, the calculated output waveform of the inner hair cell has a DC component, as the resting point of the inner hair cell lies not in a linear region of the input–output curve but on its upward curving foot (Geisler, 1992). In agreement with the model's behavior, receptor potentials recorded from inside living inner hair cells of the basal cochlea do indeed show substantial DC components in response to weak tones, components that grow rapidly with the strength of the tone (Patuzzi and Sellick, 1983).

The currents that flow through the inner hair cells also flow through the scala resistances and therefore contribute to the sensory potentials recorded in the scalae. Studies involving differential damage to inner and outer hair cells have shown that the outer hair cells produce almost all of the cochlear microphonic potential (Dallos, 1973). The DC component of the sensory potentials recorded in the scalae and beyond is known as the *summating potential*, composed of contributions from both inner and outer hair cells.

Intracellular measurements, similar to those made in the basal turn of the cochlea, have also been recorded from hair cells in the apical turns. Both types of hair cell located in the cochlear apex display asymmetrical input–output curves (Dallos, 1986) of the type possessed by inner hair cells in the base.

High-Frequency Stimulation

To change a hair cell's transmembrane potential, the net charge concentration within the thin ion sheets bordering the cell's basolateral plasma membrane must be changed. At low frequencies of stimulation, the portion of the transduction current needed to effect this change in charge density is small compared to the portion that flows through the membrane's ion channels. Ignoring the small membrane-charging component that flows at these low frequencies allows the use of a single resistor to represent the basolateral membrane with good accuracy, as in Figure 8.2. Ohm's law informs us that the amplitude of the receptor potential is proportional to the transduction current at these low frequencies.

As the frequency of the tone rises, however, the portion of the transduction current devoted to charging the ion layer rises proportionately. At some frequency this membrane-charging component becomes comparable to the ion-channel component, and the purely resistive model is no longer adequate: The membrane's charge-storing capacity, its capacitance, must be included in the picture. With further increases in frequency, the membrane-charging current comes to dominate; and the receptor potential created across the basolateral membrane by the transduction current drops off inversely with frequency. Roughly speaking, this reduction occurs because the higher the frequency, the less time the current has to deliver charge within each stimulus cycle. The frequency at which the membrane-charging component of the current becomes comparable to the ion-channel component is known as the "corner frequency." In an ideal circuit containing parallel conductance (G) and capacitance (C) elements, this frequency is determined by the ratio G/C.

For isolated outer hair cells, a systematic relation exists between their corner frequencies and their lengths: the shorter the hair cell, the higher is its corner frequency (Fig. 8.4A). This relation is somewhat surprising, for simply reducing the size of a cell does not change its corner frequency. That invariance occurs because the conductance and the capacitance of a cell both vary linearly with its surface area, keeping the ratio G/C unchanged throughout any changes in cell size provided the characteristics of the included membrane do not change. The capacitive nature of the different hair cell

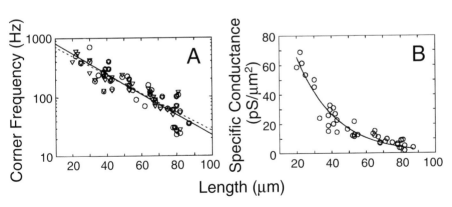

Figure 8.4. Corner frequencies (*A*) and specific conductances (i.e., conductances for a unit area of plasma membrane) (*B*) of outer hair cells in the guinea pig cochlea, plotted as functions of hair cell length. The shorter the hair cell, the higher is its corner frequency, as befits its more basal position in the cochlea. (From Preyer et al., 1996, with permission*.)

membranes was indeed found to be more or less invariant at a "specific capacitance" (i.e., capacitance for a unit area of plasma membrane) of about 2 $\mu F/cm^2$. It was the conductive nature of these hair cells that varied with length (Fig. 8.4B), from "specific conductances" of 70 $pS/\mu m^2$ for the shortest (basal) hair cells to < 10 $pS/\mu m^2$ for the longest (apical) ones.

Of relevance for Chapter 9, note that despite its systemic increase with decreasing cell length (Fig. 8.4A) the corner frequency of each isolated outer hair cell fell far below the characteristic frequency of the cochlear partition location from which it was taken.

MOTILITY OF OUTER HAIR CELLS ("REVERSE TRANSDUCTION")

Physiology

Of great significance was the discovery that outer hair cells are capable of mechanical deformations at acoustic frequencies when electrically stimulated (Brownell, 1983; Brownell et al., 1985). Many studies since then have verified that depolarization of isolated outer hair cells produces axial contractions, and hyperpolarizations produce elongations. These deformations (sometimes called "reverse transduction") are relatively small—only a few percent of the cell's length at most—yet they are in the same amplitude range as sound-evoked basilar membrane vibrations (e.g., 1% of a 30 μm hair cell is 300 nm).

This electromotility is complex, a mixture of at least two processes: "slow" and "rapid" (acoustic frequency). The magnitudes of the rapid length changes caused in a typical isolated outer hair cell by various transmembrane voltages are shown in Figure 8.5A. The sensitivity of this process, determined from the slope of a Boltzmann curve fitted to the points, is shown in Figure 8.5B. It reaches a value as high as 20 nm/mV. Therefore if 0.1 mV is taken as the magnitude of the hair cell's receptor potential at perceptual threshold (as it is in the basal part of the cochlea, according to Russell et al., 1995), these cells would exhibit axial displacements of up to 2 nm, depending on the resting potential of the cell.

An upper limit to the speed of the outer hair cells' electromotility has not yet been established. In isolated voltage-clamped cells, it easily follows sinusoidal electrical commands at frequencies up to 1 kHz, the technical limit of the present apparatus (Santos-Sacchi, 1992). Externally applied electrical signals have been observed to drive the cells at frequencies up to 24 kHz (Dallos et al., 1993). Even that may not be the limit, because in order to account for the high-frequency sensitivity of some bat species with presently

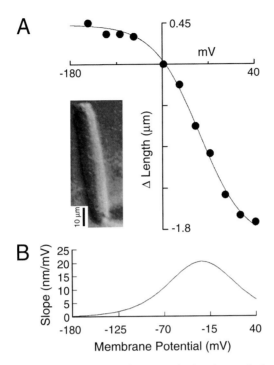

Figure 8.5. *A*. Changes in the length (ΔL) of an isolated outer hair cell in response to various transmembrane voltage steps. Hyperpolarizations elicited elongations; depolarizations caused contractions. The solid curve is the Boltzmann function which best fits the data. *Insert*. Hair cell. *B*. Slope of the fitted Boltzmann curve, giving the sensitivity of the mechanical response as a function of cell potential. (From Santos-Sacchi, 1992, with permission*.)

dominant theory (see Chapter 9) the speed of electromotility in the outer hair cells of those species would have to extend into the 100 kHz range.

These rapid hair cell deformations have unique properties. Unlike muscle cell movements, they occur even after ATP and Ca^{2+} stores within the cell are depleted (Holley and Ashmore, 1988b; Brownell, 1990). Moreover, the electromotility operates far more rapidly than allowed by the approximately 1 ms activation time estimated for actin–myosin interaction cycles (Holley, 1991). There is ample evidence to conclude that it is the voltage across the outer hair cell's plasma membrane, not the current through it, that causes the cellular deformations. This relation and the rapidity of outer hair cell movements suggest the involvement of molecules within the plasma membrane itself or in its immediate vicinity. This conclusion is consistent with several experiments demonstrating that the cell's motile elements are located more or less uniformly along its lateral surface (Dallos et al., 1991; Santos-Sacchi, 1992).

Ultrastructural Anatomy

The cortical structures of an outer hair cell are shown in Figure 8.6 (Dallos, 1992). Between the plasma membrane and the lateral cisternae (Fig. 8.1B) lie what appear to be an array of cytoskeletal filaments (actin), running more or less circumferentially around the cell. A thinner type of filament (spectrin) forms crosslinks between neighboring circumferential filaments. An orderly array of "pillars" joins the filamental framework to the plasma membrane, the latter connections apparently made to large particles embedded within that membrane. It appears that this filament array is not uniformly oriented throughout the basolateral membrane but is composed of many small patches, each patch promoting movement in a slightly different direction

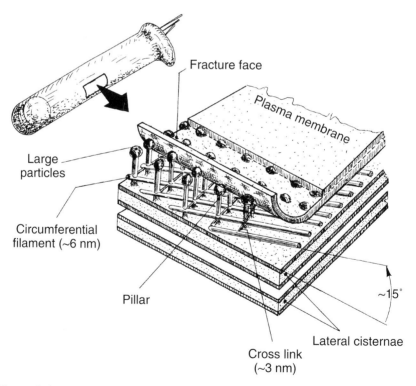

Figure 8.6. Cortical structures of the outer hair cell's lateral surface. The helical circumferential filaments, which are slightly pitched with respect to the cell's cross section (ca. 15° on average) are crosslinked by thinner strands and attached by pillars to the outermost lateral cistern and to large particles in the inner leaf of the plasma membrane. (From Dallos, 1992, with permission*.)

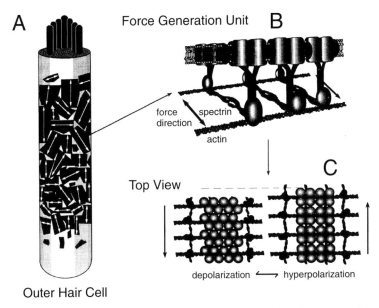

Figure 8.7. *A.* Outer hair cell, showing the existence on its plasma membrane of many functional domains, each with its own axis of elongation. *B.* Tangential view of the hair cell's lateral surface, showing circumferential filaments (actin), their crosslinks (spectrin), and the pillars. *C.* Top view of the lateral surface, showing the changes in pillar packing postulated to account for the hair cell's motility: Upon depolarization, square packing (right) is replaced by the tighter hexagonal packing. (From Kalinec and Kachar, 1995, with permission*.)

(Kalinec and Kachar, 1995). The average orientation of movement for these patches is about 75° with respect to the axis of the cell (Fig. 8.7A).

Possible Mechanisms

The roles of the outer hair cell's various cortical elements in cell motility are unclear. Because of their unique occurrence in outer hair cells and their strategic position within the cytoplasm, it is tempting to conclude that the lateral cisternae are somehow responsible for the cell's movements. That situation seems unlikely because the number of cisternae can vary widely among species with similar hearing sensitivities. For example, guinea pigs may have up to 12 cisternae, whereas rats have but one (Holley, 1991).

Widely held is a theory that attributes outer hair cell movement to the array of large particles bound in the plasma membrane (Kalinec and Kachar, 1995). According to this idea, all of these membrane-bound particles are assumed, in a hyperpolarized cell, to be packed together in one particular configuration (Fig. 8.8C, right). With increasing levels of depolarization, increasing numbers of these particles would undergo conformational changes that reduce their effective diameters or increase their packing density (Fig. 8.8C, left), and the surface area of the cell would accordingly shrink.

Strong support for this hypothesis has been provided by the sustained motility of outer hair cells in which the lateral cisternae and cortical lattices had been effectively dissolved by internal perfusion with trypsin, resulting in nearly spherical cell shapes (Kalinec et al., 1992). Also consistent with the hypothesis of conformal changes within the plasma membrane are the changes in an outer hair cell's capacitance, interpreted as charge movements within its outer membrane, which accompany the cell's mechanical deformations (Ashmore, 1989; Santos-Sacchi, 1991). Moreover, it has been found that the reductions in outer hair cell motility that occur when aspirin (salicylate) is administered are accompanied by corresponding reductions in membrane capacitance changes (Ashmore et al., 1995).

Another hypothesis (not necessarily incompatible with the first) assumes that the cell's transmembrane voltage is *directly* involved (Jen and Steele, 1987; Jerry et al., 1995). With this scheme, variations in the electrical forces known to exist between any two electrically conducting objects (or sheets of ions) maintained at different voltage levels would modulate the thickness of the plasma membrane as the transmembrane voltage was varied. Assuming no volume changes within the membrane itself, its area would have to increase when its thickness decreased and vice versa.

With either scenario, a change in the surface area of the outer hair cell would have to be translated into a change in its length. This appears to be accomplished by means of the cell's positive hydrostatic pressure, or *turgor* (Brownell, 1990). Such positive pressure exerts forces on the cell walls that tend to deform the cell into a sphere (as does the positive air pressure within a balloon). On the other hand, the circumferential filament matrix tends to preserve the cell's cylindrical shape. In fact, even a demembranated outer hair cell in which the cytoskeletal proteins are stabilized keeps its shape (Holley and Ashmore, 1988). This sheet of circumferential filaments, however, is not oriented so as to oppose *any* cellular deformation. Rather, by virtue of its slight average pitch relative to the cell's cross-sectional plane, this filamentous array behaves like a system of helical springs, displaying appreciable flexibility in the axial direction (Holley and Ashmore, 1988a). Thus the outer hair cell seems to be dynamically balanced between the forces of expansion (turgor) and compression (tension in the filaments) (Fig. 8.8). Changes in the cell surface area would clearly modulate this balance and hence the cell length (and width).

Perhaps the "slow" motility of the outer hair cells is related to maintenance of this balance. Operating on time scales that cover seconds, these

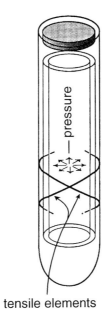

pressure

tensile elements

Figure 8.8. Outer hair cell illustrating the mechanisms that maintain its shape. Positive internal hydrostatic pressure ("turgor") stretches the lateral membrane, and the filament matrix provides the opposing tensile forces needed to create the cylindrical shape. This arrangement of forces transforms changes in the hair cell's surface area (see Fig. 8.7C) into changes in cell length. (From Brownell, 1990, with permission*.)

slow contractions can be induced by means of chemical, mechanical, and osmotic stimuli (for review see Dulon and Schacht, 1992; Schacht et al., 1995). Of particular interest are the changes brought about by changes in the concentrations of Ca^{2+} and ATP (Zenner, 1988; Housley et al., 1995) because along with the presence of many movement-related proteins (Fig. 6.5) they suggest the existence of mechanisms analogous to muscle cell contractions.

Functional Role of Electromotility

The exact role of outer hair cell motility in cochlear function is not clear at this time. What *is* clear is that the presence of normally functioning outer hair cells is necessary for the exquisite vibration sensitivity of the entire cochlear partition (see Chapter 16). An understanding of just how the internally produced vibrations of the outer hair cells are coupled back to their substrate has been the goal of auditory scientists for a decade. Experimental findings relevant to this remarkable effect are reviewed in Chapter 9, along with one of several extant theories.

NOTE

1. Potassium ions, the major charge carriers for a cochlear hair cell, appear in large concentrations on both sides of the cell's apical surface. Thus only a small *concentration*-driven component of potassium current flows across the hair cell's apical surface (reflected in its near-zero Nernst potential for K^+ ions).

9

COCHLEAR AMPLIFIER

HISTORICAL BACKGROUND

Displacements of the basilar membrane at threshold sound pressures are measured in fractions of a nanometer (Russell et al., 1995). The wavelengths of visible light, on the other hand, are about half a micrometer, three orders of magnitude greater. As displacement measurements made with ordinary (mixed-wavelength) light are limited in resolution to magnitudes on the order of the wavelengths used, von Békésy, who employed ordinary visible light in his experiments, was forced to use sound pressures intense enough to produce basilar membrane displacements in that same micrometer range. We now know that such sound levels (> 100 dB SPL) are high enough to eliminate the effects of the ''cochlear amplifier,''[1] indeed high enough to damage cochleas quickly. Measurements of cochlear motions produced by sounds in the normal physiological range had to wait therefore for the invention of submicron measurement techniques.

The first of these techniques was based on the Mössbauer effect, a quantum mechanical phenomenon of γ-rays (photons with wavelengths much shorter than those of visible light), whereby the velocity of a moving γ-ray source modulates the frequency of its emitted photons. Johnstone and Boyle (1967) were the first to use this new Doppler shift technique to measure basilar membrane displacements, a lead quickly followed up by the extensive investigations of Rhode. It was a summary paper of Rhode's early work (1978) that indicated the basilar membrane in the "best" preparations was well tuned in frequency at low sound levels, perhaps as sharply tuned as auditory nerve fibers (see Chapter 12). Several confirming and extending reports appeared during the next few years (Khanna and Leonard, 1982; Sellick et al., 1982). The paper of Khanna and Leonard is noteworthy, as it was the first to utilize laser interferometry, a superior submicron measurement technique.

From a theoretical point of view, these revelations had two important consequences. First, they eliminated the need for a conjectured "second cochlear filter," a frequency-sharpening device hypothesized to transform poorly tuned basilar membrane vibrations (the only kind observed up until then) into the beautifully tuned responses of the primary auditory neurons. As is often the case, a second yet more formidable unknown stood in place of the vanquished. What mechanism could possibly account for the newly revealed behavior of the basilar membrane itself? Finely tuned at low sound levels, it reverted to poor tuning when faced with higher sound pressures, trauma, or death (e.g., Fig. 5.8).

The second conceptual consequence of the new basilar membrane data was to underline the inadequacies of the then extant theory. To obtain large response peaks with magnitudes comparable to those measured experimentally, the friction (damping) in then existing cochlear models had to be reduced to extremely low values, much less than for the "lower damping" curve of Figure 5.6. Yet in a "Catch-22" situation, when the models' dampings were reduced to those values their frequency tunings became *much* sharper and more needle-like than had been observed experimentally. Clearly something basic was missing in those early models.

Even as the characteristics of the cochlear amplifier were being established, the first clue to its identity was independently published. In 1978 Kemp reported that faint sounds could be recorded coming *out* of some human ears, in response to brief clicks. Weak though they were, the existence of those *evoked otoacoustic emissions* (see Chapter 10) was highly significant. Although dismissed by some as "merely" echoes, these emissions suggested to Kemp that they might be by-products of cochlear transduction processes, perhaps involving the type of energy *generation* by the basilar membrane boldly envisioned decades before by Gold (1948). Supporting Kemp's conjecture was a report he published the next year (1979) that documented the existence of tone-like sounds coming "spontaneously" (i.e., *un*evoked by deliberately presented sounds) from the ears of some normal subjects, a phenomenon not unknown to clinicians.

The following year Mountain (1980) demonstrated that the "distortion product" form of evoked otoacoustic emissions (see Chapter 10) could be altered by changing the endocochlear potential directly or by stimulating the brain stem's *crossed olivocochlear bundle*, part of the cochlea's efferent system (see Chapter 15). Previous experiments had already demonstrated that electrical stimulation of this same crossed efferent bundle degraded the frequency tuning of primary auditory neurons in the same manner that raising the stimulus level degraded the frequency tuning of the basilar membrane (Wiederhold and Kiang, 1970). Because this efferent bundle was known to innervate primarily the outer hair cells, these cells were suspected as being somehow involved in both the neural and mechanical responses of the inner ear. Close correlations obtained between afferent neuron sensitivities and selective outer hair cell damage produced by the ototoxic drug kanamycin (see Chapter 16) also pointed strongly in that direction.

Such experiments prompted Neely, Kim, and colleagues (1980, 1983) to create a revolutionary model of the cochlea, which possessed, for the first time, frictional elements that supplied energy rather than absorbed it.[2] Their model was greeted with great skepticism, but arguing in its favor was the fact that its frequency tuning looked similar to that observed experimentally: steep-sided but not too sharply pointed. Also supporting the model's basic concept was an independent mathematical study indicating that to account for the observed attributes of low-level cochlear vibrations with firmly established hydrodynamic theory required the presence of energy-producing elements somewhere within the organ of Corti (de Boer, 1983).

During the same fruitful year Mountain et al. (1983) showed that a simple model of a passive, poorly tuned cochlear slice could, with the addition of feedback from the outer hair cells, produce sharply tuned frequency responses. Although the responses they reported were not realistically shaped (still too sharp), the demonstrated defeat of friction by feedback further supported Gold's hypothesis that the latter might be involved in highly tuned cochlear vibrations. Also supporting the feedback idea was the existence of spontaneous otoacoustic emissions, as it had long been known that certain feedback systems can produce sinusoidal oscillations. Indeed, feedback is the basic principle used for the design of (analogue) electronic oscillators. It was against this backdrop that Brownell and colleagues (1983, 1985) made the dramatic discovery that outer hair cells are capable of mechanical deformations at acoustic frequencies when electrically stimulated.

ROLE OF OUTER HAIR CELLS IN COCHLEAR PARTITION VIBRATIONS

In Vitro Preparations

The small size and complex geometry of the mammalian cochlea make it extremely difficult to measure its vibrations in vivo. In consequence, as work with excised parts has proved useful for studying other complicated biological systems, considerable effort has been expended on recordings from excised cochleas and cochlear sections. Of course, data obtained from such preparations do not give the whole story about how the cochlea operates when incorporated into the living animal, but considerable insight into its intrinsic properties has been gained.

Consider, for example, the mechanical responses measured in the third turn of an excised guinea pig cochlea using laser interferometry (Fig. 9.1A). When subjected to a brief "step" of applied current (Fig. 9.1B, top trace), the reticular lamina and basilar membrane moved toward each other, the former (Fig. 9.1B, middle trace) being displaced 5–10 times farther than the latter (Fig. 9.1B, bottom trace). Evidently the outer hair cells had contracted, squeezing the organ of Corti together, a conclusion consistent with the fact that those cells were depolarized by the applied current (as shown by other measurements). These data show clearly that the organ of Corti is indeed deformable to a physiologically significant extent.

Because the basilar membrane moved upward relatively little compared to the downward movement of the outer edge of the reticular lamina, it appears that the whole reticular lamina must have rotated as a plate around a longitudinal hinge formed by the tops of the rigid pillar cells (see Fig.

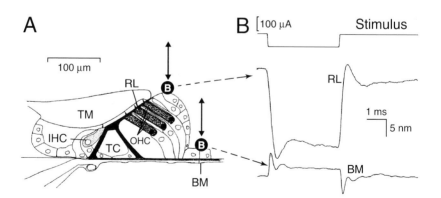

Figure 9.1. Motions of the basilar membrane and reticular lamina elicited with extracellular electrical excitation in the apical portion of an excised guinea pig cochlea. *A*. Cochlear partition in cross section, showing placement of the reflecting beads (dark circles, *B*) used for these laser interferometric measurements (made in the direction of the double-headed arrows). *B*. In response to stepwise current excitation (top trace) the reticular lamina (RL) was pulled downward nearly 25 nm (middle trace), and the basilar membrane (BM) was pulled upward a much smaller distance (bottom trace). IHC, OHC, inner and outer hair cell; TC, tunnel of Corti; TM, tectorial membrane. (From Mammano and Ashmore, 1993, with permission*.)

9.4). The peculiar anatomy of the organ of Corti seems to allow such movement, as illustrated in Figure 9.2A, a longitudinal view of the organ of Corti
as seen from its outer edge, looking in toward the modiolus (as in Fig. 6.4).
It can be seen in Figure 9.2 that the basilar membrane is made up of many
parallel fibers, providing a sturdy platform for the organ of Corti. The reticular lamina, by contrast, is simply the tightly joined tops of the outer hair
cells and the phalangeal processes of the Deiters' cells. Not only are the
lateral sides of both of these elements basically free of cellular contacts, they
are tilted at opposing angles relative to the vertical. Thus the entire outer
hair cell–phalangeal process complex seems readily deformable, easily moving the reticular lamina up and down as the outer hair cells contract and
elongate (Fig. 9.2B).

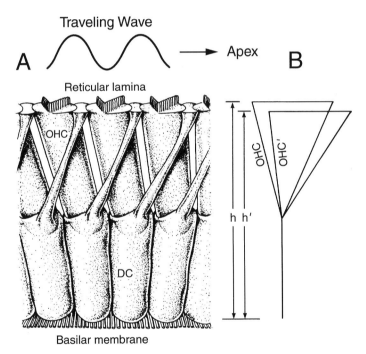

Figure 9.2. *A.* Microarchitecture of the lateral cochlear partition, looking in toward
the modiolus. The base of each outer hair cell (OHC) in the row is supported by
the cup of a single Deiters' cell (DC). The outer hair cells are tipped longitudinally,
so an acoustic traveling wave (top trace) reaches first their apices and then their
bases. *B.* Hypothesized response of the OHC–Deiters' cell complex. With the outer
hair cells at rest, the height of the complex is h; when the outer hair cells contract
(OHC'), the relative movement between the outer hair cells and the phalangeal
processes allows the organ of Corti to be slightly deformed, producing a reduced
height (h'). (From Brownell et al., 1985, with permission*.)

Illuminating in vitro experiments have also been done on excised apical portions of the cochlea (e.g., ITER, 1989; Gummer et al., 1995). Generally speaking, mechanical displacements similar to those seen in isolated whole cochleas were obtained. Radial motions of the apical surfaces of the outer hair cells were also observed, motions that were coupled mechanically to the apical surfaces of the inner hair cells via the reticular lamina (Reuter et al., 1992).

In Vivo Operation

Experimental Data

Some relevant displacement measurements have also been successfully completed in vivo. In those experiments electrical current was injected directly into scala media of the basal turn. Because of the corkscrew geometry of the cochlea, displacement measurements could be made only from the scala tympani side. That is, only the responses of the basilar membrane could be obtained.

In one type of study, sinusoidal (AC) electrical stimulation was used at frequencies ranging from less than 10 Hz to more than 40 kHz (Nuttall and Dolan, 1993; Xue et al., 1995). Basilar membrane displacements resulted whose attributes were similar to those evoked in the same measurement spot by acoustic stimulation at those same frequencies. Clearly *something* on the cochlear partition was responding to the AC electrical stimulation and successfully driving the whole cochlear partition.

Variations of these experiments provided further evidence that this ''something'' was indeed the set of outer hair cells. Specifically, when their motility forces were reduced, either by dropping the endocochlear potential (Xue et al., 1995) or pharmacologically eliminating the outer hair cells (Nuttall and Ren, 1995), the electrically driven responses of the cochlear partition essentially vanished.

In another group of similar experiments, direct electrical current (DC) was applied to scala vestibuli while the sound-evoked responses of the basilar membrane were measured (Nuttall et al., 1995). As can be seen from Figure 9.3, positive current enhanced the membrane's responsiveness near 18 kHz, the characteristic frequency of that location, whereas negative current decreased it. The farther the acoustic frequency was from the membrane's characteristic frequency, the less was the effect of applied currents. Why should *DC* electrical currents affect membrane responsiveness to *AC* acoustic signals and in such a frequency-selective manner? To account for this phenomenon and for the more general characteristics of the cochlear amplifier, further development of the simple cochlear model presented in Chapter 5 is needed.

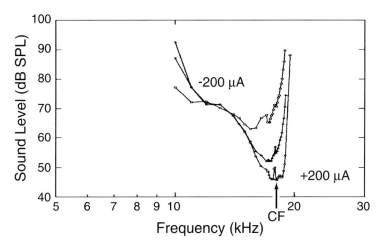

Figure 9.3. Frequency tuning curves for a point on the basal basilar membrane of the living guinea pig cochlea, showing the strong influence of electrical biasing (middle trace is normal). Positive extracellular DC current (causing increased endocochlear potential) increased sensitivity near the characteristic frequency (lower trace). Negative current (causing decreased endocochlear potential) produced the opposite effects (top trace). Weak effects occur at frequencies well below the characteristic frequency (CF) of 18 kHz. A 50 μm/sec criterion was used to construct all tuning curves. (From Nuttall et al., 1995, with permission*.)

Likely Mode of Action for Outer Hair Cells

One of the chief features of the cochlear amplifier in the basal cochlea is that it enhances the responses of the basilar membrane in the same frequency-selective fashion demonstrated in Figure 9.3: Tones with frequencies near the characteristic frequency are somehow favored (see Fig. 5.8A). From a theoretical point of view, such selectivity is revealing, as one of the attributes of a resonant mechanical system is that the impedance it presents to driving forces (Eq. 5.1) is undergoing drastic changes at frequencies near its resonant frequency. In the vicinity of resonance the impedance of the stiffness is nearly equal in magnitude to that of the mass, but the two impedances are of opposite phase. Thus these two ''reactive'' impedances nearly cancel each other out, leaving the system's resistance as the principal impediment to motion (see Fig. 5.7). If somehow that resistance could be reduced, larger responses would occur near resonance (e.g., Fig. 5.6).

Assuming that the axial changes of the outer hair cells are the ''active'' agents involved in the cochlear amplifier, their task is illustrated in Figure 9.4. This ''snapshot'' sketch catches the vibrating cochlear partition just as it is passing upward through its rest position, heading toward scala vestibuli. For sinusoidal oscillations, this position occurs at the moment of maximum

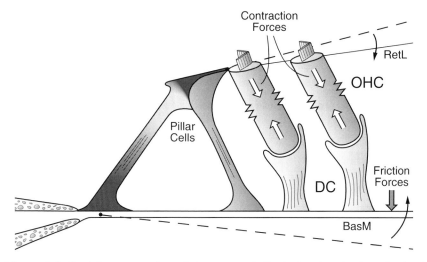

Figure 9.4. Partial cross section of the organ of Corti showing the hypothesized effects of outer hair cell (OHC) contractions. As the basilar membrane (BasM) moves upward, friction forces oppose that motion, absorbing sound energy. The outer hair cell contractions exert, through the interposing trunks of the Deiters' cells (DC), upward forces that counteract the downward friction forces.

upward velocity. Because the forces generated by viscous friction are proportional to velocity, the friction forces are also maximum at that moment, resisting the upward movement. If the movements of the outer hair cells were timed such that they were contracting at that same instant, the upward hair cell forces on the basilar membrane would counterbalance, perhaps even overshadow, the downward friction forces, and larger deflections would result. This overcompensation of friction (i.e., *negative damping*[2]) is fundamental to almost all recent cochlear models (de Boer, 1995a).

Note that this arrangement does indeed form a feedback system (Fig. 9.5). The motions of the cochlear partition generate forces that deflect the cilia of an outer hair cell $x(t)$, producing in turn the cell's transduction current $i(t)$ (see Eq. 8.1) and its receptor potential $E_{rec}(t)$. The latter serves as the generator potential for the cell's force-generating mechanisms, which accordingly modulate the length of the hair cell, pushing (or pulling) with a force, $F(t)$, on its two supports: a Deiters' cell at its base and the reticular lamina at its apex. Thus the outer hair cell feeds forces back onto the very structure that drives it, partially determining its own excitation (Mountain, 1986; Patuzzi and Robertson, 1988). Note that the microtubule-reinforced base of the Deiters' cell (see Fig. 6.5) is admirably suited to transmit forces between the outer hair cell and the basilar membrane.

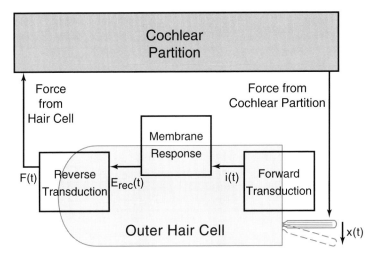

Figure 9.5. Feedback system involved in outer hair cell motility. Cochlear partition forces deflect the cilia, creating a transduction current, $i(t)$, which in turn produces the receptor potential, $E_{rec}(t)$, which changes the hair cell's length. Completing the loop, these length changes exert a force $F(t)$ on the cochlear partition, moving it and modifying the forces which it exerts on the cilia, and so on. (Adapted from Patuzzi and Robertson, 1988; Hubbard et al., 1990.)

COCHLEAR MODEL

As the precise behavior of the outer hair cells in vivo is largely unknown, cochlear models have had to incorporate various assumptions about how those cells work (for review see de Boer, 1995a; Hubbard and Mountain, 1996). One of those models is presented here (Geisler and Sang, 1995). It assumes that the tilting of the outer hair cells in the longitudinal direction is important (Fig. 9.2). With its apical end tilted toward the stapes, each outer hair cell senses an acoustic wave traveling along the cochlear partition an instant before the wave reaches the basilar membrane underneath the hair cells' basal end. The major effect of this slight delay in timing permits the outer hair cell to feed forces ''forward'' (i.e., in the direction of wave travel) to the basilar membrane at just the right phase to counteract, among other factors, the friction forces that occur there. The need for such precise timing indicates why the feedback in these models must be ''rapid'' (at the stimulating frequency) and not ''slow.'' This mode of amplification has an eerie similarity to that of the ''traveling wave'' amplifier used in microwave technology (Hubbard, 1993).

Responses of the Model to Tones

The displacements of this model's basilar membrane evoked by a 5 kHz pure tone presented at various intensities are shown in Figure 9.6A. These displacement waveforms have many of the characteristics seen in physiological recordings (see Fig. 5.8A): huge peaks (ca. two orders of magnitude) with moderate bandwidths at low stimulus levels that gradually shift leftward and lose their sharpness as the stimulus level is increased.[3] This trend is even clearer in Figure 9.6D, which normalizes these responses to the linear ones of the extreme basal basilar membrane (see Fig. 5.8D). The phases

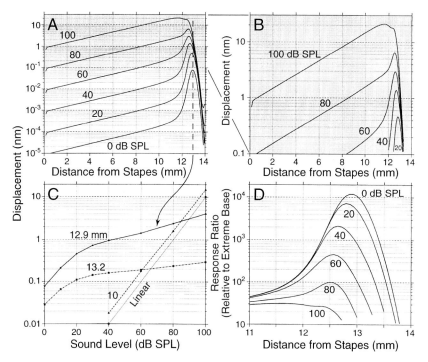

Figure 9.6. Responses of a feed-forward model to 5 kHz tones of various intensities. Compare with the experimental data in Figure 5.8, whose format is similar. *A.* Responses to tones of the indicated sound levels as a function of distance from the stapes. Only the cochlear region yielding appreciable responses (0–14 mm) is shown, though the simulation was of the entire 25 mm cat cochlea. *B.* Expanded version of the responses in *A* that exceeded 0.1 nm (putative neural threshold). *C.* Level-response functions derived from the data in *A* at the characteristic place (12.9 mm) (i.e., along the vertical dotted line), basal to it (10 mm), and apical to it (13.2 mm). *D.* Responses of *A* normalized to the (linear) responses of the basilar membrane immediately adjacent to the stapes. (From a nonlinear version of the Geisler-Sang model, 1995.)

(not shown here, but see Fig. 10.11) indicate that the responses are in fact traveling waves.

The responses shown in Figure 9.6A that exceed 0.1 nm in amplitude are shown on an expanded amplitude scale in Figure 9.6B. Assuming that the threshold for excitation of afferent neurons is at about the 0.1 nm level of displacement (see Chapter 12), the curves in Figure 9.6B show the spatial extent predicted for neural excitation. At low stimulus levels (e.g., 20 dB SPL) only a small group of neurons located near the 13 mm point would be excited, whereas at high levels more than half of the afferent neurons would be stimulated.

Amplitudes of the responses elicited by 5 kHz stimulation at three model segments are shown in Figure 9.6C. Although the 12.9 mm point (the "characteristic place"[4] for 5 kHz stimulation) displayed suitably compressed responses, even more strongly compressed responses occurred only 0.3 mm farther apically. Closer to the stapes (e.g., the 10 mm point) the responses grew linearly. This same pattern of behavior is observed in the living cochlea (see Fig. 5.8C).

Calculations regarding the responses seen in Figure 9.6 show that forces generated by the simulated outer hair cells immediately basal to the peak were indeed strong enough to override the friction forces present, providing the propagating acoustic energy with *added* energy. According to this model (and to most other recent ones), the sketch used previously to illustrate energy flow within the cochlea at high intensities (see Fig. 5.1) should be revised to include the *addition* of energy to the incoming acoustic signal during its travel to the resonance point. This revision (Fig. 9.7) shows that true amplification of the acoustic signal occurs, at least in this model.

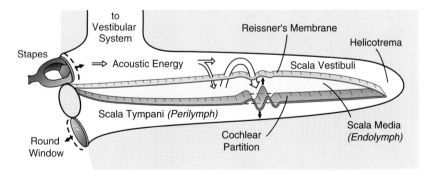

Figure 9.7. Stylized mammalian cochlea, showing the flow of acoustic energy thought to be produced by weak tones of high frequency (e.g., 5 kHz). The region of the cochlea immediately basal to the characteristic place generates more acoustic energy than it absorbs, creating amplification of the traveling sound energy, which then produces enormous, sharply tuned deflections of the cochlear partition.

The theory of energy amplification by the cochlear partition is supported by several mathematical analyses that have supported de Boer's (1983) original contention that the presence of *some* negative damping by the cochlear partition is required to account theoretically for the observed attributes of basilar membrane responses (Diependaal et al., 1987; Zweig, 1991; Brass and Kemp, 1993; de Boer, 1995b).

Other Attributes of the Model

Most recent models mimic reasonably well the basilar membrane vibrations to single tones that occur in basal sections of the cochlea. Such models, including this one, can account for a wide variety of other cochlear phenomena as well. For example, reductions of outer hair cell motility reduce the effectiveness of the models' cochlear amplifier, just as it does in living cochleas whose outer hair cells are damaged or destroyed (see Chapter 16). Moreover, some of the models can generate realistic otoacoustic emissions and create traveling distortion product waves within the cochlea (see Chapter 10).

When the endocochlear potential is increased, greater hair cell receptor potentials occur for a given amount of ciliary deflection (see Eq. 8.1). In that case, according to most recent models, the forces exerted by the outer hair cells should be strengthened, and increased signal amplification should occur in the living cochlea. Indeed it does, as does decreased amplification when the endocochlear potential is reduced (Fig. 9.3).

These models do not do a good job of representing the responses of the apical cochlea. This discrepancy reflects the fact that the apical and basal regions of the cochlea appear to have significantly different properties (see Chapters 5, 12). Efforts, both experimental and theoretical, to understand apical processes more fully are currently in progress.

Reservations About This Class of Model

Receptor Potentials

The available experimental evidence indicates that an outer hair cell's axial deformations are determined by its receptor potential (see Fig. 8.5). Yet the cell's plasma membrane acts as a ''low-pass'' filter, attenuating the receptor potentials produced by high-frequency transducer currents: the higher the frequency, the more the attenuation. How can the small voltages that are presumed to occur at high frequency generate axial movements?

Actually, those voltages may not be so small. Appreciable receptor potentials (ca. 0.1 mV amplitude) have been measured in the outer hair cells of the cochlear base in vivo when a tone at the cells' characteristic frequency of 18 kHz was presented at a level of 20 dB SPL, near behavioral threshold (Russell et al., 1995). A possible explanation for these unexpectedly large voltages is that the voltage-dependent capacitance changes of the plasma membrane associated with electromotility (see Chapter 8) appear to reduce the effective capacitance of the vibrating hair cell, thereby extending considerably its corner frequency (Hassan, 1997). Moreover, the electrical characteristics of an outer hair cell in vivo may well be influenced by its frequency-tuned mechanical supporting system (Mountain and Hubbard, 1994). In short, the receptor potentials of the outer hair cells in vivo may indeed be suitable for driving their electromotility, even at high frequencies.

Other Tuning Mechanisms

The realistic distribution of characteristic frequencies displayed by the type of model used in this chapter is obtained by assuming a basilar membrane stiffness that decreases by about four orders of magnitude from base to apex. However, preliminary evidence suggests such large changes in membrane stiffness do not occur, at least in the excised gerbil cochlea (Naidu and Mountain, 1997). It may be that the assumed stiffness gradient actually exists in the living cochlea, achieved by such means as radial forces exerted on the basilar membrane by the tension fibroblasts located in the spiral ligament (see Chapter 6). Perhaps other tuning mechanisms, presently unknown, are also at work. In any case, modifications to theory loom ahead.

ANOTHER POSSIBLE AMPLIFICATION PROCESS

It has been suggested that it is through their *cilia* whereby the outer hair cells ''amplify'' incoming sound waves. It was demonstrated some time ago that the cilia of turtle hair cells oscillate when they are subjected to applied step currents (Art et al., 1986). Moreover, it has been demonstrated in experiments on the hair cells of the frog sacculus that changes in membrane potential cause changes in the effective stiffness of the stereocilia (Assad et al., 1989). Perhaps the cilia of mammalian outer hair cells undergo oscillations of motion or stiffness in just the right timing sequence to counteract the forces of friction through some sort of feedback arrangement (e.g., Mountain et al., 1983).

However, free oscillations have not yet been observed in the cilia of mammalian hair cells, and there is convincing experimental evidence indicating that axial movements of the outer hair cells can indeed displace the basilar membrane (e.g., Fig. 9.1). It thus seems most unlikely that ciliary processes power the cochlear amplifier.

SUMMARY

There is multifaceted evidence to indicate that acoustic signals are amplified within the living cochlea, amplification that varies in extent and character in different parts of the cochlea. At the present time, the axial contractions of the outer hair cells appear to be the motor of this cochlear amplifier, although both measurement techniques and theory are still immature and struggling to make definitive judgments.

The transduction currents of the outer hair cells seem seminal to this signal amplification, and they are strongly nonlinear in nature (see Fig. 8.3). Thus the whole signal-amplification process is intrinsically nonlinear, capable of producing novel effects. Before considering the responses generated in the cochlea's afferent neurons by hair cell receptor potentials, we consider some important side effects attributable to the cochlear amplifier's compressive nature (Chapter 10).

NOTES

1. Although amplification of sound energy within the cochlea has not been *proved* to occur in vivo, the evidence for it is strong (Dallos, 1992). Accordingly, it is assumed hereafter in this book that such amplification does indeed occur, and thus the term *cochlear amplifier*, without quotation marks, is used to designate the amplifying agent(s).

2. It was shown in Chapter 7 (Note 4) that the power absorbed by an ideal friction element with damping coefficient D is equal to $v^2 * D$. If the value of D is positive, so is the power absorbed by the element, regardless of the direction of motion. By the same token, if D is negative, so is the power absorbed. In other words, the friction element *loses* power when D is negative. Because power is never destroyed, only transmuted, the power lost by the friction element must have been broadcast into its environment. Thus friction elements with negative damping constants ("negative friction" elements), such as those in the Neely–Kim model, *generate* rather than absorb energy.

3. The changes in the shapes of the responses are due to the compressive nature of the input–output characteristic that was incorporated into all of the model's outer hair cells (see Fig. 8.3). At low displacements that characteristic is essentially linear, and so the outer hair cells' receptor potentials and their resulting motile forces increase linearly with the stimulus level, as do the friction forces. As displacements increase, the transducer potentials of the outer hair cells become increasingly compressed; and the outer hair cells' motile forces accordingly become progressively smaller relative to the linearly increasing friction forces. In effect, the compressively limited feedback forces are increasingly less able to compensate the linearly growing friction forces as the stimulus level is increased.

4. When plotted as a function of cochlear location, the basilar membrane's response to a tonal stimulus of any particular frequency has a single peak (see Fig. 9.6A). When determined at low intensity, the location of that peak is known as the "characteristic place" of that frequency.

10

NONLINEAR RESPONSES OF THE COCHLEAR PARTITION: SUPPRESSIONS AND OTOACOUSTIC EMISSIONS

The nonlinear attributes of cochlear vibrations are fascinating. Response waveforms are compressed but with surprisingly little distortion; different stimulus components interact with each other in competitive ways; and new tones are created. Moreover, because of their dynamism, these nonlinear phenomena have provided us with invaluable means for probing and understanding cochlear mechanisms.

In this chapter we consider only two of the most prominent expressions of the cochlea's nonlinearities, response suppressions and otoacoustic emissions. At first sight, these two phenomena may seem to be unconnected, but it is clear from work with cochlear models that both classes of these nonlinear responses can be attributed to the same amplitude-limited motile forces of the outer hair cells widely held responsible for the compressive nature of pure-tone responses. As a case in point, the model introduced in Chapter 9 produces both realistic suppressions and life-like emissions. Accordingly, that model is referred to at appropriate points in this chapter to account for various response characteristics. Before proceeding, a brief review of *linear* responses is called for to highlight what is *not* linear about the cochlea's responses.

REVIEW OF LINEAR SYSTEMS

As mentioned previously, a linear system is one that can be described completely by *linear* equations. Such equations have many explicitly defined characteristics, of which we need to review only two.

First, a linear system, when subjected to a sinusoidal input, can respond *only* with a single sinusoid of the same frequency (see Appendix C for plausibility argument). Second, a linear system manifests "superposition"; that is, it responds to the sum of several simultaneously presented input signals as if each of those signals had been presented by itself. As discussed with respect to Fourier analysis in Chapter 2, the response to any *sum of inputs* is equal to the *sum of the responses* generated by the individual inputs acting one at a time. It follows from the latter attribute that the magnitude of a linear system's output always increases by exactly the same factor by which the magnitude of the input is increased (i.e., the output always scales with the input).

It also follows from the superposition property that different input signals cannot interact within a linear system. For example, when the input to a linear system is the sum of two sinusoids having different frequencies (e.g., f_L and f_H), the system output cannot contain any components having "cross-term" frequencies, such as ($f_L + f_H$). Moreover, when added to the first property, superposition requires that the system's output be composed *only* of sinusoidal components having the frequencies of stimulation. Components having other frequencies *cannot* be created.

The living cochlea violates not just one but all of these rules governing linear systems: Its output does *not* scale with the input, one tone *can* affect the response to another, and two tones presented together *can* create entirely new tones. The cochlea richly deserves its "nonlinear" label.

"TWO-TONE" SUPPRESSIONS

In the living cochlea, various components of an input signal often interact, almost always in a suppressive manner. As the usual paradigm for investigating such suppressions has utilized two simultaneously presented tones, this interaction phenomenon has become known as "two-tone" suppression, although there is clearly no such limitation on the number of stimulus components that can interact within the cochlea. Nevertheless, because most of the relevant experimental data exist in this two-tone format, our attention is focused on that particular manifestation of suppression.

Mutual Suppression

Experimental Data

In a common two-tone experiment one of the tones is presented at a constant amplitude, and the companion tone is varied over a series of intensities. Shown in Figure 10.1A are data from one such experiment in which the frequency of the fixed-level (or "probe") tone was set at the characteristic frequency (34 kHz) of the measurement point located at the extreme base of the cat basilar membrane. The second (or "suppressor") tone was assigned a number of frequencies, each of which was used to generate one of the probe-response[1] curves in Figure 10.1A. The pattern of probe-response suppression was much the same, regardless of the suppressor's frequency. If presented at too low a level (< 50 dB SPL), the suppressor had no influence on the response component evoked by the fixed probe tone. However, once the suppressor tone exceeded a certain "threshold" amplitude, it suppressed the 34 kHz response component—more so as the suppressor amplitude was further increased.

Close attention to the frequencies associated with the different curves shows that the second tone was suppressive to the first whether its frequency was above or below that of the probe tone. Although there was a higher limit (ca. 41 kHz) to the frequency an effective suppressor could have in

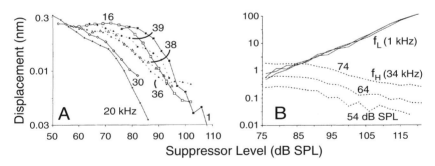

Figure 10.1. Two-tone suppression of responses of the basilar membrane in the extreme base of the cat cochlea. *A.* Amplitude of the response component evoked by a tone of 34 kHz (the characteristic frequency of the measurement point) presented at 54 dB SPL. It is plotted as a function of the level of a second simultaneously presented tone (frequency, in kiloHertz, is indicated). Type of suppression is indicated by the type of line used: solid for "low side," dashed for "high side." *B.* Amplitude of the 34 kHz response component evoked by a tone of 34 kHz (f_H), presented at three indicated levels, plotted as a function of level of a simultaneously presented 1 kHz (f_L) tone (dotted curves). The amplitude of the corresponding 1 kHz response component is also shown (solid curves). Note that the onset ("threshold") of suppression was little affected by the level of the 34 kHz tone. (From Rhode and Cooper, 1996, with permission.*)

this case, there was virtually no lower limit. Figure 10.1B, for example, shows the strong suppression exercised by a 1 kHz suppressor on the responses elicited by the probe tone presented at several levels (dotted curves). The 1 kHz tone was also excitatory, generating its own response components (Fig. 10.1B, solid curves). Note for future reference that essentially no suppression occurred until the amplitude of the 1 kHz response component exceeded that produced by the 34 kHz tone acting alone.

The most general case of suppression is when each tone reduces the response to the other (i.e., mutual suppression). That is, just as the 30 kHz tone in this experiment suppressed the response to a 34 kHz tone, so did the 34 kHz tone suppress the response to a 30 kHz tone (Rhode and Cooper, 1996).

Model Responses.

The model described in Chapter 9 also exhibits mutual suppression, as demonstrated in Figure 10.2. Shown in the dot-dashed curves in both panels are the respective response components generated by tones of 5.0 and 5.4 kHz, presented simultaneously. For ease of comparisons, the levels of these tones were adjusted so that initially the two response peaks were of approximately equal size (ca. 1.1 nm). Even these responses had been mutually suppressed, each being smaller than that produced by the tone acting alone.

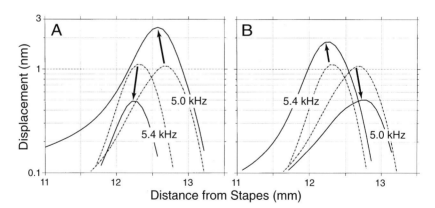

Figure 10.2. Mutual suppression produced in a cochlear model by two tones with frequencies of 5.0 and 5.4 kHz, respectively. *A.* Dot-dashed lines show the corresponding response components when stimulus levels were adjusted to generate approximately equal peaks (ca. 1 nm). Solid lines show the responses when the sound level of the 5.0 kHz tone *only* was increased by 10 dB (about threefold); the level of the 5.4 kHz tone remaining fixed. *B.* Reverse situation, in which the sound level of the 5.4 kHz tone *only* was increased, also by 10 dB. Note the strong dominance given either tone by the 10 dB increase in its strength. (From a nonlinear version of the Geisler–Sang model, 1995.)

The solid curves in Figure 10.2A show the response components produced by the same two tones when the level of the 5 kHz tone *only* was changed, increased by 10 dB. The 5.0 kHz response component more than doubled in amplitude, whereas the 5.4 kHz component was reduced to less than half of its previous size. Note the dominance thus accorded the 5.0 kHz component: It surpassed in size the 5.4 kHz component by at least a factor of 2 throughout this entire section of the model.

When the level of the 5.4 kHz tone *only* was increased, the tables were turned. As shown by the solid curves in Figure 10.2B, it was the 5.4 kHz response component that then rose in stature, and the 5.0 kHz component that shriveled.

Clearly the two tones were suppressing each other's response components. Moreover, because the only nonlinear elements in the cochlear model are the input–output curves of the outer hair cells, those compressive curves must have been the agents responsible for that mutual suppression (see next section for an explanation). It was stated in Chapter 9 that suppression may be considered a side effect of the clearly beneficial amplification processes provided by the outer hair cells. That may be so, but note that the dominance accorded to the more powerful tone by this mutual suppression may have beneficial effects all its own (see Chapter 14).

"Low-Side" Suppression

Experimental Data

When the suppressor tone has a frequency below that of a characteristic-frequency probe tone, "low-side" suppression is said to occur. If the frequency of the suppressor tone is low enough (< 4 kHz), *phasic* suppression of the probe tone responses is observed as well as *tonic* (average value) suppression.

Both phasic and tonic suppression occur in the displacements of the basilar membrane at the extreme basal end of the cat cochlea when 1 kHz and 34 kHz tones are sounded simultaneously (Rhode and Cooper, 1993). The average displacement waveforms recorded there over a 1 msec time window synchronized with the period of the 1 kHz tone, are shown in Figure 10.3 (the 1 kHz components have been filtered out). When the probe tone was presented alone, the amplitude of the response was steady at about 0.4 nm (Fig. 10.3, top left panel). When the suppressor tone was added at moderate levels (79–85 dB SPL), the amplitude of the response became modulated at 1 kHz. At even higher suppressor levels, two phases of modulation occurred within each millisecond. At its highest level (100 dB SPL), the 1 kHz tone reduced the probe-tone's response to such an extent that only once

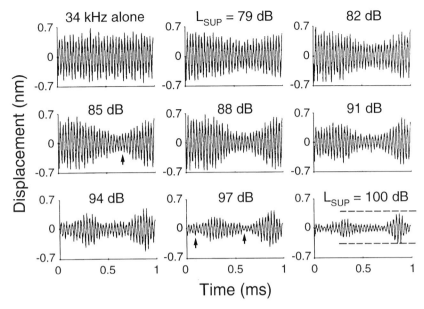

Figure 10.3. Waveforms of "low side" suppression in the extreme base of the cat cochlea. The suppressor tone, with a frequency of 1 kHz, was set at various sound pressure levels, indicated in each panel. The tone of characteristic frequency (34 kHz) had a fixed strength of 64 dB SPL. For clarity, the 1 kHz component was filtered out. The time base of all responses is 1 msec (the period of the suppressor tone). As suppressor level (L_{sup}) grew, the 34 kHz response component became phasically suppressed, first with one dip (e.g., arrow in 85 dB panel) occurring shortly after 0.5 msec, the moment of maximum deflection toward scala tympani, and then with two dips (pair of arrows in the 97 dB panel). At the highest suppressor intensity, recovery to the presuppression amplitude (dashed lines) was never achieved. (From Rhode and Cooper, 1993, with permission.*)

in the entire 1 msec window did it even approach its single-tone amplitude (Fig. 10.3, bottom right panel).

Model Responses

Low-side suppression is also a property of the model. If presented by itself, a weak 5.0 kHz tone produced a response whose peak reached almost 0.9 nm (Fig. 10.4A, dash-dotted curve). However, when presented along with a 2.4 kHz tone, the peak amplitude of this 5.0 kHz response component dropped to about 0.5 nm (Fig. 10.4A, left solid curve). It is important to note that even while acting as a suppressor the low-frequency tone also acted as an exciter, producing its own response component (Fig. 10.4A, right solid curve).

The rather small suppression exhibited in Figure 10.4A (ca. 40%) was

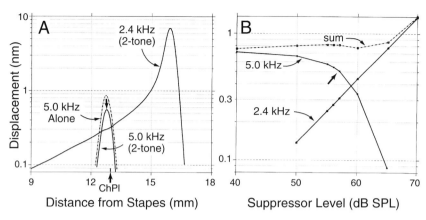

Figure 10.4. "Low-side" suppression in a cochlear model. *A*. Response waveforms produced with a 5.0 kHz tone alone at 30 dB SPL (dot-dashed line) and with a 2.4 kHz tone added at 57 dB SPL (solid lines). *B*. Magnitudes of the 2.4 kHz tone and 5.0 kHz response components in the two-tone responses at the characteristic place (ChPl) of the 5.0 kHz tone (12.9 mm), plotted as a function of the suppressor tone's stimulus level. As the suppressor intensity rose, the 5.0 kHz response component was progressively suppressed, whereas the 2.4 kHz component grew essentially linearly. Note that the sum of the two components (dot-dashed line) never fell below the amplitude of the unsuppressed 5.0 kHz component (ca. 0.7 nm). Compare with the experimental data in Figure 10.1B. Arrow indicates the 5.0 kHz data point for *A*. (From a nonlinear version of the Geisler–Sang model, 1995.)

due to the relatively low amplitude of the suppressor tone (57 dB SPL). As that magnitude was increased, the probe-tone component recorded at the 12.9 mm point (its characteristic place) rapidly diminished, losing almost 99% of its amplitude at a suppressor strength of 65 dB SPL (Fig. 10.4B, falling solid curve). By contrast, the response component produced at the 5.0 kHz place by the 2.4 kHz tone increased with suppressor level (Fig. 10.4B, rising solid line). In fact, that increase was virtually linear, as the recording location lay in an effectively linear region of the cochlea for 2.4 kHz excitation, outside the (nonlinear) amplification zone for that frequency (see Chapter 9). Note that the *sum* of the two response components was always greater than the response to the 5 kHz tone by itself (ca. 0.7 nm), as in the physiological data (Fig. 10.1B).

The behavior of the model can be readily accounted for by referring to the transfer function of the model's outer hair cells, represented in Figure 10.5A (see Fig. 8.3). Stimulation with the low-level 5.0 kHz tone alone (Fig. 10.5C, shaded) causes the input displacement of an outer hair cell located near the 5.0 kHz place to fall within the slightly curved central zone of its transfer function (Fig. 10.5A). A nearly sinusoidal receptor potential of constant amplitude results (Fig. 10.5B, shaded).

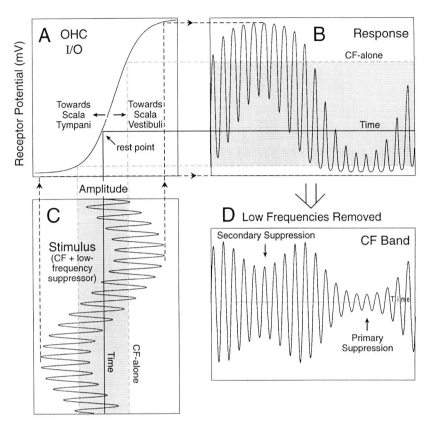

Figure 10.5. Explanation of ''low side'' suppression in the model. Used as input to the outer hair cell's (OHC) input–output (I/O) curve (*A*), the waveform in *C* produces the output waveform of *B*. Note that two-tone stimulation *always* produces, during some segment of the suppressor tone's period, peak response amplitudes that exceed the amplitude achieved with the characteristic frequency tone alone (shaded band). *D*. When the low-frequency component is filtered out, the response waveform to the characteristic frequency tone has two epochs of suppression (arrows), the primary suppression occurring with maximum basilar membrane deflection toward scala tympani. Compare with the experimental data in Figure 10.3. (From Geisler and Nuttall, 1997a, with permission.*)

When a low-frequency tone (250 Hz) is added (Fig. 10.5C), the larger excursions produced by the combined tones periodically force the transduction mechanism farther into its compressive regions (Fig. 10.5A). The resulting receptor potential is ''clipped'' on both extremes (Fig. 10.5B). When the low-frequency component is filtered out (it does not affect the amplification of the 5.0 kHz tone), it is seen that the amplitude of the 5.0 kHz response component is now modulated by the low-frequency tone (Fig. 10.5D). Because this 5.0 kHz receptor potential determines the ''gain'' of the model's amplification process at this frequency, the response of the whole cochlear partition to the 5.0 kHz tone is likewise modulated (i.e., phasically suppressed). The relative strengths of the two phases of suppression that occur during each cycle of the low-frequency tone depend on the degree of asymmetry in the location of the hair cell's "rest" point.

Comparison of the model's output with the experimental data (Fig. 10.3) shows that the model has captured at least the qualitative aspects of low-side suppression. Strong additional support for the model has just been reported in several experimental studies (Cooper, 1996; Geisler and Nuttall, 1997a,b). As in the model, both studies found that maximum suppression occurred at approximately those instants when the basilar membrane had its greatest deflection in the direction of scala tympani, and that the sum of the two response amplitudes was always greater in magnitude than the response to the characteristic frequency tone when presented alone.

This same basic phenomenon underlies the model's mutual suppression as well. Whenever another tone, of whatever frequency, reduces the probe-tone components of the relevant outer hair cells' receptor potentials, the probe tone's response is suppressed. If both tones are amplified over the same stretch of the cochlear partition, each tone acts as both a probe and a suppressor tone, and the suppression is mutual.

"High-side" Suppression

Experimental Data

Responses of the basilar membrane to a characteristic frequency tone can also be suppressed by an added tone that has a frequency greater than the characteristic frequency ("high-side" suppression). Figure 10.6 depicts some typical high-side suppressions for both basal and apical locations. Shown in each panel are the sound-level/response curves for the characteristic-frequency tone in the presence of a high-side suppressor held at one of several levels. Without the suppressor, each probe-response curve showed a classical compressive response (Fig. 10.6, dashed or dotted lines). With the addition of the suppressor tone held at one particular level, the lower segments of those response curves were systematically suppressed. As the suppressor level was increased, greater reductions occurred; and the response curves became progressively more nearly linear.

An important distinction of these data is that often *both* the probe-tone and suppressor-tone responses to the two-tone complex were considerably smaller than the unsuppressed probe-tone response. Thus in contrast to low-side suppression, the sum of the two amplitudes in high-side suppression is regularly *smaller* in amplitude than the unsuppressed response to the characteristic-frequency tone.

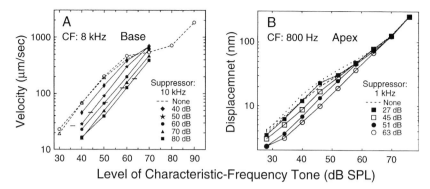

Figure 10.6. ''High-side'' suppression of cochlear partition responses in the base (*A*) and apex (*B*) of the chinchilla cochlea. *A*. Level response curves for the velocity responses of the basal basilar membrane to characteristic-frequency (8 kHz) tones presented simultaneously with a 10 kHz suppressor tone held fixed at various levels (indicated by symbols). With increasing suppressor level, the level-response curve moved progressively to the right. *B*. Level-response curves for the displacement responses of the apical cochlear partition for characteristic-frequency (800 Hz) tones presented along with a 1.0 kHz suppressor tone of various levels (indicated by symbols). The same pattern is seen in both panels, suggesting similar suppressive mechanisms. (*A*: From Ruggero et al., 1992, with permission.* *B*: From Cooper and Rhode, 1996, with permission.*)

Model Responses

The cochlear model exhibits suppression of the same type. When a high-side tone of 5.9 kHz was added to one of 5.0 kHz, the peak of the model's response to the 5.0 kHz component dropped by about 85% (Fig. 10.7A). Yet the response to the 5.9 kHz tone near the 13 mm spot was negligible. The cause for this behavior in the model is the same as that invoked to account for low-side suppression: reduction of the outer hair cell receptor potentials that drive the cell's motile processes. The difference in this case is that the outer hair cells most affected clearly lay basal to the place where the 5.0 kHz response peaked. Recall that this basal region forms the amplification zone for the 5.0 kHz tone (see Chapter 9). Thus by reducing the 5.0 kHz receptor potentials in the outer hair cells of the 11- to 13-mm region, the 5.9 kHz tone reduced the amplification process for the 5.0 kHz traveling wave as it passed through that region. A large reduction in overall amplification of the 5.0 kHz response resulted without the 5.9 kHz tone ever reaching the 5.0 kHz characteristic place.

The sound-level/response curves for this 5.0 kHz probe tone are shown in Figure 10.7B for three levels of that high-side suppressor. Note that at each of its levels the suppressor tone reduced the probe-tone response in a

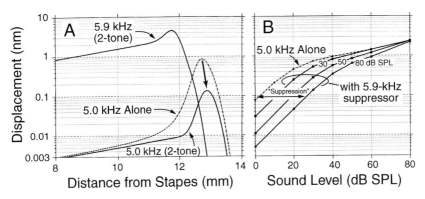

Figure 10.7. "High-side" suppression in the cochlear model. *A.* Response wave-forms produced with a 5.0 kHz tone alone at 30 dB SPL (dot-dashed line) and with an added 5.9 kHz tone presented at 80 dB SPL (solid lines). *B.* Level-response curves of the 5.0 kHz response component occurring at that tone's characteristic place (12.9 mm), plotted for various levels of the suppressor tone. As the suppressor intensity rose, the 5.0 kHz response component was progressively suppressed; the 5.9 kHz response component (not shown) was negligible throughout. Compare with the experimental data in Figure 10.6A. (From a nonlinear version of the Geisler–Sang model, 1995.)

manner similar to that seen in the basal region of the living cochlea (Fig. 10.6A). The higher the suppressor level, the greater is the probe-response reduction.

Confining attention to the lower-amplitude portions of these curves in Figure 10.7B (< 0.3 nm), the suppressor tone at any one sound level can be said to have shifted the entire probe-tone's response curve horizontally by a certain amount. For historical reasons, the magnitude of this horizontal shift is the measure traditionally assigned to two-tone suppression (see Chapter 13). As shown in Figure 10.7B, an 80 dB suppressor tone produced a little more than 20 dB of "suppression." One can think of this number as a tenfold reduction in the "effective" level of the probe tone. Obviously, such an effective attenuation does not apply at the higher probe-tone levels, where the curves merge.

Clearly, the frequency separation of the two tones is crucial. Only to the extent that the suppressor's response peak lies within the amplification zone of the probe tone is the suppressor able to affect the probe tone's amplification process. Figure 10.8A, for example, shows that a 6.7 kHz suppressor presented at 80 dB SPL caused only a small reduction in the response of a 5.0 kHz probe tone. As registered in Figure 10.8B, suppression of that 5.0 kHz response weakened as the suppressor frequency increased, becoming negligible at suppressor-tone frequencies above 8 kHz (frequency ratio of

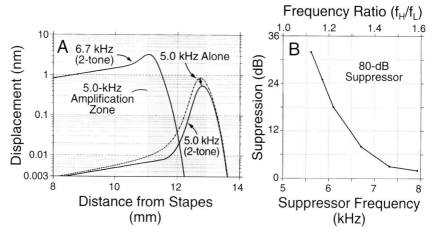

Figure 10.8. Effect of suppressor frequency on "high-side" suppression in the cochlear model. *A.* Amplitude of the response components produced by a 30 dB 5.0 kHz tone presented alone (dot-dashed line) and with an added 6.7 kHz tone of 80 dB SPL (solid lines). In contrast to the large suppression seen in Figure 10.7A, the peak magnitude of the 5.0 kHz response component was only slightly reduced. *B.* Magnitude of the suppression of the 5.0 kHz (f_L) response component provided by an 80 dB suppressor tone, plotted as a function of the suppressor's frequency (f_H). The upper abscissa scale shows the ratio of the two frequencies. For ratios greater than 1.6, there was negligible suppression. The data indicate that the "amplification zone" for the 5.0 kHz tone is about 2 mm wide (shaded in *A*). (From a nonlinear version of the Geisler–Sang model, 1995.)

1.6). From these data, it can be estimated that the model's amplification zone for a 5.0 kHz tone (Fig. 10.8A, shaded area) extends about 2 mm basally from that tone's characteristic place at 12.9 mm (see Patuzzi, 1996).

A similar dependence of high-side suppression on frequency separation is also observed on the living basilar membrane (Rhode, 1977; Robles et al., 1989; Cooper, 1996). Some evidence of this dependence is given in Figure 10.9, which shows the suppressor response/probe-tone response *ratio* measured at the threshold of suppression for apical points on five chinchilla basilar membranes having characteristic frequencies in the 600- to 800-Hz range. For almost all low-side suppressors that ratio was near or greater than unity. In other words, the sum of the two response amplitudes at suppression threshold was always greater than that of the probe tone presented alone (compare with Fig. 10.4B). By contrast, the response ratio for high-side suppressors dropped steadily with progressively higher frequencies. In fact, for suppressor frequencies between 2 and 3 kHz the response to the suppressing tone was sometimes three orders of magnitude *smaller* than the characteristic-frequency response at suppression threshold. No probe-

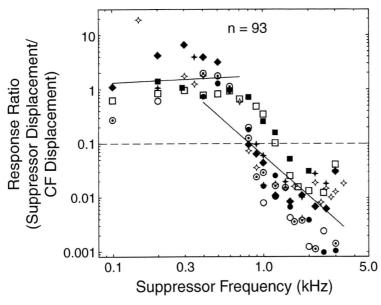

Figure 10.9. Frequency dependence of two-tone suppression in the apical portion of the chinchilla cochlea (combined data from five animals). Each point shows the amplitude of the suppressor's response at the threshold of suppressing the response component with the characteristic frequency (CF), expressed as the ratio of those two amplitudes. Solid lines show least-squares fits to two subsets of data: "low-side" suppression (nearly horizontal line) and "high-side" suppression (slope −2.5 decades/decade). For *all* "low-side" suppression the sum of the two amplitudes at suppression threshold was always greater than the response to the CF tone alone: Criterion level is 0.1 (because the amplitude of the CF component at the "threshold" of suppression was defined as 0.9 times its unsuppressed amplitude). By contrast, the tiny responses to most "high-side" suppressors did not come near meeting that criterion. Compare with the model data in Figures 10.4 and 10.8. (From Cooper and Rhode, 1996, with permission.*)

response suppressions were reported for any of these points using second tones with frequencies above 3.3 kHz.

Summary of Suppressions

The responses evoked by a tone from a location on the basilar membrane lying within that tone's amplification region can be reduced in amplitude by the simultaneous presentation of a second tone. The frequency of the second tone relative to that of the first determines the particular form that suppression takes. Regardless of its form, the basic characteristics of that suppression can be accounted for by the compressive nature of the outer hair cells' motile forces.

OTOACOUSTIC EMISSIONS

Sounds *not* generated by the acoustic stimulating equipment have been recorded in the external ear canals of virtually all vertebrates studied to date. The great weight of evidence indicates that these *otoacoustic emissions* are generated *within* the cochlea. As direct access to the cochlea is nonexistent in human patients and fraught with severe technical difficulties in experimental animals, having a noninvasive probe of the inner ear's workings is important. These emissions have become useful experimental and diagnostic tools (for reviews see Probst et al., 1991; Whitehead et al., 1996).

Otoacoustic emissions are diverse in nature. Although it is likely that they are produced by common mechanisms, for convenience they have been placed in four categories, each defined by the particular type of acoustic stimulus (or lack thereof) that evokes them: distortion-product, spontaneous, transiently evoked, and stimulus-frequency.

Distortion Product Emissions

General Characteristics

As somewhat distinct from the others in its characteristics, and because it is the easiest to account for theoretically, let us consider *distortion product emissions* first. This type of emission is produced, for instance, when two externally applied tones, of frequencies f_L (lower) and f_H (higher), excite the ear simultaneously. Analysis of the acoustic pressures recorded from the ear canal with this two-tone stimulus reveals the presence of energy not only at those two "primary" frequencies but also at some of the "cross-product"[2] frequencies, most notably at $(2f_L - f_H)$. As these cross-product tones are not present in the applied signal, they must have been generated within the ear itself.

In humans these "cubic distortion product"[2] emissions have their frequencies in the 0.5- to 5.0-kHz range and are typically small in amplitude, usually about three orders of magnitude below those of the primary tones. Much larger magnitudes are sometimes observed, however, through interactions with other types of emission (see below). The combinations of the two primary tones that can produce these emissions are limited: Their frequencies and amplitudes must be similar. In humans (Harris et al., 1989) and rhesus monkeys (Park et al., 1995) maximum emission amplitudes occur when the ratio of the primary frequencies, f_H/f_L, just slightly exceeds 1.2. A larger frequency ratio, about 1.35, works best in cats (Kim, 1980).

An example of the frequency spectrum[3] measured in a human ear excited by two tones having a frequency ratio of 1.22 is shown in Figure 10.10A.

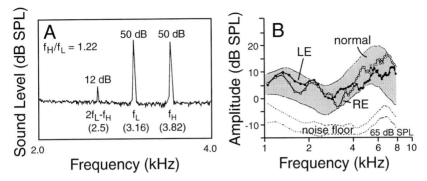

Figure 10.10. *A*. Frequency spectrum of the ear canal signal recorded from a normal human ear when excited by two equal-amplitude "primary" tones of frequency 3.16 kHz (f_L) and 3.82 kHz (f_H), respectively. In addition to the large peaks at those frequencies, there is a small distortion-product otoacoustic emission at 2.5 kHz, the frequency of the cubic distortion product $2f_L - f_H$. *B*. Amplitude of one subject's distortion product emissions, as a function of the (mean geometric) frequency of the two primary tones, each pair having a frequency ratio of 1.22. The band of amplitudes (average $\pm$ 1 standard deviation) recorded from 44 normal ears is shaded. (From Lonsbury-Martin and Martin, 1990, with permission.*)

The three narrow spikes rising above the noise floor indicate that three tones were present in the ear canal: the two applied tones (frequencies of 3.16 and 3.82 kHz, respectively) and a distortion product emission. The latter, with a frequency of 2.5 kHz, had an amplitude of 12 dB SPL, about 40 dB below those of the equal-amplitude primaries. When the emission amplitude for many frequency combinations (but the same f_H/f_L ratio) is plotted as a function of mean frequency, curves such as those shown in Figure 10.10B are obtained from normal ears. Such curves are sometimes labeled "audio-grams," although that designation is somewhat misleading. These emissions are the direct reflection of cochlear electromechanics only, not behavioral responses. Thus the presence of an emission does not always mean that the person has normal hearing in that ear (see Chapter 16).

Distortion product emissions can be manipulated in a number of ways that testify to their cochlear origin. For example, the administration of fu-rosemide, known to reduce the amplitude of both basilar membrane and afferent neuron responses (see Chapter 16), induces a similar reduction in these emissions. Such reductions are so consistent that they have even been used to track the severity of cochlear poisoning produced by the antibiotic gentamicin (Brown et al., 1989). Aspirin, which is known to affect outer hair cells (see Chapter 8), also suppresses human distortion product emis-sions, although the effects are less pronounced than those displayed by the other types of emission (Wier et al., 1988). Aspirin had little effect on the distortion product emissions of monkeys, but it abolished their emissions of other types (Martin et al., 1988).

As distortion product emissions could theoretically be generated by almost any type of nonlinearity, it is not surprising that there seem to be several mechanisms contributing to the cubic distortion product emissions. Those produced with low-level primary tones are physiologically vulnerable, diminishing with mild outer hair cell disturbance (Brown et al., 1989) and disappearing within a few minutes of death. On the other hand, distortion product emissions evoked by high-level tones can persist in the presence of outer hair cell damage and even for some hours after death. Thus it appears that (at least) two sources contribute to these emissions.

Model Responses

The generally accepted cause of distortion product emissions produced at low levels can be illustrated with the cochlear model. When equal-amplitude sinusoids of 5.0 and 5.9 kHz were simultaneously applied to it, a sinusoidal response component at a frequency of $2f_L - f_H$ (4.1 kHz) was created (Fig. 10.11A). The phase curve for this response component (Fig. 10.11B) is particularly revealing: It is not monotonic but has a *peak* near the 12 mm point. Because phases that decrease monotonically in one direction are the signature of a wave traveling in that direction (see Chapter 5), this phase peak indicates that *two* sinusoidal traveling waves with that frequency existed simultaneously. One wave traveled in the normal "forward" direction toward the spot on the cochlear partition tuned to that frequency (ca. the 14 mm point), and the other traveled "backward," toward the stapes. Some of this backward-traveling wave continued on through the middle ear ossicles and out into the external canal, causing distortion product "emissions." Another portion of that backward-traveling energy was reflected from the stapes, producing a small forward-traveling wave at the distortion product frequency. The undulations in that tone's amplitude curve in the 6- to 10-mm region were caused by interactions of those two oppositely traveling waves.

It is significant that the place along the cochlea where the distortion product tone was created is located between the twin response peaks produced by the two primary tones (Fig. 10.11A, marked by a vertical line). This interpeak region is where the amplitudes of the primary-tone responses were both about 0.5 nm, which according to Figure 9.6C is the amplitude at which the model's outer hair cells began to lose their punch (operate compressively). In other words, the distortion product emissions *in the model* are a by-product of the normal (nonlinear) functioning of the cochlear amplifier in its compression region.

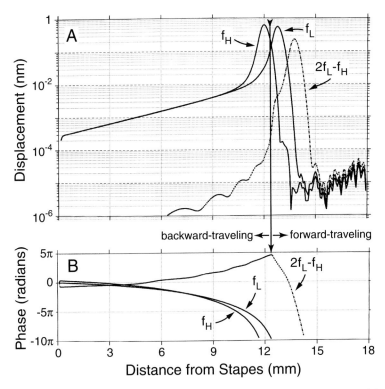

Figure 10.11. Creation of distortion product emissions in the cochlear model. The equal-amplitude primary tones, with frequencies of 5.0 kHz (f_L) and 5.85 kHz (f_H), were presented at 30 dB SPL. A sinusoidal response component at 4.15 kHz ($2f_L - f_H$) was created. A. Amplitudes of the response components at the primary and distortion product frequencies, throughout the basal two-thirds of the cochlea. B. Phases of those same components. Note that the curve for the distortion product component has a peak, indicating that sound waves of that frequency propagated in both directions from that point. (From a nonlinear version of the Geisler–Sang model, 1995.)

Much experimental evidence indicates that this situation is the case in living ears as well, although the actual site(s) of origin are still not well defined. No one seems to doubt that distortion product vibrations are generated in the cochlear region where the response components evoked by the primary tones are both strong. The difficulty is that distortion product emissions, being produced by *all* of the backward-traveling energy that reaches the stapes, likely comes from more than one location. At the very least, a whole zone of the cochlea probably contributes distortion-product energy, not just one point. Experimental evidence suggests that multiple ill-defined sites of origin are indeed involved (Stover et al., 1996; He and Schmiedt, 1997).

The distortion process illustrated in Figure 10.11 produces all manner of other cross-product components with frequencies such as $2f_H$ and $2f_H - f_L$. Why are components with these frequencies not seen in otoacoustic emissions? Algebra shows that the two frequencies just mentioned are greater than either f_L or f_H, and the frequency $2f_L - f_H$ is lower than either. Assuming that all of the distortion product components are created somewhere between the peaks of the two primary-tone responses, the tone with frequency $2f_L - f_H$ would resonate at a point apical to its birth place (as in Fig. 10.11), whereas tones with frequencies $2f_H - f_L$ and $2f_H$ would resonate at points more basal than that. Thus these higher-frequency components are born in a region that lies *beyond* their respective resonance points, in a portion of the cochlear partition where they are strongly attenuated and cannot propagate as traveling waves (see Chapter 5). By contrast, the lower-frequency distortion products are generated in a cochlear region that allows their propagation as traveling waves (in both directions).

This squelching of the higher frequency distortion products is indeed fortunate, as they comprise most of the new components created by a compressive nonlinearity. As a result, distortions of the input signal produced by the strongly compressive nature of the cochlear amplifier are limited effectively. Imagine the difficulties that would arise if the cochlear partition were constructed with the opposite polarity, such that traveling displacement waves were introduced at the low-frequency end and propagated toward the high-frequency end. With that scenario, the great bulk of the distortion products would also become traveling waves and travel on to their respective resonance points, creating extraneous neural responses.

Spontaneous Otoacoustic Emissions

General Characteristics

As stated previously, some emissions occur in the absence of any deliberate external stimulation. These *spontaneous otoacoustic emissions* are surprisingly common in humans, with more than half the population tested displaying them. Amplitudes as large as 20 dB SPL can be measured in the ear canal. For reasons unknown, these emissions occur more frequently in women (83%) than in men (68%) (Penner and Zhang, 1997), with somewhat lower but still unbalanced percentages holding even for infants and children. Puzzling is the virtual absence of this type of emission in common laboratory animals (but see below).

One illuminating characteristic of spontaneous emissions is that they are essentially pure tones or, more accurately, groups of pure tones. Figure 10.12A shows a section of the frequency spectrum of the acoustic pressure

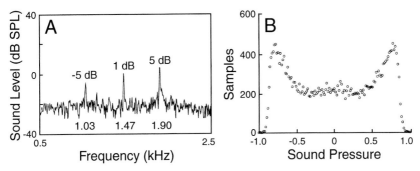

Figure 10.12. *A.* Spectrum of the ear canal signal recorded from a normal human subject in the absence of deliberate acoustic stimulation. The three narrow peaks, each labeled with its frequency and amplitude, indicate that three spontaneous otoacoustic emissions were present. Note the regular spacing of their frequencies. *B.* Probability distribution of sound pressure in the ear canal in a narrow frequency band containing a prominent spontaneous emission at 1.42 kHz obtained during 6 min of continual recording. Arbitrary units of pressure. (*A:* From Martin et al., 1990b, with permission*. *B:* From Bialek and Wit, 1984, with permission.*)

recorded from an *un*stimulated human ear canal. The three narrow spectral peaks mean not only that acoustic energy was pumped out of the middle ear into the ear canal, but that this energy was distributed among three components, each a sinusoid of almost constant frequency and amplitude (temporal variation of either of these parameters broadens the spectral peak).

It was initially argued by some scientists that even the narrow spectral peaks of these emissions do not *prove* that they are true tones (sinusoidal oscillations). Perhaps the emissions are simply sharply filtered noises, produced when random body noises excite points along the basilar membrane, which is admittedly sharply tuned. That conjecture was laid to rest by the *amplitude* histogram shown in Figure 10.12B. Obtained from one spontaneous emission, this distribution of amplitude samples is shaped like a dumbbell, meaning that the waveform of the emission spent more time at its peaks and valleys than it did near zero. Such an amplitude distribution is characteristic of a sinusoid but not of random noise, which *must* (according to theory) display a Gaussian-like distribution, no matter how sharply it is filtered. It follows that spontaneous emissions are indeed tones. Although there are still some loopholes in the argument (the random-noise theorem requires system linearity), almost all theorists consider the case closed.

The typical range of the frequencies of human spontaneous emissions is 0.5–6.0 kHz, with the largest number occurring between 1 and 2 kHz. Spontaneous emissions have also been recorded from bats (with emission frequencies in the 60 kHz region) (Kössl, 1994), primates (Martin et al., 1988), some guinea pigs (Ohyama et al., 1991), lizards, one species of bird (the barn owl) (Köppl, 1995), and many species of frogs (van Dijk et al., 1996). Especially intriguing about the latter case is the effect of body temperature on the emissions: They can be switched on and off by variations of only a few degrees.

Of special significance are the tiny amplitudes of sounds that can influence emission frequency in humans. Wit and Ritsma (1983) showed that acoustic clicks with energies as small as 1 electron-volt can affect the emission waveform. This extremely low energy level suggests that processes at the level of a few molecules might be producing (or gating) the emissions.

Another relevant feature of spontaneous emissions is that they can be reduced, even abolished, by aspirin, suggesting the involvement of outer hair cells. This suggestion is strengthened by the observation that the spontaneous emissions of one ear can be modulated by sound presented to the other ear (Mott et al., 1989), presumably via the crossed efferent system (see Chapter 15).

Source(s)

The cochlear amplifier system proposed in Chapter 9 accounts plausibly for spontaneous emissions. Indeed, the very existence of these emissions is one of the pillars supporting the theory that cochlear amplification is caused by the outer hair cells acting in feedback loops (see Fig. 9.5). It is well known that under certain conditions such a feedback system can become unstable and produce sustained oscillations. Cochlear models incorporating such feedback systems have, in fact, produced spontaneous oscillations (Zwicker, 1986; Talmadge and Tubis, 1993; Fukazawa and Tanaka, 1996).

Of particular interest here is the mathematical equation used to represent each individual basilar membrane slice in the model. It is *identical* in general form to that of the well known Van der Pol oscillator (Long et al., 1991). Comparisons between the output of that oscillator and a spontaneously emitted tone show many similarities. The amplitudes of both oscillatory waveforms, for example, can be suppressed by an externally applied sinusoid with similar frequency and magnitude. Moreover, when the frequency of the applied sinusoid is brought close to that of the spontaneous oscillation, in both mathematical and biological systems the spontaneous tone switches its frequency over to that of the applied tone.

The ability of models such as the Van der Pol oscillator to mimic spontaneous emissions so well provides strong support for the hypothesis that outer hair cell feedback produces these emissions. The damping effects of aspirin provide further support for this feedback theory, as the drug is known to have strong depressive effects on the motility of outer hair cells (see Chapter 8).

If so, why doesn't every section of the cochlea act that way and produce emissions at all frequencies? It follows that there must be something different about those cochlear sites that generate the relatively few emissions observed. Unfortunately, the search for such differences has not been successful.

For example, light microscopic histological examination of one rhesus monkey's cochlea known to have produced spontaneous emissions during life revealed no obvious pathology, only a scattered loss of both inner and outer hair cells consistent with the animal's age (Lonsbury-Martin et al., 1988). Thus the presence of low-amplitude spontaneous emissions in rhesus monkeys, as in humans, does not appear to reflect cochlear pathology. However, rhesus monkey cochleas, like those of humans, have irregular arrangements of outer hair cells, particularly in the apical regions of the cochlea. An interrupted fourth row even occurs sometimes. Perhaps those irregularities are responsible for emissions.

That conjecture is supported by the observation that spontaneous emissions are unusual in laboratory rodents, which have smooth outer hair cell arrays (Engström et al., 1966). In contrast, in chinchilla ears, which normally display no spontaneous emissions, they can be induced by exposure to noise. The frequencies of these induced emissions correlate with discrete basal-turn lesions (Clark et al., 1984). Spontaneous emissions, often of high level, have also been recorded from the ears of human subjects suffering from hearing loss (presumably caused by cochlear damage). Taken together, all of these data support the idea that spontaneous emissions are associated with cochlear irregularities, which may be congenital or the result of damage. This conjecture is also compatible with the feedback mechanism proposed above, as irregularities must be introduced into cochlear feedback models before they produce spontaneous oscillations (Fukazawa and Tanaka, 1996). Evidently, neighboring sections in such models normally serve as stabilizers of each other, preventing oscillations.

Can we account for the triple emissions of Figure 10.12A with such a feedback theory? Particularly striking about such multiple emissions, which are in fact the general rule, is the nonrandom nature of their frequency distributions: They tend to be regularly spaced. For example, the central emission in Figure 10.12A has a frequency approximately midway between those of its two neighbors. Analysis of many human spontaneous-emission spectra indicates that the difference in frequency between adjacent emissions is often in the vicinity of 50–100 Hz (about 0.4 mm in the inferred characteristic places of the two tones) (Schloth and Zwicker, 1983; Talmadge et al., 1993). It seems unlikely that such frequency regularity could be produced by spatial *ir*regularities (but see below).

Even more challenging to this proposal is the presence of spontaneous emissions in the ears of many vertebrates that do not even have outer hair cells (frogs, lizards, barn owl). The source of these emissions is not clear, but they might be produced by spontaneous oscillations of the ciliary tufts, as observed in some isolated hair cells (Crawford and Fettiplace, 1985). That same mechanism might be operating in the mammalian cochlea, but mammalian emissions have somewhat different features: They tend to have narrower frequency bandwidths (i.e., more nearly ''pure'' tones) (van Dijk and Wit, 1990), and their reactions to externally applied tones are somewhat different. More to the point, spontaneous ciliary oscillations have not been reported in mammalian hair cells. It seems likely therefore that the spontaneous emissions that occur in various vertebrate classes are generated by several mechanisms, all of which appear to require unstable feedback systems involving the hair cells.

Behavioral Correlates

The existence of spontaneous self-sustained cochlear oscillations brings to mind *tinnitus*, auditory sensations heard in the absence of deliberate acoustic stimulation (see Chapter 16). Do spontaneous emissions cause tinnitus? Not in a direct manner, it seems. Not only is there a low correlation between the occurrence of these emissions and subjective awareness of them, but in cases of coexisting tinnitus and spontaneous emissions one could be masked without affecting the other (Penner and Burns, 1987).

There *is* a subjective correlate of spontaneous emissions: acoustic sensitivity. In a normally hearing adult thresholds at the frequencies of these emissions tend to be more sensitive than at nearby frequencies (e.g., Long and Tubis, 1988). Apparently a weak applied tone can boost an existing oscillation with more effect than it can create one. The existence of spontaneous emissions in human subjects with ''normal thresholds'' (usually defined as being within 20 dB of the accepted standard) and their improved sensitivities near spontaneous-emission frequencies support the conclusion that these emissions generally do not reflect gross cochlear pathology.

Transiently Evoked Emissions

General Characteristics

Unlike spontaneous emissions, *transiently evoked emissions* (hereafter called ''transient emissions'') are responses to some short acoustic stimulus, usually a click or brief tone burst. As implied by their name these emissions eventually die out, but they sometimes take hundreds of milliseconds to do so. Examples of such long emissions, obtained from an ear that also exhibited spontaneous emissions, are seen in Figure 10.13A. The top three traces were evoked by short tone bursts at the indicated frequencies, and the fourth

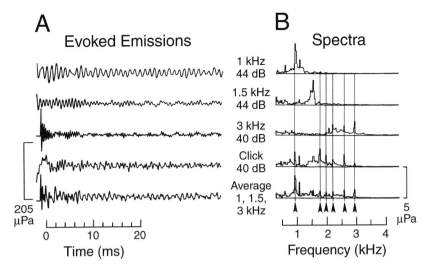

Figure 10.13. *A*. Average waveforms of the transient emissions evoked in one human ear canal by tone bursts of three frequencies (top three traces) and a click (fourth trace down). The average of the top three (tone burst) waveforms is given in the bottom trace for comparison with the click response. The much larger stimulus waveforms were deleted. *B*. Respective frequency spectra of the waveforms. The emissions evoked by each tone burst had a sharp peak at about the tonal frequency, indicating sustained ringing at that frequency (as is visible in the waveforms). The emission evoked by the click tended to produce all of those ringings simultaneously (compare bottom two traces). Six spontaneous emissions were also present, their frequencies indicated by lines and arrowheads. (From Probst et al., 1986, with permission.*)

trace resulted from clicks. (The actual acoustic stimulus, *much* larger than the emission, was deleted from the beginning of each trace). The emissions evoked by each tone burst have a spectrum restricted to a band of frequencies centered around the stimulating frequency (Fig. 10.13B), consistent with the idea that the emissions originated in the vicinity of that tone burst's resonant place. By contrast, the click, whose spectrum nominally includes *all* frequencies at equal strength, effectively excited all of those places (compare the last two traces).

Many of the characteristics of transient emissions are similar to those of spontaneous emissions. That might seem strange at first, as the two types appear to be unrelated. After all, one requires acoustic stimulation for existence, and the other does not. Nevertheless, it appears that the same mechanisms generate both types of emission. Such a situation commonly arises in feedback systems. A circuit such as that in Figure 9.5, for example, may or may not oscillate, depending on the exact nature of its elements. Just before breaking into sustained oscillations, such a circuit would tend to "ring" at the same frequency with which it would oscillate when becoming unstable. Transient emissions appear to be just such suboscillation ringings. Consistent with this view, the narrowly tuned components of human transient emissions (e.g., peaks in Fig. 10.13B) can be reduced by aspirin ingestion (Long and Tubis, 1988), like spontaneous emissions.

Because spontaneous emissions are common in human ears, we would also expect transient emissions to be prevalent. They are. In fact, virtually *all* normal human ears manifest them (Kapadia and Lutman, 1997), although some lack sharply tuned components (Probst et al., 1986). Also predictable from the incidence of spontaneous emissions, transient emissions are also found in primates, cats, frogs, and some bat species (Kössl and Vater, 1985a). They are also seen in the ears of laboratory rodents such as the guinea pig but at lower amplitudes and with much shorter latencies and durations than in humans (Whitehead et al., 1996).

Source(s)

As can be seen in Figure 10.13B, transient emissions evoked by broadband stimuli typically contain a number of tuned components. As is the case with spontaneous emissions, the frequencies of these tuned components are not randomly distributed but tend to be separated by the same 50- to 100-Hz increments (Zwicker and Schloth, 1984). Assuming that these emissions are produced by cochlear irregularities, does it not necessitate some sort of a "corrugated" cochlea? Indeed, cochlear models containing *evenly* distributed spatial irregularities do produce transient emissions with regularly spaced frequency components (Zwicker, 1986; Strube, 1989; van Hengel and Maat, 1993). However, as noted in the previous section, regularly spaced irregularities have *not* been found in the cochleas of emitting species.

Suggestively, it has been shown that cochlear models with *randomly* distributed irregularities can produce both transient emissions and spontaneous emissions that have regularly spaced spectral peaks (Talmadge and Tubis, 1993; Zweig and Shera, 1995; van Hengel, 1995). In these cases the frequency regularity of emission peaks is produced by the interaction of two oscillations: cochlear partition vibrations at the point of instability and a traveling pressure wave produced by those vibrations, partially reflected back to the point from the stapes. For some positions of the instability, the reflected wave arrives with a phase opposite to that of the intrinsic vibrations, so *destructive* interference (mutual cancellation) of the two oscillations occurs and the vibrations are attenuated. For other generation sites, however the interaction of the two oscillations is *constructive*, the intrinsic vibrations are reinforced, and appreciable emissions result. Perhaps the same interference phenomena occur in the living ear, although other possibilities exist, such as suppressive interactions between the spontaneous emissions themselves (van Hengel et al., 1996).

Diagnostic Uses

Not yet mentioned is the fact that transient emissions appear only in relatively normal cochleas: They generally do not occur at frequencies in cochlear regions where damage has resulted in more than a 20- to 30-dB hearing loss (Probst et al., 1991). This sensitivity to damage makes these emissions a valuable, noninvasive probe of cochlear mechanisms, one of the few available. Accordingly, they are used routinely in that role in both laboratory and clinical settings (see Chapter 16).

Stimulus Frequency Emissions

If a continuous acoustic stimulus is used instead of a brief one, *stimulus frequency* (or "synchronous evoked") emissions occur. The difficulty, of course, lies in detecting those emissions in the presence of the applied stimulus. Surprisingly, it can be done, at least at low levels. The technique is to compare the frequency spectra of the acoustic pressures existing in the ear canal at low and medium sound levels. As the emissions presumably saturate at low amplitudes, the difference in the *shape* of the respective spectra is a measure of the emissions that must have been present at low intensities.

As parallels between the behavior of stimulus frequency and transient emissions exist for almost every aspect compared, it is thought that the two types of emission must be produced by the same mechanisms (Probst et al., 1991). That is, expressed in terms of our models, both of these evoked emissions (low-level spontaneous emissions as well) appear to be by-products of the cochlea's amplification processes, perturbed by slight irregularities in the cochlear partition.

Electrically Evoked Emissions

Stimulation of the normal cochlea with an AC (sinusoidal) electrical current generates acoustic emissions of the same frequency in the external ear (e.g., Mountain and Hubbard, 1989). The existence of this phenomenon provides strong support for the feedback theory of cochlear amplification, according to which the AC voltages created within the outer hair cells by the applied current would cause them to generate motile forces (see Fig. 9.5). These forces would push on the cochlear partition, causing it to deflect, which in turn would initiate the backward-traveling acoustic waves that produce emissions (Fig. 10.11).

Electrically generated emissions share many of the characteristics of acoustically generated emissions. Indeed, emissions produced by the two types of stimulation interact readily: Acoustic stimulation has enhanced electrically evoked emissions (Xue et al., 1993), and electrical stimulation can modulate the amplitude of acoustically evoked emissions (Hubbard and Mountain, 1983). Consistent with the basic theory of cochlear function (see Chapter 5), electrically generated emissions can be produced only at frequencies near or below the characteristic frequency of the stimulation site (Xue et al., 1996): Higher frequency traveling waves cannot be launched at that site, since it lies apical to their characteristic places.

More than a curiosity, electrically evoked emissions are proving to be a unique way of probing basic cochlear mechanisms. According to presently accepted theory, the outer hair cells' motile forces are generated by a two-stage process that involves both forward and reverse transduction (see Fig. 9.5). It is virtually impossible to disentangle these two processes using acoustic stimulation. With electrical stimulation, the forward-transduction process is bypassed, and the reverse-transduction mechanism is stimulated directly with a known transmembrane voltage, or at least one that can be estimated using basic electrical circuit theory. Important characteristics of the reverse-transduction process are presently being establishing with this method (e.g., Nuttall and Ren, 1995; Kirk and Yates, 1996; Xue et al., 1996).

SUMMARY OF NONLINEAR PHENOMENA

The behavior of the cochlear partition is markedly nonlinear. Its responses are compressed, it creates new frequencies (sometimes from ''scratch''), and the presentation of one sound often interacts suppressively with another.

The abilities of models containing compressive amplification to mimic the full range of this behavior suggest that these nonlinear phenomena are by-products of the compressive signal-amplification processes believed to reside within the cochlear partition. As such, these nonlinear phenomena have become powerful tools for probing the electromechanical processes of the cochlea.

NOTES

1. The response of a nonlinear system to a single tone, when subjected to Fourier analysis, is usually found to contain many frequency components. In the response waveforms of the basilar membrane, the principal sinusoidal component of the response attributed to one particular tone (presented alone or in an ensemble) virtually

always occurs at the frequency of that tone. For convenience in description, the response component that occurs at the frequency of a tone (or those within a narrow frequency band centered around that frequency) is sometimes referred to as *the* response of that tone, even though other minor components may be present.

2. One of the few mathematical tools available to handle nonlinear phenomena is the ''power series.'' With this tool, the nonlinear output $y(t)$ produced by an input $x(t)$ is approximated by the sum of a series of $x(t)$ terms having increasing powers, $ax + bx^2 + cx^3 + \cdots$ (Note that only the first term in the series is linear). If the input $x(t)$ is made equal to the sum of two sinusoids, $\sin(2\pi f_L t) + \sin(2\pi f_H t)$, simple trigonometry shows that the second term in the series produces cross-product components at the ''sum'' and ''difference'' frequencies, $\cos(2\pi[f_L \pm f_H]t)$, and the third term in the series produces ''cubic'' components, such as $\sin(2\pi[2f_L \pm f_H]t)$.

3. As described in Appendix A, Fourier analysis decomposes a signal into a *frequency spectrum*, either a series of discrete sinusoidal components (a Fourier series) or a continuous density of them (a Fourier transform). In either case, the magnitudes of this frequency spectrum are usually presented as a continuous function of frequency. As each sinusoid has an initial phase, a plot of initial phase versus frequency is also required to complete the specifications of the signal's spectrum. As these initial phases are seldom of importance in physiological acoustics, they are generally ignored; and the common custom of labeling ''the plot of spectrum magnitudes'' as ''*the* spectrum'' is followed herein.

III

NEURAL RESPONSES

11

AFFERENT INNERVATION

On their way into the brain, acoustic signals must be translated from the hydromechanical world of cochlear vibrations into the electrochemical world of neural processing. The inner hair cells are the cochlea's chief agents for such translations. As discussed in Chapter 8, currents flowing through the apical ends of these hair cells owing to ciliary movements produce receptor potentials. Once established, these voltages serve as generator potentials that initiate a chain of events eventually resulting in a barrage of action potentials simultaneously coursing toward the central nervous system on thousands of parallel axons. As we shall see in Chapters 11–14, the characteristics of these two worlds are in a sense complementary to each other. Whereas the cochlea's hydromechanical mechanisms divide the incoming acoustic signals into overlapping *frequency* bands (see Chapter 5), its neural innervation seems designed for rapid, accurate encoding of *temporal* events. Both capabilities are of course important, as time and frequency are complementary dimensions of acoustic signals (see Chapter 13).

As an entry into neural representations of acoustic signals, we review in this chapter some of the basic mechanisms by which information is transmitted from the inner hair cells to their afferent innervation. Then, in the light of these transmission mechanisms, we consider in following chapters the nature of the neural responses to acoustic signals of varying complexity.

SYNAPTIC TRANSMISSION BETWEEN HAIR CELLS AND AFFERENT NEURONS

Afferent Neurons

The cochlea's afferent innervation is provided by bipolar neurons whose cell bodies lie within the aptly named *spiral ganglion*. This ganglion, depicted in Figure 11.1, runs parallel to the organ of Corti throughout its entire length. The central processes (or "modiolar axons") of these neurons entwine and form the auditory nerve. Their distal processes ("or peripheral axons") take direct (radial) courses into the organ of Corti, entering via the *habenula perforata*, holes in the bony spiral lamina. As can be seen from the included reconstructions of five spiral ganglion cells stained with horseradish peroxidase (HRP), the ganglion is "tonotopically" organized: the higher the characteristic frequency of the neuron, the more basal its location.

The total number of spiral ganglion neurons varies among species (Nadol, 1988b). Cats, with a 25 mm cochlea, average about 50,000 of these primary

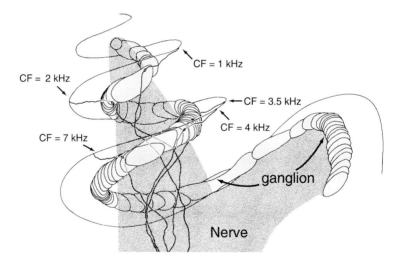

Figure 11.1. Auditory branch of the VIII cranial nerve (dark gray shading), showing the trajectories of five horseradish peroxidase (HRP)-labeled primary afferent neurons with the indicated characteristic frequencies (CF). The cell bodies (dark ovals) all lie within the helical spiral ganglion (light gray; its sliced-bread appearance represents stacked microscope slides viewed face on) from whence the peripheral axons run radially to terminate on a single inner hair cell (lying on the helical line). The modiolar axons terminate in the brain stem's cochlear nucleus (not shown). Note the orderly "tonotopic" organization of the cochlea: the more apical the axon termination of a primary neuron, the lower its characteristic frequency. (From Liberman and Oliver, 1984, with permission.*)

afferent neurons. Humans have a longer cochlea (ca. 35 mm) but fewer such neurons (25,000–30,000). Rats, with a much smaller cochlea, only have about 16,000 spiral ganglion neurons. The functional consequences of these substantial differences in numbers of hair cells (which are proportional to cochlear length) and in innervation density are unknown.

The anatomy of any particular spiral ganglion neuron indicates the destination of its distal process within the organ of Corti (Fig. 11.2). If the neuron is myelinated (therefore *type I*), as about 90% of them are (Spoendlin, 1985), its peripheral axon, shorn of its myelin sheath, runs radially to a single inner hair cell with which it forms a single synapse (Liberman, 1980b; Kiang et al., 1982). There are apparently only rare exceptions to this rule for type I neurons. If, on the other hand, the afferent neuron is one of the few unmyelinated ones (*type II*), its peripheral axon extends radially toward the rows of outer hair cells but turns before reaching them and runs spirally (longitudinally) for a distance, after which it branches and

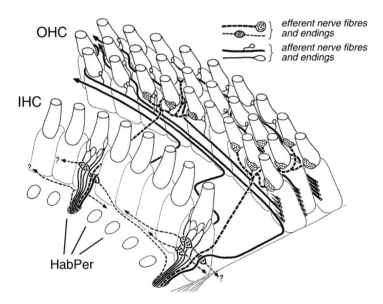

Figure 11.2. Cat organ of Corti showing the basic principles of its innervation with afferent and efferent neurons. The peripheral axon of each type I afferent neuron (thin solid line) enters through the habenula perforata (HabPer) and terminates in a single synapse on one inner hair cell (IHC). A type II afferent neuron sends its peripheral axon (thick solid line) on a spiral route that eventually innervates a group of outer hair cells (OHC). Efferent neurons (see Chapter 15) make multiple synapses with either a group of outer hair cells (thick dashed lines) or the peripheral axons of afferent neurons (thin dashed lines). Only representative examples of peripheral neurons arriving at the organ of Corti through two habenular openings are shown. (From Spoendlin, 1967, with permission.*)

forms synapses with 10–20 clustered outer hair cells. The cell bodies of these type II neurons lie off to the sides of their axons, forming pseudo-monopolar cells (Kiang et al., 1982).

Efferent innervation is provided by neurons whose cell bodies lie within the brain stem. This feedback from the central nervous system likewise has a twofold nature: After taking spiral courses, some efferent axon terminals contact the outer hair cells directly, whereas others terminate among the afferent axons servicing the inner hair cells (see Chapter 15).

Inner Hair Cells

Depending on its location within the cochlea, one inner hair cell forms a single synaptic connection with each of 10–30 afferent neurons. Figure 11.3, an electron micrograph of an inner hair cell in cross section, shows a number of these axon terminals running close to the hair cell's lateral wall. Typically, each of these axons ends in a terminal swelling that shares a single synaptic complex with the hair cell. On the hair cell side of the synapse, the specialization usually takes the form of a single synaptic *bar* or *ribbon* (e.g., Fig. 11.3, at 12 o'clock), although several closely clustered bars sometimes exist (Merchan-Perez and Liberman, 1996). Each bar is surrounded by a halo of small clear vesicles, presumably filled with neurotransmitter(s). On the neural side of the synapse, the plasma membrane is asymmetrically thickened.

From the appearance of the synapse and the need of the synapse to release neurotransmitter endlessly (see below), it appears that the synaptic bar is some sort of holding station for transmitter-filled vesicles ready to be released. Similar looking ribbon synapses are seen in visual receptors. Perhaps this similarity in appearance is related to the fact that both visual and auditory receptors must maintain a continuous efflux of neurotransmitter.

In addition to their suggestive anatomy, there is overwhelming electrophysiological evidence that hair cell synapses are chemical in nature: The postsynaptic excitatory potentials (EPSPs) recorded from afferent terminals in several acousticolateralis maculae display the benchmark characteristics of transmitter release, such as quantized amplitudes, synaptic delays, and adaptive rundown (e.g., Furukawa and Matsuura, 1978; Sewell, 1990; Siegel, 1992; Rossi et al., 1994). Some of these recordings were made from large axon terminals, such as those in the sacculus of the goldfish (Furukawa and Matsuura, 1978). Similar intracellular recordings have been made from the much smaller afferent axon terminations of the mammalian cochlea but only with great difficulty (Siegel, 1992).

One sequence of successful recordings, made ''quasi-intracellularly'' from directly underneath an inner hair cell, is shown in Figure 11.4. In traces *A*

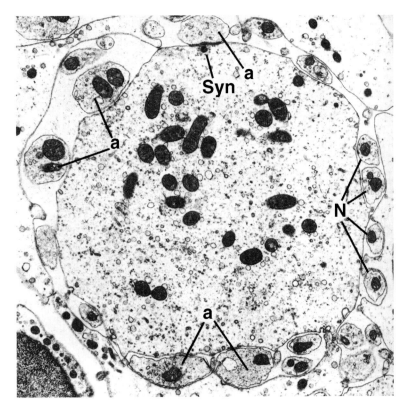

Figure 11.3. Electron micrograph of a horizontal section through the basal portion of an inner hair cell, showing the peripheral axons (N) and axon terminals (a) of many individual afferent neurons. Each nerve terminal generally forms only a single afferent synapse (Syn), characterized on the presynaptic side by a synaptic "bar." Abundant mitochondria are apparent. A small segment of an inner pillar cell is shown in the lower left corner. (From Spoendlin, 1985, with permission.*)

and *B*, small pulses of similar shape (small filled arrowheads) occur immediately following the action potential. Note their extraordinarily large amplitudes (> 1 mV) and short durations (ca. 0.5 msec). In the records obtained from this axon, only about 8% of these small pulses failed to trigger a spike, and those usually occurred during the axon's short refractory period (5–6 msec). Larger pulses, about double in size, also occurred during the neuron's refractory periods, as in traces *C* and *D*, the latter of which resulted in the generation of a second, stunted action potential (open arrowhead).

The similar shapes and indivisible amplitudes of the small subthreshold pulses suggest that they were uniquantal EPSPs (i.e., produced by the reception of a *single* quantum of neurotransmitter). When this suggestion is coupled with the fact that the size of each small pulse is approximately the

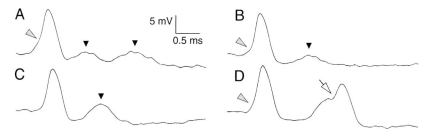

Figure 11.4. Excitatory postsynaptic potentials (EPSPs) recorded from a presumed type I afferent terminal in the guinea pig cochlea. Synaptic potentials usually triggered action potentials, but during refractory periods subthreshold potentials were recorded. Inflections indicating initiation of action potentials are shown with shaded arrowheads (*A, B, D*). Some of the ineffective EPSPs (filled arrowheads) had the same irreducible size, suggesting that a single quantum of neurotransmitter had been released from the sensory cell in those cases. An action potential triggered late on the rising phase of an EPSP is shown in *D* (open arrowhead). (From Siegel, 1992, with permission.*)

same as those that initiated action potentials (Fig. 11.4, tilted grey arrowheads), the natural conclusion emerges that action potentials are produced in these neurons by a small number of neurotransmitter quanta, perhaps only one. A similar possibility exists for some of the afferent neurons of the lateral-line organ of the African clawed toad (Sewell, 1990). Such an arrangement results in a great economy of transmitter production for the continuously emitting hair cells, as well as providing a hair trigger connection between them and each synapsing neuron.

Intracellular evidence from hair cells is also consistent with the classical picture of calcium-triggered neurotransmitter release ("exocytosis"). In hair cells of the frog sacculus, for instance, depolarization caused increases in membrane capacitance[1] that were dependent on calcium ion concentration (Parsons et al., 1994). Moreover, the Ca^{2+} channels embedded in the plasma membranes of such cells were found to be concentrated in the appropriate places, a few "hot spots" thought to coincide with the active synaptic sites (see Chapter 7).

Identification of the neurotransmitter released by inner hair cells has been extraordinarily difficult, owing at least in part to the small size and complicated geometry of the cochlea and to the relatively small total number of hair cell synapses present in any one cochlea. Nevertheless, much evidence has been accumulated suggesting that some molecule closely related to glutamate is the neurotransmitter (for reviews see Eybalin, 1993; Sewell, 1996). Glutamate itself seems unlikely because although excitatory to afferent neurons it must be applied to the cochlea in relatively high concentrations (millimolar) to cause measurable neural responses (Gleich et al., 1990).

In any case, it appears that glutamate *receptors* are involved in afferent transmission (Chmori, 1995). Such receptors are known to exist in the cochlea, and they are presumed to be the agents which mediate the neural excitation caused by applications of known glutamate receptor agonists (excitors), some in micromolar concentrations. Moreover, drugs known to block glutamate receptors partially block transmission at the afferent synapse. Thus it appears that transmission at the cochlea's principal afferent synapses involves, if not glutamate, then a glutamate agonist. A new transmitter candidate, apparently filling the latter role, has just surfaced (Sewell and Evans, 1997). Although its characterization is still incomplete, it appears to contain hydroxyphenyl glycine, which has a molecular structure resembling known glutamate agonists.

Outer Hair Cells

Different from the synaptic connections of the inner hair cells are those of outer hair cells (Fig. 11.5). The latter make few synaptic connections with afferent neurons, and those that do exist do not always display synaptic bars. On the other hand, synapses with vesicle-filled efferent terminations are plentiful. On the hair cell side of these efferent synapses are clear subsurface cisternae, perhaps for the purpose of sequestering Ca^{2+} ions involved in the cell's postsynaptic processes (see Chapter 15). Puzzling is the discovery of *reciprocal synapses* (side by side presynaptic and postsynaptic membrane specializations) in human outer hair cells but not in those of the guinea pig or normal cat (Nadol, 1988a).

NEURAL ACTIVITY IN THE ABSENCE OF DELIBERATE ACOUSTIC STIMULATION

Characteristics of Spontaneous Discharges in Type I Neurons

Microelectrode recordings of neuronal action potentials (often called "spikes") can be made from the cell bodies and axons of afferent neurons in the auditory nerve, either within the modiolus itself or along the auditory nerve as it spans the short gap between the cochlea and the brain stem. All of the reconstructions of spike-discharging spiral ganglion neurons whose axons were traced with HRP staining have proved to be of type I (Liberman, 1982a; Liberman and Oliver, 1984). Only once has a recording from a labeled type II neuron been reported (Robertson, 1984). Unfortunately, no spike activity could be recorded in that case, and so the response properties of these thin, unmyelinated neurons remain a mystery. By inference, it appears that *all* successful recordings of primary neuron spike activity have been made from type I neurons.

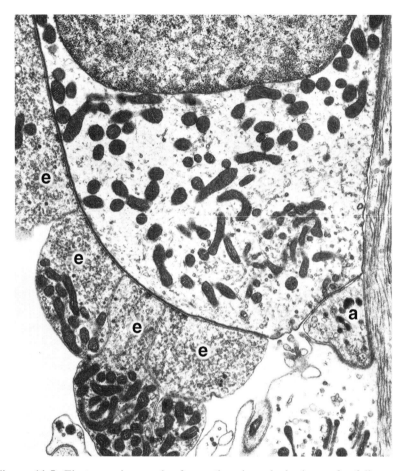

Figure 11.5. Electron micrograph of a section through the base of a feline outer hair cell, showing one afferent nerve terminal (a) and many efferent nerve terminals (e), which collectively had a large contact area with the hair cell. A slice of the hair cell's nucleus is seen at the top of the micrograph. (From Spoendlin, 1985, with permission.*)

Characteristic of almost all of the recordings from these primary afferent neurons is the presence of *spontaneous* discharge activity (i.e., spikes occurring in the absence of deliberate sound stimulation). Samples of this activity recorded from one typical axon are shown in Figure 11.6A. Note the unpredictability of the spike occurrences: Sometimes a spike is quickly followed by another, sometimes not. In fact, it has been found that occurrences of a primary neuron's spontaneous discharges are almost totally random, regardless of its average discharge rate (Kiang et al., 1965).

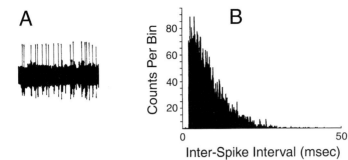

Figure 11.6. *A*. Sample of spontaneously occurring action potentials ("spikes") recorded from a single afferent neuron in guinea pig cochlea. Note the irregular timing of the spikes. *B*. An interspike interval histogram of the spontaneous activity of a sensitive afferent neuron. The distribution is nearly exponential, except for the lack of very short intervals (see Fig. 11.7). (From Robertson and Manley, 1974, with permission.*)

One traditional plot used to study such temporal characteristics is the *interspike interval histogram*, each bin of which contains the number of "interspike intervals" (i.e., the intervals between successive spikes) whose values fell within that bin's boundaries during the allotted counting period. One such histogram is seen in Figure 11.6B. If we assume that the processes generating the intervals are statistically "stationary" and that each interval is statistically independent of its predecessors,[2] the histogram can be interpreted as giving estimates of interval probabilities. For example, if 100 interspike intervals, among 5000 recorded intervals, had durations of between 20.0–21.0 msec, the probability of the next (or any) interval having a duration of 20.*x* msec is estimated at 100/5000 or 0.02, *regardless* of the discharge history.

The shape of the histogram in Figure 11.6B is remarkable. After a silent period of about 1 msec (i.e., no intervals < 1 msec), the histogram rises steeply to peak at about 5 msec and falls thereafter in a nearly exponential curve. Interpreted as a probability density function, the histogram can be thought of as indicating that the probability of any one interspike interval occurring after the next spike decreases exponentially with increasing length of that interval. That type of probability curve is characteristic of a "Poisson process."

Such a process can be illustrated with the simple model of the afferent neuron's spike-generation process shown in Figure 11.7. The neuron's transmembrane potential $V(t)$ is assumed to consist of a resting potential of -61 mV plus the EPSPs produced by the neurotransmitter released from the inner hair cell being innervated. Let us further assume that the neurotransmitter

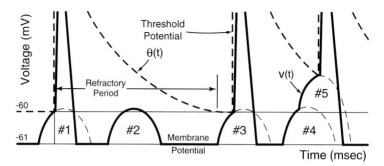

Figure 11.7. Theoretical explanation for the data in Figure 11.4, assuming that a uniquantal EPSP is large enough to reliably trigger a spike (e.g., EPSPs #1 and #3) except during refractory periods (e.g., EPSP #2). Spikes can be generated during refractory periods if several EPSPs occur nearly simultaneously (e.g., EPSPs #4 and #5). The hair cell's threshold for spike initiation, $\theta(t)$, is shown with a dashed line, and the cell's transmembrane potential, $V(t)$, is shown with a thick solid line.

occurs in quantal amounts released at totally random moments, and that the EPSP produced by each quantum is 1.2 mV in magnitude. Whenever $V(t)$ exceeds the threshold potential of the neuron $\theta(t)$, a spike occurs. At the moment of spike occurrence, the cell's threshold is assumed to jump to infinity during the absolute refractory period (< 1 ms) and then to asymptote to -60 mV during a brief relative refractory period (< 5 msec long).

Now follow the cell's behavior after the occurrence of a uniquantal EPSP (Fig. 11.7, #1) and the spike discharge it elicited. As can be seen, the spike's relative refractory period ends without the occurrence of another spike. The difference between the cell's resting potential (-61 mV) and its recovered threshold (-60 mV) is then 1 mV. Thus, the 1.2 mV EPSP produced by a single vesicle, when added to the resting potential, enables the membrane potential to cross threshold and generate the next spike. When will that next EPSP (Fig. 11.7, #3) occur?

It is a bit like flipping a coin. It is clear that on any one coin toss the probability of getting "heads" is 0.5. What is the probability of getting "heads" only after trying n times unsuccessfully to get it (i.e., after first flipping n "tails" in a row)? It can be shown that this particular probability drops approximately exponentially with the value of n; that is, the probability of flipping ten "tails" in a row (with an honest coin) is very low, less than 0.001.

The model works in the same way. The probability (p) that the model neuron will receive a randomly released vesicle is identically the same for all 1 msec time segments (though p is much lower than 0.5), so the chances that the next EPSP will occur only after many successive milliseconds of no transmission (i.e., after a long silent interval) becomes progressively smaller as the length of the interval grows longer. This type of model generates interval histograms that decay exponentially with interval length (Geisler and Goldberg, 1966). Somewhat surprisingly, this type of random vesicle release is well suited for the faithful transduction of acoustic signals (see Chapter 13).

During the model's relative refractory period, the difference between the cell's membrane and threshold potentials is greater than 1 mV (e.g., 2 mV) at a particular instant. Thus the appearance of a single uniquantal EPSP (Fig. 11.7, #2) at that moment is fruitless. To generate a spike under refractory conditions would require the near-simultaneous occurrence of at least two uniquantal EPSPs (Fig. 11.7, #4 and #5), a much less likely event than the occurrence of only one. Thus a reduced number of very short intervals should occur, as is indeed always the case in the experimental data (e.g., Fig. 11.6).

Source of Spontaneous Activity

It still might seem possible that the afferent neurons are spontaneously active themselves, generating spikes intrinsically in the absence of transmitter release by the inner hair cell. There is a great deal of convincing evidence against this supposition (recounted for acousticolateralis organs in general by Guth et al., 1991). Some of the relevant data involve manipulations of inner ear solutions in a manner that primarily affects classical neurotransmitter release. For instance, the substitution of cochlear perilymph with a solution high in Mg^{2+} and low in Ca^{2+} causes the afferent neurons to fall silent (Siegel and Relkin, 1987).

Most important from the standpoint of signal transmission, a systematic relation was found to occur between the spontaneous activity of these primary auditory neurons and scala media's endocochlear potential, as modified by injections of furosemide (Sewell, 1984a). This diuretic drug rapidly reduces the endocochlear potential and hence the resting potential of the inner hair cells (see Fig. 8.2) but is not known to affect afferent innervation directly. The relation found in that study not only strengthens the case for transmitter-initiated spontaneous activity but indicates that changes in the transmembrane potentials of the inner hair cells modify the probabilities of that transmitter release, a process essential to the faithful transmission of information through the inner hair cells (see Chapter 12).

Distribution of Spontaneous Discharge Rates

For any particular primary auditory neuron, the average rate of its spontaneously occurring spike discharges (referred to simply as its ''spontaneous rate'') is usually nearly constant, at least over normal recording times, which can extend for more than an hour. When a histogram of the spontaneous rates of a large number of spiral ganglion neurons is compiled, a clear bimodal distribution occurs (Fig. 11.8). Most of the neurons (about 60% in cats never exposed to loud sounds) fall within the upper mode, displaying spontaneous rates from 18/sec to more than 100/sec (Liberman, 1978). These neurons have been labeled ''high spontaneous.''

The remainder of the neurons, with spontaneous rates ranging from 18/sec down to virtually zero, fall within the lower mode. These neurons are sometimes lumped together into one class, but because of their differing response characteristics (see Chapter 12) most workers further subdivide them. Those neurons with the lowest rates (< 0.5/sec) are called ''low spontaneous.'' They make up about 15% of the total in undamaged ears. The remaining 25% of the primary neurons, the ''medium spontaneous,'' have intermediate spontaneous rates (0.5–18.0/sec).

It has been shown in the cat that about 60% of an inner hair cell's afferent synapses are with relatively large terminal axons (diameters averaging about 1 µm) that contain relatively large numbers of mitochondria (Liberman, 1980b). Most of these synapses occur on the pillar cell sides of the inner hair cells (far sides in Fig. 11.2). The remaining 40% of the afferent axons

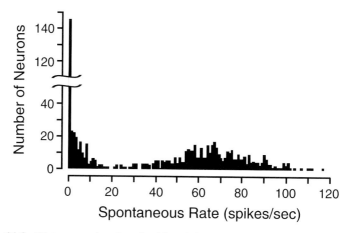

Figure 11.8. Histogram showing the bimodal distribution of spontaneous rates recorded from many type I afferent neurons of cats raised in quiet conditions. Neurons with spontaneous rates higher than 18/sec have homogeneous physiological attributes and so are lumped into one category (''high spontaneous''). The group with lower spontaneous rates is often subdivided into two categories, those with ''low'' (< 0.5/sec) and those with ''medium'' (0.5–18/sec) spontaneous rates. (From Liberman, 1978, with permission.*)

have smaller diameters and contain smaller numbers of mitochondria. These axons form synapses almost exclusively on the modiolar sides of the inner hair cells (near sides in Fig. 11.2). Three-fourths of these smaller axons (30% of the total) form synapses that are similar in appearance to those on the pillar cell sides of the inner hair cells, and the remainder (10% of the total) form "complex" synapses. It appears that the latter synapses are the ones that sometimes contain more than one synaptic bar (Merchan-Perez and Liberman, 1996).

Note that these percentages of different axon sizes are similar to those of the different classes of spontaneous activity. A decisive experiment by Liberman and Oliver (1984) showed that this similarity is no coincidence; the two phenomena are in fact intimately connected. In this experiment, individual auditory nerve axons were injected with HRP (Fig. 11.1) and their separate trajectories traced within the organ of Corti. It was found that whereas most (11/13) of the high-spontaneous neurons formed synapses on the pillar sides of the bases of inner hair cells, all of the medium-spontaneous neurons (3/3) and almost all of the low-spontaneous neurons (10/11) formed synapses on the modiolar sides of those hair cells.

When combined with Liberman's earlier neuron-labeling work (1982a), these findings led to the conclusion that all the primary auditory neurons that display low or medium spontaneous rates (e.g., < 18 spikes/sec) have rather thin terminal axons. Moreover, because all inner hair cells appear to synapse with both thick and thin axon terminations, it follows that there is probably no such thing as a "high-spontaneous" inner hair cell; apparently *each* inner hair cell forms synaptic connections with afferent neurons of all spontaneous-rate classes.

It has been suggested that the bimodal grouping of spontaneous discharge rates is due, at least in part, to the relative sizes of the respective EPSPs (Geisler, 1981). If the spike threshold is so low it can be crossed with one of the uniquantal EPSPs, each quantum received by the neuron would elicit a spike, except during refractory periods (as in Figs. 11.4 and 11.7). Such neurons would have high spontaneous rates. On the other hand, if the voltage needed to reach spike threshold were greater than the amplitude of a uniquantal EPSP, it would take the nearly simultaneous reception of two or more quanta to produce an EPSP large enough to cross threshold. These neurons would, for the same rate of quantal release, show much lower rates of spontaneous activity.

The positive correlation between spontaneous activity and axon diameter makes good physiological sense because the axons with the highest firing rates would probably undergo the greatest exchange of Na^+ and K^+ ions due to action-potential propagation. As the energy needed to maintain proper cation concentrations comes from the action of mitochondria, we would expect those axons with the greatest rates of ion exchange to have the most mitochondria and the increased volumes necessary to house them.

Speaking of energy requirements, it might be wondered what the operational justification is for the considerable amount of energy spent to maintain continuous discharges in the afferent neurons even in the absence of acoustic stimulation. As noted in Chapter 12, this spontaneous activity plays much the same role for the neural spike traffic on the auditory nerve as the ''silent current'' plays for the hair cells (see Chapter 8). It provides a steady stream of output that can be modulated both up and down, allowing the neural signals to follow both the positive *and* negative phases of AC driving signals generated by the inner hair cells in response to acoustic stimuli.

NOTES

1. The exocytosis and endocytosis encountered in a cell bearing synaptic release sites is accompanied by changes in the cell's membrane capacitance (Matthew, 1996). These changes in electrical capacitance are believed to be the result of temporary increases in the area of the cell's plasma membrane (recall that capacitance is proportional to area). As presently envisioned, when a vesicle carrying neurotransmitter docks and fuses with the cell's plasma membrane, the combined plasma–vesicle wall is punctured, allowing the vesicle's contents to diffuse into the synaptic cleft (''exocytosis''). During this process the area of the cell is increased in the same way that a new harbor or bay increases the length of a coastline. When the vesicle is absorbed back into the cell (''endocytosis''), the cell's surface membrane returns to its initial area.

2. Strictly speaking, the processes generating the spontaneous discharges of mammalian primary auditory neurons do not appear to be statistically stationary processes, as long-term fluctuations characteristic of fractal processes occur in the spontaneous spike trains (Lowen and Teich, 1992). Small but significant correlations also occur between shorter intervals. Nevertheless, for virtually all practical purposes, the generators of spontaneous activity can be treated as stationary processes, producing spikes at random moments that are not correlated with each other.

12

RESPONSES OF PRIMARY AUDITORY
NEURONS TO SINGLE TONES

After following the auditory signal through many intermediate stages, we come to its final form: The signals that are sent into the central nervous system by the spiral ganglion neurons in response to acoustic stimuli. These responses are truly remarkable. They are nonlinear, as would be predictable from the strongly nonlinear aspects of basilar membrane vibrations (see Chapter 10), yet many of their properties can be accurately predicted by linear analysis. They occur at relatively low discharge rates (usually <200/ sec) but are able to track the wave shapes of signals having kiloHertz frequencies. With action potentials lasting half a millisecond, they permit behavioral discriminations to be made in the submicrosecond range. Perhaps the best summary of the cochlea's overall behavior is that it divides the signal into many (overlapping) *frequency* bands and then simultaneously encodes the output of those bands using automatic gain control, all the while preserving the *temporal* aspects of the signal accurately.

In this chapter and those immediately following, we examine the responses of primary auditory neurons to a number of acoustic stimuli, in the order of their increasing complexity (and interest). We start in this chapter with pure tones. Exploring some of the mechanisms involved in those tonal responses provides the background for the following consideration of the discharge patterns evoked by more complex stimuli, such as noise, simultaneously presented tones, and tones that change in amplitude and frequency. Finally, in Chapter 14, the responses to speech are studied.

GENERAL PATTERN OF RESPONSES

Single tones provide a natural starting place, as they seem to possess a fundamental waveform. Not only do tones sound "pure" and unitary to us, but Fourier analysis of more complex acoustic signals provides a useful framework within which to analyze responses to a wide range of stimuli.

The responses of one primary neuron to a tone presented at two levels is shown in Figure 12.1. Shown in the form of a "poststimulus time histogram,"[1] each response goes through four basic stages (Kiang et al., 1965). First, there is an "onset" response, where the probability of discharge increases sharply for the first few milliseconds of the tone. Immediately afterward "adaptation" begins and the discharge rate gradually subsides to a new steady-state level. Investigations of this adaptation indicate that several mechanisms are probably involved (Westerman and Smith, 1987). When the tone is turned off, there is an "offset" response, in which the discharge rate drops abruptly to levels below the rate of spontaneous activity (even to zero in Fig. 12.1B). Gradual "recovery" then returns the neural discharge rate

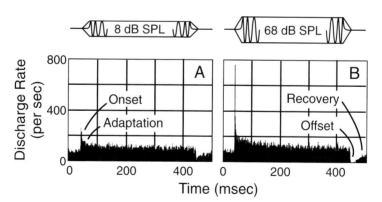

Figure 12.1. Responses of a "high-spontaneous" primary afferent neuron in the gerbil to a tone of 6.9 kHz presented at two intensities. *A.* Poststimulus time histogram, showing the response to the tone at 8 dB SPL. At tonal onset (top), there was a sudden increase in discharge rate ("onset" response) followed by a gradual decrease ("adaptation") to a new steady-state level. When the tone was terminated (at 450 msec), there was an abrupt drop in discharge rate ("offset" response), followed by "recovery" back up to the spontaneous rate. *B.* Response to the tone at 68 dB SPL. Each of the four response phases seen in *A* is emphasized, particularly the onset and offset responses. (From Westerman and Smith, 1987, with permission.*)

to its rest condition. Note that the neuron in Figure 12.1 had a spontaneous spike rate of about 60/sec, placing it squarely within the high-spontaneous class.

Despite the increase of 60 dB (1000-fold) in the sound pressure used to obtain the response in Figure 12.1B, there was only a tripling of the onset response, and the steady-state response increased by less than a factor of 2. Clearly, strong compression was at work.

The basic pattern of Figure 12.1 can be readily accounted for with "reservoir" models of hair cell neurotransmitter release. In the simplest version (Fig. 12.2) a single reservoir stores the neurotransmitter available for release at each synapse (Schroeder and Hall, 1974; Oono and Sujaku, 1975). The amount of transmitter present in the reservoir at any one time, $q(t)$, can go up or down. The release of this transmitter from the reservoir is governed by the inner hair cell's receptor potential.

That voltage is not the only factor involved, as the contents of the reservoir are also important. If the reservoir were empty, for example, no amount of hair cell depolarization would cause transmitter release. Thus transmitter release must depend on both the command to release issued by $v(t)$ (the hair cell's membrane potential) and the amount available to *be* released. In one of our models, the rate of transmitter release is related to a product of these contributing factors, $v(t) * q(t) * q(t)$ (Geisler and Greenberg, 1986). The ensuring postsynaptic discharge probability, $p(t)$, is assumed equal to this transmitter release rate, modified by brief refractory properties (see Chapter 11). A constant influx of transmitter into the reservoir and a leakage spigot ("vent") complete the model.

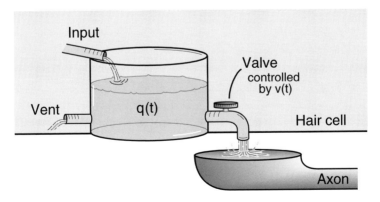

Figure 12.2. Simple reservoir model of neurotransmitter release at an inner hair cell's afferent synapse. Transmitter flows into the reservoir at a steady rate, stored for release to the afferent neuron by the joint action of reservoir contents $q(t)$ and the hair cell's membrane potential $v(t)$. A vent prevents excessive build-up of transmitter.

The output of the model to a tone pip of 1.0 kHz is shown in Figure 12.3A. The four major stages identified in the responses of neurons are all present here: onset, adaptation, offset, and recovery. The courses of the internal variables are instructive when accounting for the model's mimicry. Although the command voltage (resting plus receptor potentials) was fixed at a high level (Fig. 12.3B), the reservoir contents dropped steadily until a new steady-state level was reached (Fig. 12.3C). After cessation of the tone,

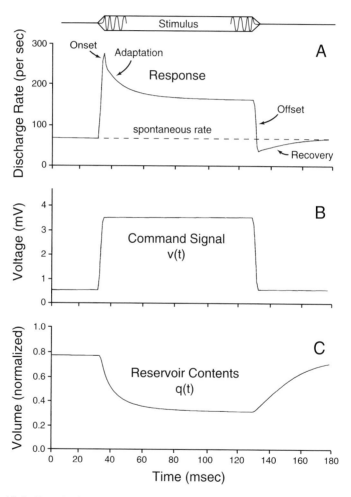

Figure 12.3. Functioning of a reservoir model when stimulated by a tone. *A.* Response of the model (i.e., amount of neurotransmitter released). Note that it has all four phases seen in the experimental data of Figure 12.1. *B.* Hair cell's membrane potential $v(t)$, the command signal for transmitter release. *C.* Contents of the reservoir, showing gradual emptying during stimulation and refilling during silence. (From a modified Geisler–Greenberg model, 1986.)

the receptor potential dropped to zero, and the reservoir slowly refilled. More complex synaptic models have been developed that involve numbers of interconnected reservoirs, but the output wave shapes do not differ fundamentally. Due to our basic ignorance about transmitter release by inner hair cells, it is difficult to know which of these models is the most realistic (for comparisons see Hewitt and Meddis, 1991; Ross, 1996).

To add to the complexity, there is increasing pharmacological evidence that the spontaneous release of neurotransmitter by inner hair cells differs somewhat in nature from their acoustically driven releases. For example, cochlear perfusions of glutamate cause reductions in the "driven" discharge activity of primary neurons but not in their spontaneous firing rates (Gleich et al., 1990), whereas applications of acetylcholine increase their spontaneous activity without affecting the driven rates (Guth et al., 1991). A different utilization of Ca^{2+} ions for vesicle release under these two conditions has been suggested as a cause for these differential effects (Guth et al., 1991).

Primary auditory neurons with low spontaneous discharge rates respond to tones much as do high-spontaneous neurons but with considerably slower recovery processes. Tone "pips" of 25 msec duration, for example, produced responses in these low-spontaneous neurons that are similar in shape to those of Figure 12.1 when 225 msec intervals of silence separated the pips. However, when there were only 75 msec rests between pips, the onset responses practically vanished (Rhode and Smith, 1985). Moreover, quantitative measurement of the recoveries from prior stimulation ("forward masking") showed that whereas high-spontaneous neurons were back to normal after about 200 msec of silence neurons with lower spontaneous discharge rates took nearly ten times that long to recover fully (Relkin and Doucet, 1991). The reservoir model of Figure 12.2 can be made to mimic such sluggish behavior by reducing its rate of transmitter inflow.

PROPERTIES OF DISCHARGE RATE RESPONSES

Dynamic Range

As can be deduced from Figure 12.3, reservoir models also have automatic gain control properties. If the command voltage of Figure 12.3B were to increase in amplitude, transmitter would initially be released at a faster rate, eventually reducing the steady-state amount of transmitter in the reservoir to a still lower level. Then, because it is a product of the command voltage and the reservoir contents that determines response probability, an increase in stimulus amplitude of, for example, twofold would produce less than a doubling of response probabilities. This compressive effect is seen in the responses of the model to the 1.0 kHz tone, presented at three strengths over a range of 20 dB (Fig. 12.4A). As stimulus strength went up, so did the steady-state response rates, but only by a factor of about 2.

The magnitudes of the model's steady-state responses, plotted as a function of stimulus strength (Fig. 12.4B), emphasize that point. In the midrange of the curve, a tenfold increase in signal strength (20 dB) barely doubled the response rate. The behavior of this curve at its extremes is also important. At low sound pressures there was virtually no response: The amount of transmitter released by the stimulus at those levels was negligible compared to that already being tonically released to maintain the spontaneous discharges (ca. 67/sec in this case). Although there is no sound pressure below which it can be stated that there was absolutely *no* increase in response probabilities, for practical purposes a "threshold" pressure can be identified. In this case, threshold would be somewhere between 0 and 10 dB SPL, depending on the criterion used.

At the other end of the sound–pressure scale, the model's response rate "saturates." This extreme form of compression is due to the fixed rate with which neurotransmitter enters the model's reservoir. No matter how high the stimulus amplitude, the steady-state rate of transmitter release cannot exceed this influx rate. The difference between the threshold and saturation pressures, the "dynamic range" of the neuron, is 30–35 dB for this model.

The responses of living spiral ganglion neurons to pure tones behave in a similar manner. The magnitudes of the steady-state responses to a wide spectrum of pure tones recorded from a primary neuron in the squirrel monkey auditory nerve are shown in Figure 12.5A. At the lowest level (30 dB

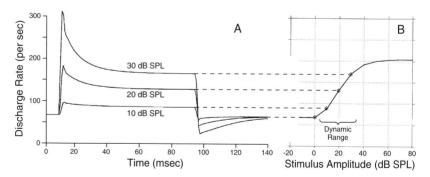

Figure 12.4. *A.* Responses of the reservoir model to a tone of 1.0 kHz presented at three levels. *B.* Steady-state discharge rate of the afferent neuron elicited by the tone over a wide range of sound levels. A "threshold" of responsiveness occurred at about 5 dB SPL; and the response saturated at sound levels greater than 50 dB SPL, giving a practical dynamic range of about 35 dB. (From a modified Geisler–Greenberg model, 1986.)

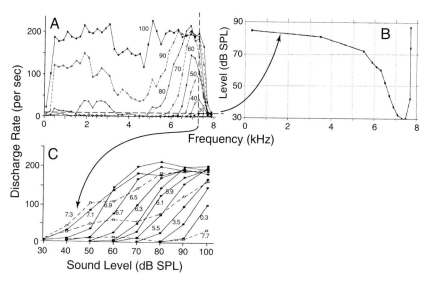

Figure 12.5. *A.* Steady-state spike rates of a primary auditory neuron in the squirrel monkey responding to tones of various frequencies and intensities. All responses obtained with a particular sound level (dB SPL) are connected by a labeled line. *B.* Threshold-level frequency tuning curve for the neuron, derived from the data in *A* (along the horizontal dashed line). *C.* Level-response functions obtained from the data in *A* at various frequencies (e.g., along the vertical dashed line at 7.3 kHz). Data obtained with frequencies above 7.1 kHz are shown with dashed lines. Compare to Figure 5.8. (From Geisler et al., 1974, with permission.*)

SPL), only tones in the immediate vicinity of 7.3 kHz excited the neuron. As stimulus strength was raised in 10 dB steps, the response rates evoked by 7.3 kHz tones increased, and the range of frequencies that excited at least some neural response also increased. For 70 dB excitation, the discharge rate produced by a 7.3 kHz tone saturated at about 200 spikes/sec. With still higher sound pressures, the frequency ranges of both responsiveness and saturation spread widely until with 100 dB stimulation the neuron was responding at its maximum rate to almost every tone with a frequency between 500 Hz and 7.5 kHz.

This pattern of responsiveness is a direct reflection of basilar membrane vibrations at the cochlear location tuned to 7.3 kHz. With 30 dB excitation, only tones whose frequencies fell in the immediate vicinity of 7.3 kHz were able to generate inner hair cell receptor potentials capable of releasing detectable amounts of transmitter (see Fig. 9.6B). With successively increased levels of stimulation, virtually all tones with frequencies lower than 7.3 kHz eventually crossed this "threshold" level. By contrast, only a restricted set of higher frequency tones became excitatory, regardless of stimulus level.

This abrupt frequency cutoff in responsiveness is seen in all neurons tuned to high frequencies. It is caused by the sharp attenuation of a tone's traveling wave once it has passed its resonance point in the basal region of the cochlea (see Fig. 9.6A).

The response rates of this neuron at several frequencies are plotted as functions of stimulus pressure in Figure 12.5C. Note the similarity in shape of all of the curves obtained with frequencies below 7.3 kHz (solid lines). This similarity reflects the same responsiveness (basically linear) of the basilar membrane at the 7.3 kHz location to tones of lower frequency (see Fig. 5.8C). For higher frequencies the slopes of the response curves become much less. These flattened response patterns are also faithful reflectors of basilar membrane vibrations, which themselves undergo strong compression at frequencies above the characteristic frequency of the measurement spot.

The neuron of Figure 12.5 had a moderately low spontaneous discharge rate, placing it within the "medium-spontaneous" category. This point is significant, as primary neurons of the different spontaneous-rate classes have different dynamic ranges. These differences can be seen clearly in Figure 12.6A, which contains sample rate-versus-pressure curves for two of those

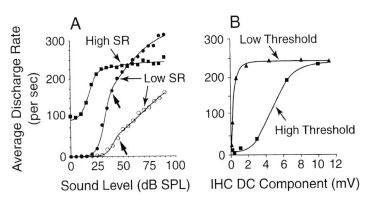

Figure 12.6. *A.* Rate-level functions for three primary afferent neurons in the guinea pig to tones of characteristic frequency. The single neuron with a high spontaneous rate (SR) coupled a low threshold with a small dynamic range (ca. 15 dB). The two low-spontaneous neurons had higher thresholds, but their response rates did not saturate, although each curve showed a slope reduction in the neighborhood of 40 dB SPL (arrows), apparently due to the onset of basilar membrane compression (see Müller and Robertson, 1991). The solid lines are fits from a quadratic equation relating rate and inferred basilar membrane displacement. *B.* Response rate versus inferred inner hair cell DC receptor potential for two basally located primary auditory neurons to tones of 525 Hz presented at various levels. The threshold to this tone was about 50 dB SPL for the "low-threshold" neuron, about 80 dB SPL for the "high-threshold" neuron. (*A:* From Müller et al., 1991, with permission.* *B:* from Zagaeski et al., 1994, with permission.*)

classes. The single high-spontaneous neuron had a threshold of about 10 dB SPL and rate saturation at all sound pressures above 25 dB SPL, making up a dynamic range of less than 20 dB. By contrast, the two low-spontaneous curves, with somewhat higher thresholds, had enormous dynamic ranges: 70 dB and climbing. As in everything else, medium-spontaneous neurons are intermediate, with dynamic ranges generally about 30 dB (Fig. 12.5).

These differences in dynamic range are important, as they highlight yet another compressive process of the auditory periphery: discharge rate saturation. The fact that the response rates of the low-spontaneous neurons kept climbing, even at stimulus strengths of 90 dB SPL, indicates that the average receptor voltages of the inner hair cells were still increasing in size at that sound pressure. Yet the high-spontaneous neuron in Figure 12.6A reached a saturation rate at about 25 dB SPL. This rather extreme compression at such low sound pressures raises the interesting signal-processing question as to how stimulus magnitudes are decoded more centrally. As might be expected from Figure 12.6A, theoretical analysis has suggested that low-spontaneous neurons (despite their relatively small numbers) play a dominant role in signaling amplitudes at high sound pressures (Delgutte, 1987; Winslow and Sachs, 1988).

Relations Between Discharge Rate and Other Cochlear Processes

The data in Figures 12.5C and 12.6A indicate that there is a generally monotonic relation between sound pressure and afferent neuron discharge rate, although an apical neuron sometimes exhibits a sharp "dip" in spike rate[2] for one particular sound level in the range between 90 and 100 dB SPL (Kiang et al., 1986). This general monotonic trend is entirely consistent with the monotonic relation observed between stimulus strength and the amplitude of EPSPs recorded intracellularly from the large primary neurons of the goldfish sacculus (Furukawa and Matsurra, 1978).

As reviewed in previous chapters, monotonic relations also exist between acoustic pressure, basilar membrane displacement, ciliary displacement, and hair cell receptor potential. It follows that there must also be a monotonic relation between inner hair cell receptor potential and afferent neuron discharge rate. Figure 12.6B shows examples of this relation, inferred from a series of non-simultaneous recordings, for two primary neurons, one with low threshold and the other with high threshold (Zagaeski et al., 1994). According to an extension of the model given in Figure 11.7, such striking differences in sensitivity can be accounted for simply because it takes more quanta to generate a particular discharge rate if a uniquantal EPSP is subthreshold (assumed for low-spontaneous neurons) than if it is suprathreshold (assumed for high-spontanous neurons) (Geisler, in press).

It also follows that there must be a monotonic relation between basilar membrane displacement and afferent neuron discharge. In fact, the latter relation has been exploited to cast light on basilar membrane displacements throughout the cochlea, most of which is inaccessible for direct mechanical measurement (Cooper and Yates, 1994). Working backward from the neural-rate versus sound–pressure curves, the degrees of basilar membrane compression affecting vibrations at the characteristic frequencies of the respective primary neurons were estimated. In agreement with existing basilar membrane measurements (see Fig. 5.8), the deduced basilar membrane compression for basal locations was large. Moreover, the analysis suggested that the breaks in the slopes of the low-spontaneous curves that occur in Figure 12.6A (arrows) reflect the onset of compression in basilar membrane responsiveness, although this compression onset has sometimes been measured at still lower pressures (see Fig. 5.8C).

By contrast, the degree of basilar membrane compression estimated to occur in the apical region was small, almost nonexistent. This conclusion is in agreement with direct vibration measurements made in that region (see Fig. 5.9), which showed only a small amount of amplification (and hence of compression). The region with characteristic frequencies between 1.5 and 3.6 kHz formed a transition zone between large and small amounts of estimated basilar membrane compression.

Frequency Tuning Curves

Returning to Figure 12.5, a frequency tuning curve for the neuron can be derived from its response curves (Fig. 12.5B) by connecting the threshold points for many frequencies (e.g., along the horizontal dashed line in Fig. 12.5A). As the resulting threshold-level tuning curve is most sensitive at 7.3 kHz, that frequency is labeled its characteristic frequency. Frequency selectivity in this ''tip'' region is sharp, particularly above the characteristic frequency: The slope on the high-frequency side is so steep as to be practically unmeasurable. By contrast, for frequencies more than half an octave below characteristic frequency, selectivity vanishes. This tuning curve ''tail'' reflects the fact that all low-frequency traveling waves must pass through this neuron's location on the way to their apical resonance locations (see Fig. 10.4). Even though just transitting the basal region, at high enough levels (> 80 dB SPL) those tones produced basilar membrane deflections there that were large enough to excite the afferent neurons.

The tip-and-tail type of tuning curve shown in Figure 12.5B is found in all (normal) neurons tuned to high frequencies, but neurons innervating the apical section of the cochlea behave differently. As examples of the diversity encountered, the tuning curves of four primary neurons, all obtained from the same cat, are shown in the top row of Figure 12.7 (plotted, as is customary, on logarithmic frequency axes). The two curves with the lowest characteristic frequencies (Fig. 12.7A,B) do not even have a tail. Note, moreover, that the most apical of these neurons had a nearly symmetrical tuning curve (Fig. 12.7A). The dividing zone between those neurons that display a tuning curve tail and those that do not is the 1.5- to 2.0-kHz region (located in the transition zone between the basal and apical types of cochlear partition responses).

The distribution of the thresholds at respective characteristic frequencies

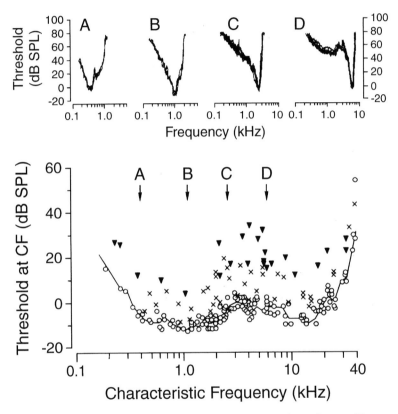

Figure 12.7. *Top.* Frequency selectivity of four representative primary afferent neurons in one cat, as shown by their (threshold level) frequency tuning curves. The neuron tuned to the highest frequency (D) showed the familiar ''tip'' and ''tail'' shape, whereas the neurons tuned to low frequencies (left panels) showed only a ''tip'' portion. *Bottom.* Thresholds of many of this cat's primary neurons at their respective characteristic frequencies (i.e., the lowest point on each frequency tuning curve), plotted as a function of those characteristic frequencies: high-spontaneous neurons (circles), medium-spontaneous neurons (X), and low spontaneous neurons (triangles). The solid line represents the average thresholds of the high-spontaneous neurons of this animal (raised in a low-noise environment). The characteristic frequencies of the four neurons (*top*) are indicated. (From Liberman and Mulroy, 1982, with permission.*)

for many primary neurons in this same cat are shown in the bottom panel of Figure 12.7. Among many remarkable features is the nearly uniform sensitivity of the ensemble of high-spontaneous neurons to tones with frequencies ranging from 500 Hz to 20 kHz—despite the frequency attenuation that occurs in the middle ear above 1 kHz (see Chapter 4). Another important feature of the data concerns the differences in the sensitivities of the various classes of primary neurons. The high-spontaneous neurons were uniformly the most sensitive. The medium-spontaneous (neurons) were 5–10 dB less sensitive, and the low-spontaneous neurons were the least sensitive.[3]

Although unobtrusive, perhaps the most stunning feature of the threshold data is the *value* of the most sensitive thresholds: near −10 dB SPL (7 μPa). These sounds are incredibly weak, producing ossicular vibrations of less than $1/1000$ the diameter of a hydrogen atom (Rhode, 1978). With all of the noise sources involved (e.g., Brownian motion of air and fluid molecules, spontaneous ciliary movements) it is difficult to determine just how this sensitivity compares to the intrinsic noise level of the system. Estimates for the first of these sources, the pressure fluctuations due to the Brownian motion of air molecules impinging on the eardrum, are about 2 μPa (−20 dB SPL), when the frequency bandwidth relevant for the detection of a 3 kHz tone is included (Harris, 1968). Calculations using this number suggest that the behavioral thresholds of humans for 3 kHz tones are not limited by this Brownian motion, but that those for the most sensitive of cats may approach it (Green, 1976).

It follows that the peripheral auditory apparatus as a whole, from external ear to afferent neurons, operates so efficiently that it is able to pick out tonal signals not much larger than the inherent acoustic static. Such sensitivity approaches that of the eye, where single photons are known to activate retinal receptors (Bialek, 1987). Finally, note that these *neural* thresholds are similar to the cat's *behavioral* thresholds (see Fig. 2.4). This close agreement in thresholds implies that the central auditory system of the cat is also highly effective: It can detect the threshold-level responses of auditory nerve neurons about as well as our present computer-based analyses.

Quantitative analysis supports the visual impression that the tuning curves for the apical neurons of Figure 12.7 are not as finely tuned as those of the basal neurons. The sharpness of tuning for a wide sample of primary neurons, as measured by the quality factor Q_{10} (see Chapter 5), is plotted versus respective characteristic frequencies in Figure 12.8. Although the data are a bit scattered, the average degree of sharpness increases markedly as the neural location approaches the stapes. (These values of sharpness should be noted, as they are important in Chapter 13.) In the apex the typical 1 kHz neuron has a relatively wide bandwidth, only half the value of its characteristic frequency ($Q_{10} = 2$), whereas a neuron tuned a decade higher, to 10 kHz, has a much narrower relative bandwidth, equal on average to about

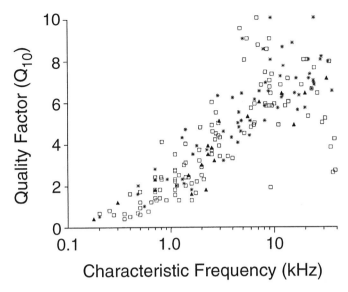

Figure 12.8. Frequency selectivities (Q_{10}) of many primary auditory neurons in the cat, plotted as a function of their respective characteristic frequencies. Note the steady increase in selectivity as the characteristic frequency is increased. Open squares, high-spontaneous neurons (SR > 16/sec); asterisks, low-spontaneous neurons (SR < 2/sec); triangles, medium-spontaneous neurons. (From Rhode and Smith, 1985, with permission.*)

one-seventh its characteristic frequency (Q_{10} = 7). The frequency tuning in certain types of bats, those whose echolocating calls contain long constant-frequency components, are more than an order of magnitude sharper than that (Suga et al., 1976).

With only rare exceptions, each primary auditory neuron innervates a single inner hair cell (see Chapter 11). Thus the characteristic frequency of one such neuron must also be that of the hair cell it innervates and presumably of the cochlear partition at that cell's location. Hence if we could locate the place along the cochlear partition where the neuron forms its synaptic connections, we would know the characteristic frequency of that particular cochlear location. Intraaxonal injections of horseradish peroxidase and subsequent tracings of the marked axons have enabled just such determinations to be made (see Fig. 11.1).

The data so obtained from many marked primary neurons have been pooled to produce a "map" of characteristic frequency versus cochlear location in several species, two of which are shown in Figure 12.9. Most prominent in the map for the cat (Liberman, 1982b) is the precise logarithmic relation that exists in the basal portion of the cochlea: To drop an octave in characteristic frequency, one must go apically 3.5 mm. This logarithmic

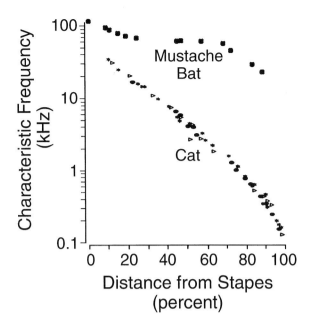

Figure 12.9. Relation between the cochlear location of an axon termination and the characteristic frequency of that neuron for many individually labeled primary auditory neurons in the cat and mustache bat. The trend for the cat is essentially logarithmic over the most basal 70% of the cochlea. For the bat, the 60- to 61-kHz region is greatly exaggerated. (Cat data: From Liberman, 1982b, with permission.* Bat data: From Kössl and Vater, 1985b.)

relation is reminiscent of the piano, where each octave occupies the same span on the keyboard (seven whole notes). However, below about 1.5 kHz (that frequency again) the curve departs from logarithmic, squeezing almost four octaves of characteristic frequencies into the most apical 7 mm. This arrangement might appear to short-change the apical neurons spatially, but their principal mode of stimulus encoding appears to be in an entirely different dimension: the synchronization of spike occurrences with the stimulus waveform (see next section).

The cat's type of logarithmic characteristic-frequency/location map is typical for mammals considered auditory ''generalists,'' those for whom sounds of any frequency composition seem equally likely and significant (Fay and Popper, 1994). However, some mammals have narrow frequency ranges of great behavioral importance, such as the 60- to 61-kHz range the mustache bat uses primarily for its sonar-guided hunting. As the cochlear map for this bat shows (Fig. 12.9, top points), the length along the cochlear partition tuned within that narrow range of frequencies is extensive, covering a full third of the cochlea (Kössl and Vater, 1985b). It follows that the central nervous systems of these animals receive massive amounts of information about returning sonar signals from the many thousands of afferent neurons that innervate this "acoustic fovea."

Several other vertebrate species also have acoustic foveae: two bat species, the barn owl, and the mole rat (Köppl and Kössl, 1997). Mole rats, which are subterranean, have cochleas specialized for acoustic signals of very low frequencies, no doubt of special importance in their tunnel domains.

TEMPORAL SYNCHRONIZATION OF DISCHARGES TO STIMULUS WAVEFORMS

Only the average discharge rates of primary neurons have been considered so far, which reflect the average (DC) components of inner hair cell receptor potentials. As these potentials also have AC components (see Fig. 8.3) and the probability of transmitter release is evidently a monotonic function of receptor potential (Fig. 12.6B), it follows that AC modulation of primary-neuron discharge rates is also expected. In fact, this AC modulation *did* occur in the output of the reservoir model (Fig. 12.3) but was hidden by the large time intervals (1 msec) used to plot the output waveforms. To study this AC modulation in physiological data, the "period histogram" is usually used, wherein a spike is binned according to the time of its occurrence within the cycle of a repetitive acoustic stimulus. That is, the timing clock is restarted at the beginning of each stimulus cycle, rather than only once at stimulus onset (as used to compile poststimulus histograms).

The period histograms obtained from one high-spontaneous primary neuron with 1 kHz tones of various strengths are shown in Figure 12.10. With no stimulus the neuron's discharges were random with respect to the stimulus' time base (Fig. 12.10I). At 14 dB SPL (Fig. 12.10G) there was clear modulation of the discharge rate in synchrony with the stimulus waveform, a process sometimes called "phase locking" or "phase synchrony" (see computer animations on our World Wide Web page). With increasing signal strength, the phase synchrony became increasingly pronounced until a level of 40 dB SPL was reached (Fig. 12.10D). Increases in stimulus strength above that level, even to 90 dB SPL (Fig. 12.10A), had little further effect on the phase synchrony.

The wave shapes of discharge probability produced at those higher sound pressures (Fig. 12.10A–C) are surprisingly faithful renditions of the stimulating sinusoidal waveform. It is true that the response probabilities can no longer follow the negative-going parts of the stimulus waveform (zero probability of spike discharge is as low as it goes), and so the bottom parts of

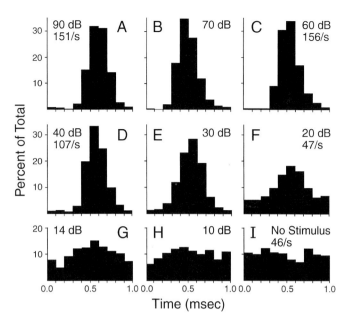

Figure 12.10. Responses (in the form of period histograms) to a tone of 1 kHz presented at various sound levels, recorded from a high-spontaneous axon in the squirrel monkey auditory nerve, with the spike rate given in selected panels. At low sound levels, discharges began to synchronize to the stimulating waveform with no noticeable change in discharge rate (F–H). At high sound levels, neither the response rate nor the fully developed synchrony varied appreciably (A–C). (From Rose et al., 1967, with permission.*)

the discharge probability waveforms become truncated ("half-wave rectified"). Even so, the accurate portrayal of at least the positive-going part of the stimulating waveform over an 80 dB range, when the neuron itself had a dynamic discharge rate range of only about 30 dB (ca. 30–60 dB SPL), is most remarkable. The distortion-limiting aspects of basilar membrane vibrations (see Chapter 10) undoubtedly played a key role in this waveform preservation.

Finally in Figure 12.10 note that appreciable phase synchrony began at a sound pressure level of about 10 dB SPL, which was at least 15 dB below the discharge rate threshold (> 25 dB SPL). This ordering of response modes is always observed with high-spontaneous neurons responding to low-frequency tones: At the lowest detectable pressures only phasic modulation of the discharge probabilities is observed (without changes in average rate), whereas at somewhat higher pressures the average rates also increase.

Reservoir models behave in exactly the same way. At low sound pressure the pattern of discharge probabilities faithfully follows the stimulus waveform throughout its complete cycle. It occurs because the model's inner hair cell is *de*polarized at some moments, which increases the probability of transmitter release, and *hyper*polarized at other moments, decreasing that probability.

It is at this point that the beauty of the hair cells' "silent current" and the continual discharge activity of the high-spontaneous afferent neurons become especially apparent. Owing to their joint presence, both negative *and* positive changes in transmitter release can occur and be represented neurally. Moreover, with the exception of brief refractory periods following each discharge, each afferent neuron sits waiting for the release of trans-mitter in a recovered state of readiness (see Fig. 11.7). Virtually *all* increases and decreases in hair cell transmitter release are tracked by the neuron's discharge probabilities (down to zero), more or less independently of when its own discharges occur. (Were the primary neurons to have long refractory periods, the discharge probabilities would be a messy mix of both stimulus and threshold recovery waveforms.)

To be sure, the *magnitude* of the discharge probabilities does not follow that of the inner hair cell's receptor potential faithfully owing to effects such as adaptation (see Fig. 12.1 for short-term effects; Javel, 1996, for long-term effects), compression (Figs. 12.4–12.6), and suppression (see Chapter 13); but the cadence of the discharge probabilities of high-spontaneous primary neurons *does* track the wave shape of the receptor potential (often half-wave rectified).

This temporal encoding of waveform holds firm even when the stimulus has a complicated wave shape. An example is in Figure 12.11, which shows period histograms produced with a stimulus composed of two low-frequency tones with frequencies in the ratio of 4:3. When the tone with the higher frequency (1064 Hz) was the stronger one, the neuron's discharges were synchronized to that tone alone (Fig. 12.11A). By the same token, when the tone with the lower frequency (798 Hz) was stronger, discharges were largely synchronized to *it* (Fig. 12.11C). When the tones were of the same amplitude, the discharge synchrony was a combination of the two tones (Fig. 12.11B), presumably reflecting a similar wave shape of the inner hair cell's receptor potential for that stimulus. In each setting in Figure 12.11 the solid curve is the simple sum of the two stimulating sinusoids, with amplitudes and phases picked for the best fit between the positive excursions of that sum and the neural data.

The picture that emerges for excitation with a single tone is shown in Figure 12.12. As the tone's traveling wave nears its resonance place, it excites a patch of primary neurons. Each of the excited neurons discharges in cadence with the stimulating waveform, but the restricted rate of this spike generation (< 200/sec) means that it does not (*cannot*) discharge on

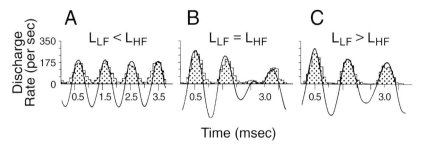

Figure 12.11. Responses to two-tone stimuli recorded from a primary afferent neuron in the squirrel monkey. The two frequencies—798 Hz (LF) and 1064 Hz (HF)—had a 3:4 ratio. When the sound level of the high-frequency tone was greater (by 20 dB), the spikes virtually synchronized to that tone alone (A). When the low-frequency tone was more intense (by 10 dB), the spikes largely synchronized to that tone (C). When the tones were of equal strength, the spikes synchronized strongly to both tones simultaneously (B). Each period histogram (plotted on the time base of the 266 Hz fundamental frequency) is fitted with a curve that is the sum of the two sine waves, arbitrarily adjusted in phases and amplitudes to achieve the best fit of its top (positive) half with the data. (From Brugge et al., 1969, with permission.*)

each cycle (except for stimuli of very low frequencies). In fact, many cycles of the stimulus usually occur between successive discharges (Rose et al., 1967). Recall, however, that each inner hair cell is innervated by ten or more afferent neurons, each apparently discharging independently (Johnson and Kiang, 1976). If we were to treat this group of neurons as a single ensemble,

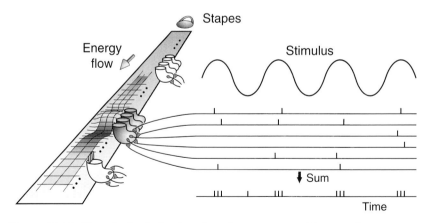

Figure 12.12. Neural stimulation by a low-frequency tone. The sound energy propagates to the characteristic place of the tone, where it causes tuned deflections of the cochlear partition (left side). Neural spikes, when they occur (right side), are synchronized to the peaks of the local deflections. The sum of these neural spikes (lower trace) tends to mimic the wave shape of the local deflections.

its summed spike rate *does* track the stimulus waveform (see World Wide Web animations). The heavy convergence of primary neurons on their targets within the brain stem's cochlear nucleus suggests that something like this summing does go on centrally.

An intriguing question about this central summing concerns the effects of the finite velocity of the acoustic traveling waves (see Chapter 5). Because neurons lying more apically are excited at later times than those lying more basally, the spike trains produced by the various afferent neurons are staggered in time. In fact, the phases of these various spike trains relative to each other are even more complicated (and confusing) than Figure 12.12 suggests (see Ruggero et al., 1996). How does the central nervous system take into account this temporal staggering when developing for us the perception of a "pure" tone, particularly at high sound pressures when much of the cochlea is responding?

As valuable as this discharge synchrony is for encoding the stimulus waveform, it does not extend to all frequencies. To quantify this effect, the "synchrony coefficient"[4] is employed. Plotted as a function of stimulus frequency (Fig. 12.13), these coefficients show that maximum discharge synchrony in the cat is uniformly strong up to about 1.0 kHz, above which it tapers off gradually. With only rare exceptions, there is an upper limit for significant synchrony of about 6 kHz for the cat and the squirrel monkey.

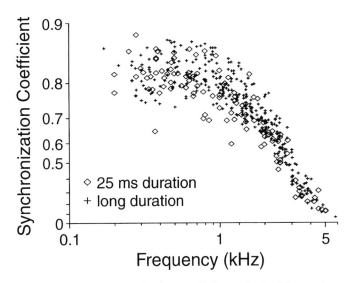

Figure 12.13. Maximum synchronization coefficients obtained from a large number of primary auditory neurons in the cat, as a function of tonal frequency. Data were obtained with tones whose durations were both long (15 or 30 sec) and short (25 msec). The ordinate is nonlinear. (From Joris et al., 1994, with permission.*)

In the guinea pig this limit is almost an octave lower (ca. 3.5 kHz). The primary auditory neurons of lizards and birds also show phase synchrony, the latter up to about 5 kHz for almost all species studied (Manley, 1990). Of special interest is the finding that secondary auditory neurons in the barn owl synchronize their discharges to frequencies as high as 9 kHz (Sullivan and Konishi, 1984), about an octave higher than those seen in comparable (cochlear nucleus) neurons of the cat (Joris et al., 1994).

One of the principal reasons for the loss of discharge synchrony at the higher frequencies is that the cell walls of the inner hair cells behave like resistor-capacitor (*RC*) circuits, which "low-pass" filter the receptor potentials created by the transduction currents (see Chapter 9). It may be that this filtering is indeed *the* limiting factor, as suggested by the observation that the "corner" frequency of inner hair cells in the guinea pig is about 600 Hz, approximately the same frequency at which auditory nerve neurons in that species begin to lose their phase-sychronizing abilities (Palmer and Russell, 1986). It is also possible that temporal "jitter" in the release of transmitter quanta also contributes to the loss of synchrony at high frequencies (Anderson et al., 1971).

The ability of primary auditory neurons to synchronize the cadences of their discharges with the waveforms of low-frequency stimuli means that the central nervous system is receiving detailed temporally coded information about those stimuli. Although this type of *wave shape* encoding is denied to high-frequency signals, the timing of primary-neuron discharges still provides important temporal information about the time structure of such signals (e.g., their onsets, offsets, and variations in amplitude). Frequency composition in these cases is encoded solely by the discharge rate profiles generated on the spatially distributed terminal axons of the basal cochlea (see Fig. 9.6B). Perhaps it is no accident therefore that the frequency at which the cat's cochlear frequency-space map begins its logarithmic course (at about 1.5 kHz) is close to the frequency at which the waveform synchronization abilities of its primary neurons begin to wane. In short, greater spatial representation along the cochlear partition is provided for those stimulus components whose frequencies are encoded only with discharge rate profiles than for those whose wave shapes are also encoded temporally.

In this connection, note that the cochleas of turtles, lizards, and birds, generally limited as they are to frequencies below 8 kHz, also employ both temporal and spatial encoding of acoustic stimuli. In fact, the frequency selectivities of the primary auditory neurons in these animals are often sharper than those of comparable neurons in the mammal (Crawford and Fettiplace, 1980; Manley, 1990). Evidently, even with spike synchronization, splitting the signal into frequency bands is useful, regardless of the size of the cochlea. It is interesting to note that despite their different sizes and the different tuning mechanisms used to obtain them (see Chapter 7), the characteristic-frequency/location "maps" for all of these smaller cochleas and papillae are approximately logarithmic in nature (Crawford and Fettiplace, 1980; Manley, 1990). What is so special about working in octaves?

NOTES

1. A *poststimulus time histogram* is formed by superimposing the responses to many presentations of the same stimulus. This form of display is necessitated by the fact that the neural response evoked by any particular presentation of a sound stimulus is different in detail from all other responses to that same stimulus. Thus some sort of averaging or trend extraction is necessary. To the extent that each response is a sample drawn from a statistically identical set of responses, the histogram can be treated as yielding estimates of spike-discharge probabilities. For example, if one time slot ("bin") in the histogram contains 15 spikes in a histogram that was compiled by summing 100 responses, the probability of a spike occurring in that particular time bin during the next response (or any other one) is estimated at 15/100, or 0.15.

2. The mechanism producing these dips, indeed the general functioning of the cochlea at high intensities, is poorly understood and so will not be covered here.

3. Different methods of determining "threshold" yield different relative sensitivities of the different spontaneous-rate classes (e.g., Geisler et al., 1985). However, the same basic order of sensitivities as that in the lower panel of Figure 12.7 is always observed.

4. The *synchrony coefficient* of a period histogram is defined as the amplitude of its fundamental (Fourier) component divided by its average (DC) value (Goldberg and Brown, 1969). This coefficient can have values anywhere between 0 and 1. With absolutely no discharge synchrony to the stimulating waveform, the coefficient's value is zero. When all discharges register in a single bin of the histogram, the value of the coefficient is unity. For a "half-wave rectified" sinusoid, the synchrony coefficient equals 0.78.

13

RESPONSES OF PRIMARY AUDITORY NEURONS TO OTHER BASIC SOUNDS

Armed with an understanding of the primary neuron's responses to tones, we can anticipate many aspects of its responses to other acoustic stimuli. However, before tackling the complex waveforms of natural sounds, it would be well to deepen basic insights by considering the responses to more structured stimuli. Accordingly, responses of the primary neurons to simplified versions of common sounds comprise the subject matter of this chapter.

RELATIONS BETWEEN TIME AND FREQUENCY

Time is of crucial importance when accounting for the responses of primary auditory neurons. This conclusion is not just a consequence of the reciprocal relation that exists between a pure tone's frequency and period but, rather, the reflection of a *fundamental* relation that exists between the temporal and frequency attributes of any tuned physical system (Licklider, 1951).

Consider for example, the performance of a simple resonant filter (Fig. 13.1). When the frequency selectivity of the filter is set to a high level, with a quality factor[1] (Q) of 10 (Fig. 13.1A), the response of that filter to excitation by a single "impulse" (roughly, a *very* brief pulse) is quite long, a lightly damped oscillation that rings at the resonant frequency for about ten

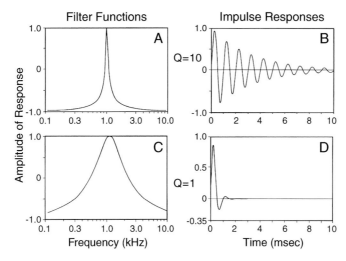

Figure 13.1. Relation between a filter's frequency selectivity (left) and its transient response (right). A sharply tuned linear filter (top row) has an "impulse" response (*B*) that "rings" at about the filter's resonant frequency for many cycles. By contrast, a broadly tuned linear filter (bottom row) has a brief impulse response (*D*). Roughly speaking, the duration of a filter's impulse response can be thought of as determining the "attention span" of the filter. (From Geisler, 1987, with permission.*)

cycles (Fig. 13.1B). However, when the frequency selectivity of the filter is decreased by an order of magnitude, to a *Q* of 1 (Fig. 13.1C), the impulse response becomes heavily damped, lasting only about one cycle of oscillation (Fig. 13.1D). In each case the agreement between these two numbers (*Q* and number of oscillations) is not accidental: the narrower the frequency selectivity, the longer *must* be the impulse response, as readily proved by Fourier theory. In fact, the frequency selectivity curve and the impulse response of a linear filter form a Fourier transform "pair," each transformable into the other with the use of a single equation.[2]

Although the stimulus used in this example was an impulse, the filter's response to *any* type of stimulus would include transients having the same time span as the impulse response. Stated differently, the impulse response can be thought of as the time window that frames the section of the incoming signal being processed at any one instant. Perhaps contrary to initial expectations, we would *not* want cochlear filters to be tuned too sharply. If they were, they would have long processing "windows," which might interfere with the cochlea's ability to track rapidly changing stimuli (see Responses to Modulated Tones, below). By the same token, the price of rapid response times (short "windows") is poorly tuned filters, something we would not want either. Cochlear construction appears to strike a balance between these conflicting requirements, a compromise that favors rapid response times.

RESPONSES TO CLICKS

Aware of the relation between spectral shape and impulse responses in linear systems, it was natural for early investigators of cochlear physiology to hope that they could utilize the relation to estimate the frequency selectivity of the cochlear partition (thought at that time to behave linearly) by measuring the "click" (impulse) responses of primary auditory neurons (e.g., Goblick and Pfeiffer, 1969). Those neurons displaying slowly decaying oscillations should possess narrow frequency bandwidths centered around the oscillation frequency, whereas those with rapidly damped oscillations should have poor frequency selectivity. To a first approximation, those expectations were fulfilled.

For example, consider the responses of an apically located primary neuron to acoustic clicks of various intensities (Fig. 13.2A–C). The temporal aspects of the responses are as expected. Each peak in the responses is separated from its neighbors by approximately 0.9 msec, the period of the neuron's characteristic frequency (1.1 kHz), and the responses do decay away with elapsed time. Note, however, that the click responses change their shape

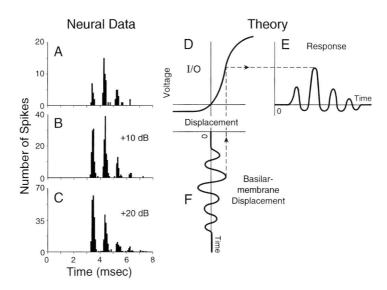

Figure 13.2. Responses of a primary auditory neuron to acoustic clicks and a theoretical explanation. *Left.* Poststimulus time histograms showing the responses of a low-spontaneous cat neuron to successively more intense clicks presented at $t = 0$. Theory: The click response of the local basilar membrane (*F*) forms the drive to the inner hair cell's input–output curve (*D*), producing the hair cell's receptor potential (*E*). This potential, which governs transmitter release, closely matches the neural response seen in *A*. (Histograms are from Cai and Geisler, unpublished data.)

with stimulus level, the unmistakable signature of a nonlinear system. Which one of those responses should we use to estimate the filter characteristics of the neural responses? More fundamentally, is it even a meaningful question as Fourier theory holds only for linear systems and so is not strictly applicable here?

Before pursuing those questions we should account for the shape of these click responses with the theory developed so far. Accordingly, let us assume that the apical cochlear partition has the response to a click shown in Figure 13.2F, and that the input–output curve of the inner hair cell driving the neuron is of the form shown in Figure 13.2D (see Fig. 8.3). The resulting output (Fig. 13.2E) is the receptor potential of the inner hair cell, a truncated ("half-wave rectified") version of the input waveform (see Fig. 12.11). If this receptor potential were imagined to modulate the release of transmitter from the hair cell, an output similar to the neural response shown in Figure 13.2A would result.

With a 10 dB increase in click strength, the neural response (Fig. 13.2B) increased in amplitude (note the different ordinate scales), but it had a relatively larger first peak. With another 10 dB increase in stimulus level, the first peak came to dominate the response (Fig. 13.2C) due probably to a combination of amplitude compression (see Chapter 10) and neural refractoriness. The latter becomes a factor when the first peak in the inner hair cell's generator potential grows so large that it almost always provokes a neural spike. When this happens, neural responsiveness to succeeding peaks is reduced for a few milliseconds by refractoriness (see Chapter 11). Despite these limitations, the general properties of the (presumed) input waveform *were* captured by the cadence of the neuron's discharge probabilities at all intensities (see Kiang et al., 1965).

Typical click responses for primary neurons innervating several sections of the cochlea are shown in Figure 13.3. So long as the neuron's characteristic frequency is below about 5 kHz, it is matched by the frequency of the oscillations in the click response, as expected (Fig. 13.3A,B). For primary neurons with higher characteristic frequencies, click responses contain no such oscillations (Fig. 13.3C). That also is expected, as the inability of primary neurons to synchronize their discharges to the waveforms of tones with frequencies above about 5 kHz (see Fig. 12.13) suggests that the mammalian cochlea's spike-generating processes cannot follow temporal variations in the stimulus waveform that take less than about 100 μsec.

Another important feature of a primary neuron's click response is that its length is inversely related to the characteristic frequency of the neuron: the higher the frequency, the shorter the response. This inverse relation is the net result of two competing factors. *Shortening* the response is the increase in the characteristic frequency itself. Even if frequency selectivity (Q_{10}) were

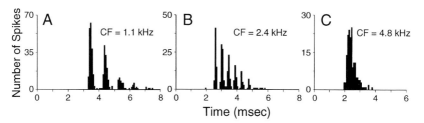

Figure 13.3. Click responses of three low-spontaneous primary afferent neurons of the cat cochlea having different characteristic frequencies (CF). For neurons whose characteristic frequencies are below about 5 kHz (*A, B*), the response waveform (expressed as a poststimulus time histogram) resembles the positive half of the local basilar membrane's click response (Fig. 13.2). For neurons tuned to higher frequencies, synchrony to the individual transient oscillations of the cochlear partition is lost, but the time interval between click and response onset becomes remarkably precise. (From Cai and Geisler, unpublished data.)

identical at all neural locations, thereby generating click responses with the same number of oscillations, the higher the frequency of those oscillations, the less time they would take. *Lengthening* the responses are the observed increases in frequency selectivity that accompany increases in characteristic frequency (see Fig. 12.8). As can be seen from Figure 13.3, the duration-shortening factor won. Primary neurons tuned to high frequencies show brief click responses, often just a single spike, accurately marking the arrival of the click at that cochlear location.

Because of the complications with neural refractoriness already mentioned, click responses are only infrequently used to estimate (via Fourier theory) a primary neuron's frequency selectivity (Evans, 1985). Surprisingly, such estimates can also be made from that neuron's responses to random noise, without the complications of refractoriness.

RESPONSES TO RANDOM NOISE

A primary auditory neuron responds to ''wide-band'' random noise[3] vigorously (Ruggero, 1973), in a manner predictable from basic cochlear physiology. The filtering action of the cochlear partition creates from the noise an inner hair cell receptor potential with an quasioscillatory waveform that resembles the waveform of a characteristic-frequency tone whose amplitude is randomly waxing and waning, and the reservoir properties of the synapse provide a compressive stimulus-response curve, similar to that seen with pure-tone stimuli (see Fig. 12.6A). Of course, direct manifestations of these inner hair cell oscillations can be observed only in the discharge cadences of primary neurons with characteristic frequencies below about 5 kHz (see Fig. 12.13).

The shared ability of click and noise stimuli to provide estimates of cochlear partition tuning may seem odd, as their waveforms are certainly different from one another. From a frequency-content point of view, these two stimuli are similar. Recall that brief pulses can by synthesized from a large ensemble of pure tones, each in cosine phase (see Fig. 2.3). Randomize the phases of those same tones, and the resulting waveform is virtually indistinguishable from that of random noise. In effect therefore a noise signal can be thought of as a sum of randomized sinusoids. Comparing one frequency component of the output waveform with the same component of the input signal determines the filter's response at that frequency. This comparison can be done at all frequencies simultaneously by ''cross-correlating'' the input and output waveforms. The end result is a waveform that is identical with the response of the filter to an impulse (Oppenheim et al., 1983).

It has been shown that this procedure works not only when the different frequency components of the stimulus do not interact (e.g., in a linear system) but also in a class of nonlinear filters whose mechanisms are compressive in nature. That class seems to include the cochlea, as the random noise technique has been successfully adapted for use with neural spike trains (de Boer and de Jongh, 1978). Examples of the *reverse correlation* (''revcor'') responses obtained with this technique from a primary neuron are shown in Figure 13.4B for several levels of noise. Note that these revcor responses, like a neuron's click responses, differ in shape. Yet these responses are quite useful.

For example, the neuronal frequency selectivity predicted by the theory from the revcor responses obtained with the lowest levels of noise (30 and 50 dB SPL) compare favorably with the threshold-level frequency tuning curve of the same neuron measured frequency by frequency with a sequence of pure tones (Fig. 13.4A). With still higher noise levels, the revcor responses in this case became increasingly shorter and so the inferred frequency selectivity of the neuron became wider, reflecting the same loss of frequency selectivity the basilar membrane undergoes at higher sound pressures (see Fig. 5.8).

For primary neurons with characteristic frequencies below about 1.5 kHz, there is little variation in the revcor responses obtained at various noise levels; good correspondence between the pure-tone frequency tuning curve and the frequency selectivity predicted from a revcor response is maintained for noise levels over a 40- to 60-dB range of intensities (Evans, 1977). This relative invariance of the revcor responses for neurons of low characteristic frequencies is expected, as the frequency selectivity of the cochlear partition in the apical region is also relatively level invariant (see Fig. 5.9).

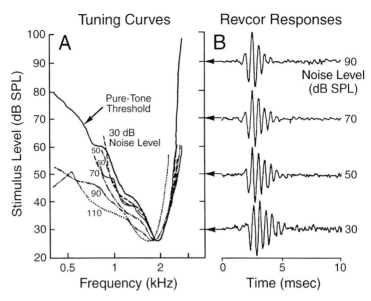

Figure 13.4. "Revcor" responses and frequency spectra obtained from a primary auditory neuron in the cat. *B*. Revcor responses obtained at four noise levels. As the noise level increased, the associated revcor response became shorter and more highly damped. *A*. Comparison between the neuron's pure-tone frequency tuning curve (thick solid line) and the (inverted) shapes of the frequency spectra of the revcor responses obtained at various noise levels. At low noise levels (e.g., 30–50 dB SPL), the tonal tuning and the noise tuning were remarkably similar. At high noise levels (e.g., above 70 dB SPL), the noise tuning became much broader. (From Evans, 1977, with permission.*)

All things considered, it appears from the nature of the revcor responses obtained from its primary neurons that the apical cochlea is behaving in a partially predictable fashion. Although the random-noise technique does not yield a single impulse response that characterizes the system at all stimulus levels (as it would in a linear system), it does provide estimates of the *effective* frequency selectivity operative at the particular stimulus level of the noise used to obtain that estimate. In fact, the revcor functions can be employed to generate fairly accurate predictions of response wave shapes evoked by other stimuli of the same strength (Carney and Yin, 1988). Because of the inability of the neural discharge patterns to track the wave shapes of high-frequency stimuli (see Fig. 12.13), this technique is applicable only to primary neurons with characteristic frequencies of less than 5 kHz. Another related technique that is independent of neural synchrony, "spectrotemporal receptive fields," can be applied to all primary neurons (Kim and Young, 1994).

RESPONSES TO MODULATED TONES

A pure tone is not very interesting and, once initiated, does not convey much information. It is *modulation* of the tone that carries information (and catches interest). Of the three parameters that define a tone—amplitude, frequency, initial phase—the first two are particularly important in acoustic communication. It is not surprising therefore that the cochlea encodes variations of those parameters robustly.

Amplitude Modulation

Let us consider *amplitude modulation* (AM) first. The simplest case, mathematically speaking, is when the amplitude of one sinusoid, called the "carrier," is modulated by another sinusoid, known as the "modulator." The equation for such a signal is

$$p(t) = A[1 + m * \cos(2\pi f_m t)]\cos(2\pi f_c t), \qquad f_c \gg f_m \qquad (13.1)$$

where f_c is the frequency of the carrier wave, f_m is the frequency of the modulating signal, and m is the "depth of modulation," which varies between 0 (no modulation) and 1 ("100% modulation"). The term $A[\cdots]$, which oscillates in a sinusoidal fashion between the extremes of $A[1 \pm m]$, is considered to be the time-varying amplitude (or "envelope") of the carrier wave.

Using our knowledge that the average discharge rates of primary neurons are monotonically related to the stimulus level of tones (see Fig. 12.6A), we would expect these rates to encode faithfully the amplitude variations in the stimulus. Indeed they do. At the right of Figure 13.5A, the stimulus waveforms (positive halves only) are shown for two depths of modulation. The left side shows the corresponding neural responses, which in each case has a deeper modulation depth. The synchrony of these various waveforms to the modulating sinusoid was quantified for the entire range of modulation depths ($0 \leq m \leq 1$) using the synchronization coefficient (see Chapter 12). The results (Fig. 13.5B) show that, in all cases, the neural response pattern displayed greater modulation depth than did the stimulus, particularly for small depths of modulation.

This enhanced ability of primary neurons to encode amplitude modulations seems due, at least in part, to the adaptation properties of the afferent synapses. According to the single-reservoir model of adaptation (see Fig. 12.2), the amount of neurotransmitter in the reservoir level would drop initially to a more or less fixed level appropriate for the stimulus' *average*

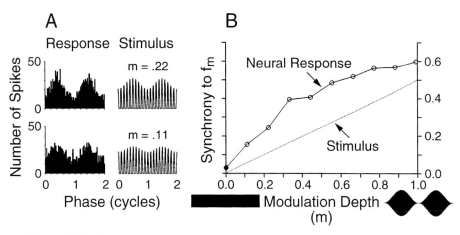

Figure 13.5. Responses of a cat primary afferent neuron to amplitude-modulated tones. *A*. Neural responses are at left (in period histograms with a time base equal to two periods of the modulating sinusoid). Corresponding stimulus waveforms are at right (only positive halves shown). Carrier frequency was 20 kHz (the neuron's characteristic frequency); modulating frequency was 100 Hz. At either level of modulation (m = 0.11 or 0.22), the neural discharge pattern follows the stimulus' amplitude variations but with even deeper modulations. *B*. Depths of these modulations, as measured by the synchronization coefficient calculated at the modulating frequency f_m. The neural histogram is more deeply modulated than the stimulus waveform at all modulation depths. Stimulus envelopes at modulation depths of 0 and 1 are sketched just below the abscissa. (From Joris and Yin, 1992, with permission.*)

amplitude (except at modulation rates slow enough for the reservoir level to follow). Then, roughly speaking, the rising phase of each modulation cycle (i.e., when the carrier's amplitude approaches $A[1 + m]$) would be treated as an abrupt increase in amplitude. The equivalent of an ''onset'' response would thus occur, as it does for stepwise increases in amplitude (Smith and Zwislocki, 1975). The main difference in this case is that *each* modulation cycle would provoke an onset response. Similarly, each falling phase of the AM wave would be treated as an abrupt decrease in stimulus amplitude, and an ''offset'' response would result (Smith et al., 1985).

Consistent with this picture, the high-spontaneous primary neurons, which have the largest ''onset'' responses (see Chapter 12), showed the greatest enhancement of modulation amplitudes (Cooper et al., 1993), at least for moderately low intensities. For higher intensities (> 70 dB SPL), the discharge apparatus of these high-spontaneous neurons became deeply saturated (see Fig. 12.6A), and registration of all but the deepest amplitude modulations (e.g. $m \approx 1$) became negligible (Joris and Yin, 1992; Cooper et al., 1993).

For their part, low-spontaneous primary neurons, which show weaker

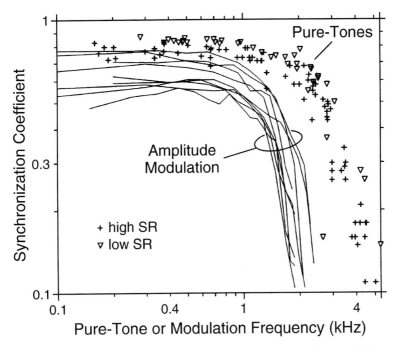

Figure 13.6. Maximum discharge synchrony of responses to the modulating frequency f_m of amplitude-modulated tones, plotted as a function of modulating frequency, for basally located primary neurons. Each solid line shows the modulation depths of a primary neuron's responses. There is little effect so long as f_m is less than 1 kHz. For comparison, the synchrony coefficients of the responses of many primary neurons of both high and low spontaneous rates (SR) to their respective characteristic frequency tones are shown as data points (see Fig. 12.13). (From Joris and Yin, 1992, with permission.*)

"onset" responses (see Chapter 12), had lesser enhancements of their amplitude-modulation encoding (Cooper et al., 1993). Although less sensitive to the envelope modulations, these low-spontaneous neurons were able to encode them over an almost unlimited range of intensities, even up to 100 dB SPL (the highest level used in that study). It is this ability to encode amplitude changes at high sound pressures that has singled out low-spontaneous neurons, despite their relatively small numbers, as being the probable providers of amplitude information at high intensities (see Chapter 12, Properties of Discharge Rate Responses). They appear to play other unique roles as well (see Chapter 14).

At high modulation frequencies, all primary auditory neurons lose their ability to encode amplitude modulations with their discharge cadences, as shown by the solid curves in Figure 13.6. This limitation was expected from the neurons' demonstrated inability to synchronize to sinusoidal waveforms that had frequencies higher than about 5 kHz (see Fig. 12.13). What *is* surprising is that the "cutoff" frequency for temporally encoding amplitude modulations in the cat ear is only about 1 kHz, almost an octave lower than that for encoding pure tones (Fig. 13.6, data points). No satisfactory theoretical explanation has been given for this difference.

Variation in Tone Frequency

The other principal way to encode information with a tone is by varying its frequency. The equation of such frequency variation can be written approximately[4] as

$$p(t) = A * \cos[2\pi f_v(t) * t] \tag{13.2}$$

where $f_v(t)$ is the time-varying frequency. Clearly, the receiving system must track this changing frequency to obtain the information it carries. The auditory periphery is well suited for that task, practically regardless of the speed with which these frequency changes are made.

Consider, for example, the responses of a primary neuron whose threshold-level tuning curve is shown in Figure 13.7A (characteristic frequency 3.2

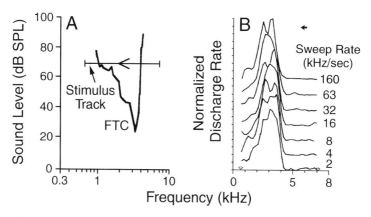

Figure 13.7. Responses of a cat primary auditory neuron to a tone whose instantaneous frequency was swept linearly from 7.0 kHz down to 0.65 kHz. *A.* Parameter track of the constant-amplitude variable-frequency tone is shown, along with the neuron's pure-tone frequency tuning curve (FTC). *B.* Responses of the neuron, plotted as (time-reversed) poststimulus time histograms for various sweep speeds. Responses are offset vertically for display clarity. As shown, sweep speed had little effect on the neural response rate, indicating that the neuron (CF = 3.2 kHz) had rapid response times. (From Sinex and Geisler, 1981, with permission.*)

kHz). In this experiment the instantaneous frequency of a tone having a fixed amplitude of 70 dB SPL was swept at constant speed from 650 Hz up to 7 kHz and then, after a momentary pause, back down again to 650 Hz (parameter path indicated by the horizontal bar). The instantaneous discharge rates of the neuron measured during the downward sweep are shown in Figure 13.7B for seven sweep rates. Almost independent of sweep rate, these neural spike-rate profiles traced out the neuron's sensitivity to *pure* tones of various frequencies; that is, discharges began when the instantaneous frequency crossed the threshold curve into the neuron's pure-tone "response area" at about 4 kHz, increased to a maximum discharge rate for 3 kHz excitation, and the gradually decreased as the lower boundary of the response area was approached. A similar set of responses (not shown here) was obtained during the upward frequency sweeps.

The ability of this neuron to respond to the instantaneous frequency of the stimulus, even at the top sweep rate of 160 kHz/sec (i.e., frequency changed by 1 kHz in about 6 msec), is the practical result of the rapid transient response (short stimulus "window") of the peripheral system at this neuron's location (see Responses to Clicks, above).

If the frequencies involved are low enough, the neural spikes synchronize to the instantaneous waveform of a variable-frequency tone. For example, consider the discharge cadences of another low-frequency primary neuron, also responding to a tone having linearly varying frequency. In this case the *intervals* between successive discharges were measured, as shown in Figure 13.8A. As in the previous case, the neuron did not discharge until the instantaneous frequency entered the neuron's (pure-tone) "response area" (ca. 200–400 Hz). When discharges did occur, they displayed strikingly precise interspike intervals of T, $2T \cdots NT$ (Fig. 13.8B), providing all the information needed to reconstruct the stimulating waveform (e.g., with a post-stimulus time histogram).

Recapitulation

The inner ear seems beautifully adapted for encoding both amplitude and frequency variations of the tone-like components of acoustic signals. Provided these variations occur at modulating frequencies below some limit (about 2 kHz in the cat), the discharges of the primary neurons become entrained by the stimulus waveform. For more rapid variations of instantaneous frequency, the response rates of the primary neurons keep pace, up to some limit as yet undetermined. Whether the incoming signals are faint or intense, with transitions that are slow or fast, some of the primary neurons are poised, ready and able to encode essential features of the stimulus waveform.

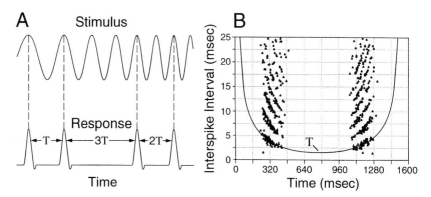

Figure 13.8. Synchrony of a cat primary neuron's discharges to the waveform of a low-frequency tone whose instantaneous frequency was swept linearly from 20 to 690 Hz and then, with a brief pause, back to 20 Hz again. *A.* The stimulus (top trace) and a hypothesized response pattern in which neural discharges are synchronized to the stimulating waveform (bottom trace). *B.* Interspike intervals of the neuron's discharges evoked by the variable-frequency tone. The reciprocal of the tone's *instantaneous* frequency is indicated by the solid line (*T*). Note that when the neuron discharged the intervals between spikes had values of the then-current T, $2T \cdots NT$ (i.e., the neural discharges were synchronized to the stimulating waveform). (Neural data from Sinex and Geisler, 1981, with permission.*)

RESPONSES TO PAIRS OF TONES

When two-tone stimuli are used, the tones usually interact suppressively in producing vibrational responses of the cochlear partition (see Chapter 10). Responses of primary auditory neurons to these same acoustic stimuli of course reflect such cochlear partition interactions. Therefore a primary neuron's response to multitone stimuli can be estimated roughly by imagining how an automatic gain control system would treat the stimulus waveform: The discharge rate would be greater than that evoked by either of the tones acting alone (unless one causes spike-rate saturation); and if the tones were to have frequencies below about 5 kHz, the discharge cadences would be dominated by the more effective of the two tones. Examples of this dominance are provided in Figure 12.11, first by one tone (panel A) and then by the other (panel C).

General Suppression

A generalized scheme for considering primary-neuron responses to paired tones is encapsulated in Figure 13.9, a sketch of tonal parameter space applicable to a basally located primary neuron (characteristic frequency > 4

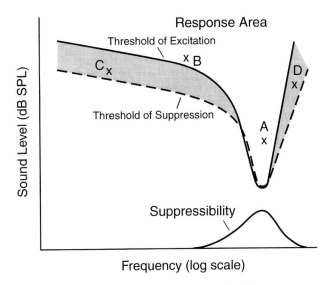

Figure 13.9. Interplay of excitation and suppression in the responses of a primary auditory neuron innervating the basal cochlea. The top traces show the parameter spaces of tones that excite the neuron and tones that suppress an excitatory response. Any point above the threshold of excitation is excitatory; any point above the suppression threshold is potentially suppressive. Suppressibility (bottom trace) depends primarily on the frequency of the excitatory tone. Because only responses to tones in the "tip" of the response area are suppressible, reduction of cochlear-amplifier gain by the suppressor is implied. Tones A–D are discussed in the text. (Modified from Geisler and Sinex, 1980, with permission.*)

kHz). In the upper half of Figure 13.9 are two "threshold" curves, the uppermost of which is the familiar threshold-level excitation curve for single tones (see Fig. 12.5B). Because virtually all tones whose amplitudes exceed the threshold level are excitatory for a primary neuron (see Fig. 12.6A), the area above its threshold excitation curve is often referred to as its "response area."

The lower of the two threshold curves is the line connecting the points at which a second tone just-noticeably suppresses the discharge rate evoked by an excitatory first tone. In general, the farther the second tone's sound pressure lies above that suppression threshold curve, the greater is its suppression of the first tone's response. Note that for most frequencies the suppression threshold lies below (i.e., is *more* sensitive than) the excitation threshold. It follows that any one excitatory tone might also be suppressive of the response evoked by another excitatory tone.

The *degree* of suppression exerted by one tone on the other depends on other factors, chief among which is the relation of the tonal frequencies to the neuron's own characteristic frequency. If, on the one hand, a tone has a frequency in the "tip" region of the neural response area (e.g., point A), its response is vulnerable to suppression, as also is seen on the basilar membrane (see Fig. 10.1). This vulnerability is represented by a correspondingly high value in the lowest curve, one that expresses "suppressibility." If, on the other hand, a tone has a frequency in the "tail" region of the response area (e.g., point B), its response cannot be suppressed at all, also a reflection of basilar membrane behavior (see Fig. 10.1B). Hence tones with "tail" frequencies are represented in the lowest curve as having negligible suppressibility. These general features of suppression can be accounted for, at least qualitatively, by the attenuation of cochlear amplification, which is attributed to localized reductions in the relevant response components of the outer hair cells (see Chapter 10).

As discussed, the response of a primary neuron to a two-tone stimulus is usually a complex mixture of excitation and mutual suppression. Particularly welcome for investigative purposes therefore are those cases where the sounding of a *non*excitatory second tone suppresses the response to an excitatory tone (Sachs, 1969). To do so, the parameters of the second tone must fall within one of the two narrow "suppressive" zones that flank the tip of the excitatory threshold curve. Should the frequency of such a purely suppressing tone be less than that of the characteristic frequency (e.g., point C in Fig. 13.9), the suppression is colloquially described as "low-side"; "high-side" suppression is said to occur when the frequency of the suppressor is greater than the characteristic frequency (e.g., point D). These forms of "pure" suppression are particularly illuminating, so each is worth a brief description.

Before proceeding, however, the two ways in which the word "suppression" is applied to neural responses must be made clear. On the one hand, when the *average* discharge rate of a neuron responding to one tone is reduced by the sounding of a second tone, *rate suppression* is said to have occurred. It was this spike rate criterion, for instance, that was used to determine the "threshold of suppression" in Figure 13.9. On the other hand, when the response *component* due to one tone is reduced by the second, the reduction is called *synchrony suppression*. This form of suppression, which is applicable only to synchronized response components, differs principally from the former in ignoring totally the excitation provided by the suppressor tone. Although these two types of suppression are not mutually exclusive, it was in the latter sense that the word usually was employed in the preceding paragraphs.

The excitation–suppression pattern for apically located neurons resembles that of the "tip" region shown in Figure 13.9, but the corresponding suppressibility curve has not yet been worked out.

"High-Side" Suppression

Typical examples of high-side *rate* suppression are given in Figure 13.10, which shows the stimulus-response curves of a primary neuron responding to its characteristic-frequency tone (9.6 kHz) in the presence of a nonexcitatory 12 kHz tone, presented at various strengths. Addition of the purely suppressive tone almost always resulted in a reduction in the neuron's discharge rate. The higher the sound pressure of the suppressor, the greater was the rate suppression.

In a now familiar pattern, the responses were reduced in such a manner that the suppressor tone, presented at any one level, shifted the entire stimulus-response curve for the characteristic-frequency tone to the right by a certain amount, sometimes by more than 20 dB. This rightward shift is basically a desensitization, similar to that produced in basilar membrane vibrations with comparable two-tone stimuli (see Fig. 10.6). That is, the neural suppression appears to be simply a reflection of the reduced amplification the 9.6 kHz hydroacoustic wave obtained in its passage through the 12 kHz region (see Fig. 10.7).

This desensitization interpretation is further supported by the data in Fig-

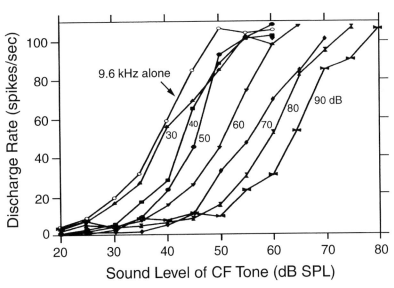

Figure 13.10. "High-side" suppression of the response rates of a cat primary neuron evoked by a characteristic frequency (CF) tone. The level-response curves for the neuron are shown as the intensity of the CF (9.6 kHz) tone was increased. Each curve was obtained in the presence of a 12 kHz tone with the indicated sound level. This pattern of suppressions is similar to that seen with "high-side" suppression of the basilar membrane's responses (see Fig. 10.6A). The 12 kHz tone by itself did not excite the neuron. (From Javel et al., 1978, with permission.*)

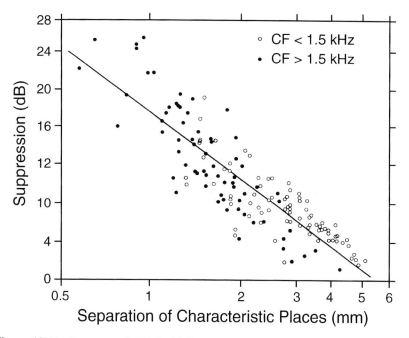

Figure 13.11. Summary of ''high-side'' suppressions obtained with 80 dB suppressors of many frequencies in the cat. The magnitude of suppression (i.e., the rightward shift of the rate-level curve) is plotted as a function of the *difference* between the frequencies of the two tones, expressed as the separation (in millimeters) between their respective characteristic places. For neurons having a CF above 1.5 kHz (solid circles), the suppressor frequency had to be within one octave of the CF (3.5 mm separation). For neurons having a CF below 1.5 kHz (open circles), the suppressor frequency could be anywhere within two octaves of CF (see Fig. 12.9). (From Javel et al., 1978, with permission.*)

ure 13.11, which show the amounts of suppression (rightward shifts) produced by high-side suppressor tones of different frequencies presented at a level of 80 dB SPL. The unusual abscissa scale used for these data, pooled from observations on many animals, is the spatial *separation* between the domains of the two tones, expressed as the distance (in millimeters) between their respective characteristic places on the cochlear partition. From the plot it is obvious that suppression decreases rapidly as the suppressor tone's vibration pattern becomes increasingly separated spatially from that of the characteristic-frequency tone, as happens on the basilar membrane (see Fig. 10.8).

For the apical neurons (open dots), those with characteristic frequencies below 1.5 kHz, the suppression region was about 5 mm wide, a width corresponding to about two octaves on the cat's frequency-place map (see Fig. 12.9). In other words, suppression occurred so long as the suppressor's frequency was within *two* octaves of the characteristic frequency. This is almost the same ratio observed in apical cochlear-partition suppressions (see Fig. 10.9). By contrast, for more basally placed neurons (Fig. 13.11 solid dots), the suppressor zone was about 3.5 mm wide, the distance separating the characteristic places of two tones differing in frequency by a single octave (see Fig. 12.9). Thus in the cochlea's base the two frequencies had to be within *one* octave of each other for the high-side tone to suppress the responses of the excitatory tone. This difference in the width of high-side suppression regions is taken to reflect differences in the widths of the amplification zones active in the various cochlear regions (see Chapter 9).

The effects of the efferent system also suppress the responses of primary neurons to tones with near characteristic frequency (see Chapter 15). However, these efferent effects take many milliseconds to develop, in marked contrast with the almost instantaneous onset of two-tone suppression (Arthur et al., 1971). It seems evident therefore, that the type of suppression discussed here must be caused largely by processes located within the cochlea itself.

"Low-Side" Suppression

As indicated in Figure 13.9, suppression of the responses evoked by a characteristic-frequency tone can also be achieved by adding certain lower frequency tones. These low-side rate suppressions behave somewhat like high-side suppressions but with some unique features. An example of low-side suppression is given in the top curve of Figure 13.12, which shows the average discharge rates of a primary neuron produced in response to a fixed characteristic-frequency tone (14 kHz) in the presence of various levels of a 1 kHz suppressor. The spike rates produced by the 1 kHz tone sounded alone are also shown for comparison. At the lowest level of suppressor tone used (60 dB SPL), there was essentially no suppressive effect: The spike rate of about 50/sec was nearly the same as that produced by the 14 kHz tone alone. As the suppressor strength was progressively increased, the discharge rate dropped precipitously, becoming a mere shadow of itself (ca. 8/sec) at suppressor levels of 75 and 80 dB SPL.

For still higher levels of the suppressor the downward trend reversed, and the average discharge rate began to climb, producing essentially the same rates as the suppressor acting alone. It appears therefore that the 14 kHz tone made virtually no contribution to the neural response at these higher suppressor levels. This conclusion is supported by the discharge patterns produced in similar experiments but at frequencies low enough to produce discharge synchrony. Fourier analysis of these low-frequency responses indicates that the characteristic frequency component continued to be increasingly reduced as the sound pressure of the suppressor was increased, even in the region of increasing spike rate (Javel, 1981; Hill and Geisler, 1992).

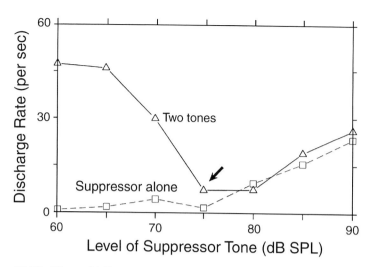

Figure 13.12. ''Low-side'' suppression of the response rates of a cat primary neuron to a characteristic frequency (CF) tone. The CF (14 kHz) tone by itself evoked a discharge rate of about 47 spikes/sec from that medium-spontaneous neuron. As the intensity of an accompanying 1 kHz suppressor tone was progressively increased, the discharge rate first dropped sharply and then grew (solid curve). Above 75 dB SPL, the two-tone curve is nearly identical to that of the suppressor alone (dashed curve), indicating that in both cases the neuron is responding solely to the suppressor tone. This behavior differs markedly from ''low-side'' suppression of basilar membrane responses (e.g., see Fig. 10.1B). (From Cai and Geisler, 1996, with permission.*)

Thus at those high suppressor levels (e.g., 85 and 90 dB in Fig. 13.12), the responses to the combined tones were essentially those produced by the suppressor tone alone; the influence of the characteristic-frequency tone had been virtually eliminated.

The general behavior of the rate-suppression curve of Figure 13.12 reflects the known effects of the suppressor tone on the basilar membrane (see Fig. 10.1B): simultaneous suppression (of the characteristic-frequency component) and excitation (at the suppressor frequency). What is unexpected in the data of Figure 13.12 is the virtual absence of a response to the suppressor tone when it was presented alone at 75 dB SPL, a level that produced an 80% reduction in the neuron's average response rate (arrow). Such suppressor reduction of the *overall* response has not been observed in basilar membrane vibrations, where the sum of the two response components has always exceeded that of the single-tone response (see Fig. 10.4B).

The unexpectedly large magnitude of low-side suppression is further illustrated in the top row of Figure 13.13, which presents both the suppressed and unsuppressed responses of another primary neuron. These responses,

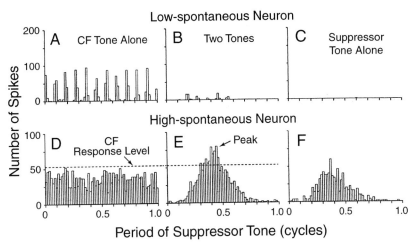

Figure 13.13. Temporal responses of ''low-side'' suppression in cat primary neurons having low and high rates of spontaneous activity. *Top row.* Responses of a low-spontaneous neuron evoked by a characteristic frequency (CF) 1.1 kHz tone alone (*A*), a 100 Hz suppressor tone alone (*C*), and the simultaneous presentation of the two tones (*B*). *Bottom row.* Corresponding responses of a high-spontaneous neuron: Characteristic frequency (CF) was 18 kHz and the suppressor frequency 1 kHz. The two-tone response (*E*) is for the case of maximum rate suppression. The differing heights of the peaks in the two-tone responses are significant. Displays are all period histograms, calculated on the period of the respective suppressor tone. (From Cai and Geisler, 1996, with permission.*)

presented as period histograms (with the suppressor-tone's period used as the time base), show that the neuron's response to the combined tones was virtually *zero* (Fig. 13.13B), even though the characteristic-frequency tone by itself produced a robust response (Fig. 13.13A). There was no response at all to the suppressor tone presented alone (Fig. 13.13C).

Not all primary neurons behave in this manner. A different pattern is seen in the comparable responses of still another primary neuron, shown in the bottom row of Figure 13.13. At the suppressor level that caused maximum suppression of the *average* discharge rate, the maximum *instantaneous* rate produced by the two simultaneously presented tones (Fig. 13.13E) was greater than that produced by the characteristic-frequency tone alone (Fig. 13.13D). Unlike those of the top-row neuron, the responses of this neuron *do* seem to share the basic characteristics of both basilar membrane and inner hair cell low-side suppressions, in which the peak of the two-tone response is always greater than that of the unsuppressed response (see Fig. 10.4) (Russell and Kössl, 1992).

Why the difference in the two-tone responses? It is the spontaneous-discharge rate. The neuron of the top row in Figure 13.13 was a low-spontaneous neuron (0.5 spikes/sec), whereas that of the bottom row was a high-spontaneous one (42 spikes/sec). More generally, it has been shown that the types of low-side suppression exhibited by these two neurons are characteristic of their respective spontaneous-rate classes (Cai and Geisler, 1996). Maximum suppression in lower-spontaneous primary neurons almost always produced peak rates that were below rates produced by the characteristic-frequency tone alone. Indeed, *all* discharges of low-spontaneous neurons were sometimes virtually eliminated (as in Fig. 13.13B). By contrast, high-spontaneous neurons usually showed increased peak rates, even when their average discharge rates were maximally suppressed (as in Fig. 13.13E).

The conclusion reached in the latter study was that because the low-side suppression of lower-spontaneous primary neurons is much more severe than that seen on the basilar membrane there must be some additional suppressive factor acting on neurons of this class (and perhaps to a lesser extent on the high-spontaneous neurons). Just what this factor might be is unclear, although extracellular potentials, which would change the *transmembrane* potentials of both hair cells and afferent terminals, have been suggested (Hill et al., 1989). This possibility is explored further in our discussion of efferent effects (see Chapter 15). Another hypothesis is that the suppressor's response is somehow filtered out between the basilar membrane and the neuron (Pfeiffer, 1970), but no clear trace of such a filter has ever been found.

The view that low-side suppression is of a different nature than high-side suppression is further supported by the differences that occur in the *rate of growth* of suppression strength as the suppression level is increased. Such data, pooled from many primary neurons, are given in Figure 13.14; they are divided into two groups based on the respective characteristic frequencies of the neurons. Note that the suppressor frequency in each panel is normalized to the characteristic frequency (i.e., the *ratio* of the suppressor frequency to the neuron's characteristic frequency is plotted on the horizontal axis).

Trends are clearest for neurons that had characteristic frequencies above 2 kHz (Fig. 13.14B); suppression (rightward shift of the stimulus-response curve) grew by an average of about 2 dB with each 1 dB increase in suppressor level for low-side suppressors, whereas high-side suppression grew much more slowly. Incidentally, note that the high-side suppression for these basal neurons dropped off steeply with increasing suppressor frequency, ceasing entirely at frequency separations of more than an octave. This same highly localized frequency dependence was also observed in Figure 13.11. More apical neurons were suppressed in fundamentally the same manner (Fig. 13.14A), except in a more subdued manner. The growth rate of their low-side suppressions was considerably weaker, and their high-side sup-

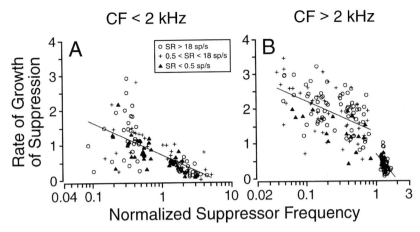

Figure 13.14. Rate of growth of discharge rate suppression as a function of suppressor frequency for cat primary auditory neurons having characteristic frequencies below 2 kHz (*A*) and above 2 kHz (*B*). Each point represents one neuron's rate of suppression *growth* (i.e., the increase in rate suppression, in decibels, brought about by a 1 dB increase in suppressor level). The abscissa shows the ratio of suppressor frequency to the relevant neuron's characteristic frequency (CF). The category of each neuron's spontaneous spike rate (SR) is indicated. (From Delgutte, 1990, with permission.*)

pressors had a much wider permissible frequency range, stretching two octaves above the characteristic frequency.

Recapitulation

The two-tone suppressions observed in the responses of mammalian primary neurons are largely accounted for by basilar membrane suppressions, which themselves appear to be consequences of the basic cochlear-amplifier mechanisms. The one glaring exception is the unexpectedly strong rate suppressions produced by low-side suppressors.

The functional consequence of these suppressions is to desensitize (not silence) the primary neurons. For instance, the neuron of Figure 13.10 had its dynamic range for characteristic frequency tones shifted up the sound level scale as much as 25 dB by the suppressor tone. Thus even though nonexcitatory, at each of its strengths the suppressor tone pulled the neuron's dynamic range upward toward its own level. In essence therefore suppression is acting as automatic gain control (Lyon, 1990)—all the better to cope with more intense signals.

Two-Tone Suppressions in Other Vertebrates

Somewhat surprising in view of the principal role in two-tone suppression just attributed to the cochlear amplifier is the realization that two-tone suppression occurs in the primary auditory neurons of many species of vertebrates that have no outer hair cells. Some do not even have a basilar membrane. For our purposes, the suppressions exhibited by lizards, birds, and frogs are the most informative.

A number of species of lizards display two-tone suppression in a variety of styles (for a summary see Manley, 1990). In some species, notably the alligator lizard (Holton and Weiss, 1978) and the Tokay gecko (Eatock et al., 1981), high-side and low-side suppression are seen. However, only high-side suppression is seen in some lizards, such as the bobtail skink and European lizards of the family Lacertidae, and then only from primary neurons tuned to low and intermediate frequencies (Manley, 1990). No compelling reasons for this variability have been given. In one suggestive case (the alligator lizard) neurons innervating the papillar region devoid of a tectorial membrane (see Fig. 6.9) did not show suppression. Yet the mere presence of a tectorial membrane does not guarantee suppression, as the unsuppressible primary neurons of the bobtail skink originate in a papillar region that has a tectorial membrane.

Avian primary neurons also display suppression (Manley, 1990), not only of the two-tone variety but sometimes even ''single-tone'' suppression (i.e., the presentation of a *single* tone reduced discharge activity to a rate below that which occurred spontaneously). It is not clear if this single-tone suppression is fundamentally different from two-tone suppression. It may be, for instance, that the ''spontaneous'' activity exhibited in such cases is excited acoustically by noises originating from within the animals themselves. There are scattered reports of such single-tone suppression in the primary-neuron discharges of a number of vertebrate species, some mammalian.

Two-tone suppression is especially interesting in the bullfrog, as it is observed only in primary neurons innervating the amphibian papilla (Feng et al., 1975). Neither this low-frequency papilla nor the high-frequency one (the basilar papilla) even has a basilar membrane: In each papilla the hair cells rest on an apparently rigid platform and thus must be excited by the tectorial membrane. Is the tectorial membrane also responsible for suppression? If so, it is pretty selective, as no neurons of the basilar papilla and only some of the amphibian papilla (the lower-frequency ones) exhibit two-tone suppression. Many neurons of the amphibian papilla show single-tone suppression as well (Christensen-Dalsgaard and Jørgensen, 1996).

The existence of two-tone suppression in these various nonmammlian vertebrates is not only important in its own right, it shows that suppressive mechanisms exist that are more general than those attributed to the mammalian cochlea's amplification processes. It is therefore not beyond the realm of possibility that these general mechanisms also flourish within mammalian ears. Perhaps the same enigmatic suppressive mechanism that produces suppression in lizards and frogs is the still unknown "additional suppressive factor" that was invoked above to account for the unexplained strength of low-side suppression in mammalian cochleas.

CODA

We have investigated the responses of primary auditory neurons to simplified versions of naturally occurring sounds. Encouragingly, most attributes of these responses can be accounted for with current theory. This knowledge forms a solid base from which we now proceed to explore the responses of primary neurons to one representative class of natural sounds, speech.

NOTES

1. The "quality factor" (Q) of a filter is defined as the filter's resonant ("characteristic") frequency divided by its bandwidth. In electrical circuitry the bandwidth is customarily measured on the filter's spectral *response* curve (e.g., Fig. 13.1A), between the two points on either side of the peak whose amplitudes have seven-tenths the amplitude (half the power) of the peak. In auditory physiology the practice is to measure frequency selectivity on the threshold-level *tuning* curve, between the two points on either side of the tip whose stimulus levels are 10 dB greater than that of the tip. For clarity, the latter quality factor is usually written as Q_{10}.

2. It is the predictive relation between a linear system's "impulse response" and its response to *any* stimulus, including pure tones, that makes the former of such great use in many fields. If we could measure a linear system's impulse response (often easy to obtain), we then could calculate that system's response at any and all frequencies (laborious and often difficult to obtain by direct frequency measurements). That seems a bit like magic at first, but reference to Figure 2.3 makes it plausible. In Figure 2.3 we saw how a train of brief pulses could be constructed by adding together many harmonically related sinusoids. From a Fourier theory point of view, a linear system's response to a train of brief periodic pulses is simply the sum of its responses to sinusoids of many different frequencies (see Appendix A). In fact, this method was used to obtain the frequency-response functions of the cat external ear shown in Figure 3.8B.

3. *Random noise* refers to a nonrepetitive signal possessing a randomly varying amplitude, usually with a (nominally) Gaussian distribution. Such noise has an initial-phase spectrum that is randomly distributed and an amplitude spectrum that can have almost any shape, depending on the application. "Wide-band" noise has a "flat" amplitude distribution (i.e., equal power density at all frequencies) within

a wide band of frequencies. "White noise" is wide-band noise whose frequency band is (nominally) unlimited.

4. The *instantaneous frequency* of a sinusoid is defined as the time derivative of its phase angle (Oppenheim et al., 1983). Thus the proper expression for a sinusoid with a time-varying radian frequency $\omega_v(t)$ is $\cos\{\int[\omega_v(t)dt]\}$. The approximation used for this expression in Eq. 13.2 yields a phase derivative of $\omega_v + t(d\omega_v/dt)$ and so is in error with the inclusion of the continually growing term $t(d\omega_v/dt)$. For present purposes, that error can be ignored.

14

RESPONSES OF PRIMARY AUDITORY NEURONS TO SPEECH SOUNDS

We depend on speech to an extent not often appreciated for both physical well-being (''watch out'') and emotional health (solitary confinement is a dreaded punishment). Therefore knowledge about how the inner ear responds to speech has much practical value—for the design of prosthetic devices—as well as being of great theoretical interest. It would be convenient if we could obtain that information in an easy manner, such as predicting it from the responses to simple stimuli such as tones or clicks (see Chapters 12, 13). Unfortunately, because of the ear's strong nonlinearities and our limited understanding of them, accurate predictions are currently impossible. There is no choice but to measure those responses directly, using the speech sounds themselves as the acoustic stimuli.

Consideration of the neural responses to speech sounds also serves the more general purpose of providing us with exemplars of responses to a wide variety of sounds, as speech contains long sounds and short, shouts and whispers, amplitude modulations and frequency shifts, abrupt starts and long-term effects. Moreover, speech covers most of the frequency spectrum to which we are sensitive (see Fig. 2.4). In short, for its practical and theoretical importance, and for the great variety of its waveforms, speech provides us with some of our most interesting sounds.

For obvious ethical reasons, we have virtually no direct information about how the primary auditory neurons of humans encode speech. Of necessity, therefore, essentially all of our knowledge on the subject is obtained from laboratory mammals, an area into which we now delve (for summaries see Greenberg, 1988; Delgutte, 1997). Because our cochleas are similar to those of laboratory mammals in terms of basic structure and, from all external indications (e.g., cochlear emissions), appear to operate on the same fundamental mechanisms, it is expected that we have gained from these animal studies at least a qualitative picture of how the human ear responds to speech.

SPEECH ACOUSTICS

An appreciation for speech waveforms is provided by the acoustic theory of speech production[1] (see introductory books by Lieberman, 1977; Pickett, 1980). In an overview of this theory, the picture is straightforward. As shown in Figure 14.1, air is forced from the lungs into the hollow vocal tract through the *glottis*, the narrow opening between a pair of muscular half-moon-shaped flaps, the *vocal folds* (or *cords*). As the air jets through the narrow opening of the glottis, a time-varying pressure (i.e., a sound) is created that then propagates acoustically along the length of the vocal tract and emerges from the mouth or nose (or both). During its journey through the vocal tract, the tonal qualities of this sound wave are established, just as the length and width of an organ pipe determine the tone it generates. However,

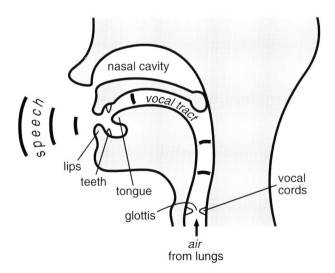

Figure 14.1. Cross section of the head, showing features of the vocal tract important for speech production. (Adapted from Pickett, 1980.)

unlike the organ pipe with its fixed dimensions, the vocal tract has different cross-sectional areas at different points along its length, dimensions that are under dynamic control. For instance, the position of the tongue determines tract areas in the region of the mouth. Thus we may compare the vocal tract to an organ pipe made up of many small sections connected end to end, each of which has a changeable length and shape.

The resulting speech wave has one of several basic types of tonality, depending on the state of the vocal cords. If, on the one hand, the two vocal cords are strongly tensed, they press together, closing the glottis—only momentarily, however, as lung pressure pushing on the abutting vocal cords soon forces some air between them, separating them again. Muscle tension and aerodynamic pressures quickly re-close the gap; the cycle then rapidly repeats, over and over again. Hence in this tensed state of the vocal cords, the glottis is rhythmically opened and closed, a vibration that creates a quasi-periodic, pulsed pressure wave at the base of the vocal tract. (Making the "Bronx cheer" is analogous.) These repetitively pulsed (or "voiced") sounds are used to utter vowels and some consonants (e.g., /v/ and /z/).

If, on the other hand, the cords are held just slightly open, the air rushing between them creates turbulence, and a noisy wind-in-the-trees sort of sound is thereby produced (as when blowing out birthday candles). Actually, this noisy pressure wave can be created anywhere along the vocal tract if the local cross-sectional area is made narrow enough to produce air turbulence. The sounds produced by such turbulence do not have regularly recurring peaks and so are known as "unvoiced" sounds. They are used for the production of many consonants (e.g., /f/ and /s/) and in whispered speech.

There are also two other recognized modes of vocal tract excitation, the more prominent of which is designated "breathy." This mode, not uncommon among women, can be thought of as a combination of the two just described: partially touching vocal folds result in the simultaneous presence of both turbulent ("unvoiced") and pulsed ("voiced") excitation. The fourth mode, known as "modal," occurs when the vocal folds are only lightly touching along their entire length (Stevens, 1981).

Vowel Sounds

Let us assume that the glottal-pressure pulse train is periodic with a period equal to T (Fig. 14.2), the reciprocal of which yields the "fundamental" frequency, F_0. Fourier series analysis shows that this pulse train waveform is composed of only a limited number of frequencies, the fundamental frequency and its harmonics (see Fig. 2.3). An idealized version of this frequency spectrum, for a fundamental frequency of 100 Hz, is shown in the bottom-left panel of Figure 14.2. The strongest component is the fundamen-

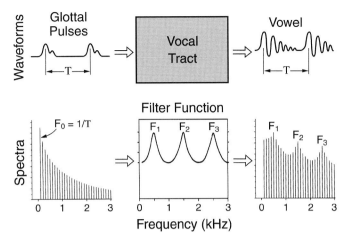

Figure 14.2. Production of the vowel "uh" according to the dominant acoustic theory. *Top row*: Acoustic waveforms that occur at the glottis (left) and in the emitted vowel (right). *Bottom row*: In corresponding graphs are the spectra of those two waveforms, along with the frequency-filtering function of the vocal tract (middle). The filter imprints its signature on the smooth spectrum of the glottal-pulse waveform. Sound radiation from the mouth (not included in the "vocal tract" filter function) affected final vowel spectrum. (*Bottom row*: From Pickett, 1980, with permission.*)

tal frequency, and the amplitudes of the harmonics decrease monotonically from that point at a rate of about -12 dB/octave.

As this pulsed sound wave makes its way through the vocal tract, its frequency spectrum is modified (e.g., the wave is "filtered"). Because of various tract resonances some components are attenuated more than others, as in an organ pipe. An idealization of the filter function of the vocal tract when configured for the vowel "uh" (as in the phrase "a h*u*t") is shown in Figure 14.2 (lower middle). The peaks in this filter function, called "formants," are the acoustic fingerprint of the vocal tract when uttering this particular vowel. In this sketch, the first three of these formants (labeled F1, F2, and F3, respectively) occur at 500, 1500, and 2500 Hz. Other vowels have formants of different frequencies.

The spectrum of the resulting speech signal is shown in Figure 14.2 (lower right). Because of the filtering action of the vocal tract, the peaks in the speech spectrum's profile now occur at (or close to[2]) the formants of the vocal tract's filter function. The frequencies of these peaks can usually be used to identify the vowels, although ambiguities do arise. Vowel identification in those cases is aided by other factors, such as "pitch" (see below).

Consonant Sounds

Consonants, in the English language at least, are a varied lot. Some are voiced (e.g., /v/) and some are unvoiced (e.g., /f/). Some are caused by partially obstructing the vocal tract (as for /s/), some by total closure followed by abrupt reopening (as for /d/). Still others reroute some of the sound energy through the nasal passages (as for /m/ and /n/). We have room in this chapter to consider only a small sample of such sounds.

RESPONSES TO VOWEL SOUNDS

Discharge Rate Encoding

Vowel sounds presented to the mammalian ear are encoded along both of the dimensions known for the representation of low-frequency signals: spike rate and synchrony (see Chapter 12). A prime example of spike rate encoding is given in Figure 14.3, which plots the average discharge rates of a large set of primary neurons responding to the vowel "eh" (as in "head"), as a function of the neurons' respective characteristic frequencies. At a low sound level, the peaks in the response rate profile (Fig. 14.3C) correspond closely with the vowel's formants (Fig. 14.3A, vertical lines). At a higher sound level, that of normal speech (Fig. 14.3B), the peaks in the response rate profile have pretty much washed out (Fig. 14.3D) due in part to the large number of neurons driven into saturation.

Careful examination of Figure 14.3D shows that across-the-board saturation did not apply to the low-spontaneous neurons. Even at this sound level (and higher), their rate profile has two clear peaks that align roughly with the first two formants. Thus whether at low or moderately high intensities at least some groups of primary neurons are able to encode vowel formants with their rate profiles. This ability to encode level differences at high intensities illustrates, in a concrete way, the virtue of the extended dynamic ranges exhibited by low-spontaneous primary neurons. You may recall that this capability was purchased at the expense of reduced sensitivity (see Fig. 12.6A). For instance, some of these neurons were negligibly excited by the higher formants when the vowel was presented at the lower sound level (Fig. 14.3C).

Although not so obvious, the responses of Figure 14.3 also show evidence of strong automatic gain control. For example, the vowel's second formant is about 16 dB smaller in amplitude (a factor of 6) than the first formant (Fig. 14.3A,B), yet the amplitudes of the corresponding peaks in the neural rate profiles are nearly equal (they differed by less than a factor of 2 at all intensities used). It seems that amplitude per se is not nearly as important

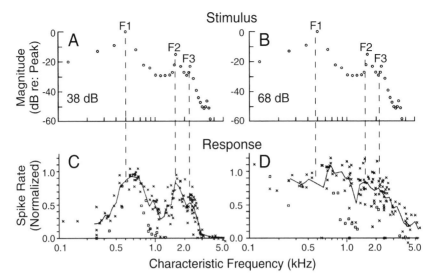

Figure 14.3. Discharge-rate responses of cat primary auditory neurons to the vowel "eh" presented at two sound levels. *A,B.* Spectrum of the vowel, with formants (F1–F3) at 38 dB SPL (*A*) and 68 dB SPL (*B*). *C,D.* Corresponding "driven" discharge-rate responses of a large family of primary neurons, plotted according to respective characteristic frequency. Responses were normalized to estimated value of maximum driven response rate evokable by respective characteristic-frequency tones. *C.* Ensemble of discharge rates evoked by the 38 dB vowel. The peaks in the responses of the high-spontaneous and medium-spontaneous neurons (x with solid-line average) accurately represent the vowel's formant frequencies. *D.* Ensemble of discharge rates evoked by the 68 dB vowel. Although the group of high-spontaneous and medium-spontaneous neurons no longer encoded the formant frequencies (solid-line average), the ensemble of low-spontaneous neurons (squares) still showed one peak near F1 and another near F2 and F3. (From Sachs and Young, 1979, with permission.*)

to the cochlea as are local amplitude *differences* (i.e., the differences between a peak and its adjacent troughs). We encounter this automatic gain control throughout our consideration of speech responses, though in a subliminal fashion: The amplitudes of the acoustic stimuli are plotted on logarithmic (decibel) scales, whereas the magnitudes of the neural response rates are plotted on linear scales.

Discharge Synchrony Encoding

In addition to setting the average values of the neural discharges, vowel stimuli dictate the temporal cadences of those firings. This entrainment is strikingly illustrated in Figure 14.4A, which contains the massed responses of primary neurons in the process of responding to the vowel in the syllable

Responses

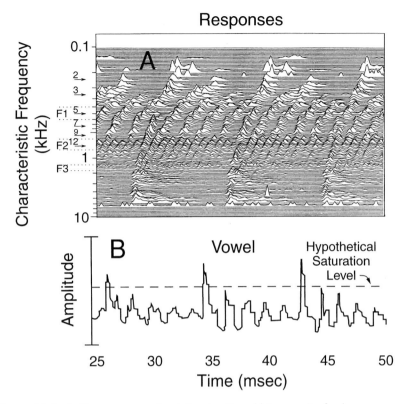

Figure 14.4. *A.* The responses (poststimulus time histograms) of a large group of primary auditory neurons evoked by a segment of the vowel in the syllable /da/, arranged vertically according to the respective characteristic frequency, top to bottom. Various harmonics of the fundamental frequency are indicated on the ordinate, as are the frequency ranges of the vowel's three formants. *B.* The acoustic waveform of that vowel segment. Note the increasing delays with which the primary neurons, from base to apex, responded to the vowel's main peaks. The hypothetical saturation intensity for high-spontaneous neurons is shown by dotted line. (Vowel waveform: From Miller and Sachs, 1983, with permission.* Neural data: From Shamma, 1985, with permission.*)

/da/ (Fig. 14.4B). A three-dimensional plot, Figure 14.4A contains the responses of hundreds of neurons, ordered vertically according to their respective characteristic frequencies (lowest at the top).

Among the vast amount of information contained in this plot, several patterns stand out. First, the vowel's basic glottal-pulse period (8.3 msec) is strongly represented in two groups of neurons, those with high characteristic frequencies (bottom traces) and those with very low ones (top traces). This response pattern is expected for the low-frequency group of neurons because they were situated in the extreme apex of the cochlea and thereby received only the syllable's lowest frequency component (i.e., the fundamental frequency). The strongly cadenced responses of the neurons tuned to high frequencies are perhaps unanticipated. These response shapes can be accounted for by the pulsatile waveform of the vowel waveform. Its main peaks evidently stimulated the basal region of the cochlea in a manner similar to that of a train of clicks (see Chapter 13, Responses to Clicks).

Another feature of the responses in Figure 14.4 is the manner in which one or another of the various glottal-pulse harmonics captured the discharge cadences of a group of primary neurons (see Chapter 13, Responses to Pairs of Tones). For example, those whose characteristic frequencies were in the broad range from 500 to 1000 Hz synchronized primarily to the vowel's first formant (ca. 600 Hz: the fifth harmonic), whereas neurons tuned to frequencies near the second formant (ca. 1.3 kHz) discharged in steady synchrony with the appropriate glottal-pulse harmonic (11th or 12th). By contrast, neurons with characteristic frequencies in the vicinity of the third formant (2.4 kHz) generated damped oscillations of that approximate frequency on each glottal pulse. This dominance of neural cadences by single harmonics is likely aided by the mutual suppressions the various harmonic components exert on each other (see Chapter 13, Responses to Pairs of Tones).

Because human subjects can almost always identify a vowel on the basis of its first two formants (Lieberman, 1977), although the third formant is also of use when it is present, just the basic synchronies of the neural discharges in Figure 14.4A alone most likely provide us with the information we need for perceptual recognition of this vowel. This temporal encoding of vowels, when combined with its spatial encoding (e.g., Fig. 14.3), produces a robust transmission of information regarding formant frequencies.

Encoding of the Glottal Pulse Period

The perceptual "pitch" of vowel sounds is due to the quasiperiodic nature of their waveforms. This basic periodicity, which is important for word identification (e.g., in Mandarin Chinese) and intonation (e.g., in English), is encoded in the discharge cadences of virtually all responding neurons regardless of characteristic frequency; not only do primary neurons tuned to both high and very low frequencies tend to fire in direct synchrony with the glottal pulses (Fig. 14.4), the ensemble of primary neurons collectively carries information on the fundamental periodicity in their response waveforms, extractable by several analysis methods (e.g., Miller and Sachs, 1984; Geisler and Silkes, 1991). How these various cues are used to determine musical pitch is still a matter of heated debate (Lyon and Shamma, 1996).

Comparisons between the discharges of various classes of primary neurons indicate that the neurons with "lower" spontaneous rates (< 20/sec) generally signal this basic glottal-pulse periodicity more strongly and robustly than do the high-spontaneous neurons (Geisler and Silkes, 1991). It appears that this enhanced ability of the lower-spontaneous neurons is related to their much wider dynamic ranges. As a consequence, they are able to register clearly the main peaks in the vowel waveform with increased discharge rates, whereas the high-spontaneous neurons often cannot, their spike rates having become saturated at lesser amplitudes (e.g., at the dashed line in Fig. 14.4B).

RESPONSES TO CERTAIN "VOICELESS" CONSONANTS

Consonants formed by nearly occluding the vocal tract at locations above the vocal cords are known as "fricatives." This important class of consonants includes voiced consonants such as /z/ and /v/ and voiceless ones such as /s/ and /f/. Frequency spectra of the latter pair of consonants are shown in the top row of Figure 14.5. Composed mostly of high-frequency energy, the peaks (formants) of these two spectra occur at different frequencies. The

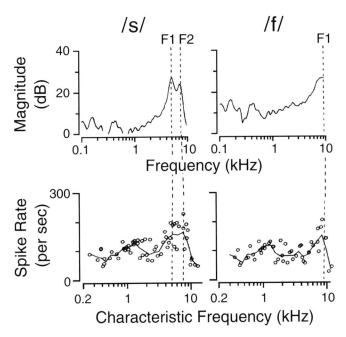

Figure 14.5. Discharge rate responses of primary auditory neurons to the fricative consonants /s/ and /f/. *Top.* Spectra of the two consonants, with formants labeled. *Bottom.* Corresponding steady-state discharge rates of a family of primary neurons, plotted according to their respective characteristic frequencies. For both syllables the peaks in the response-rate profile encode formant frequencies. (From Delgutte and Kiang, 1984a, with permission.*)

spectra of the voiced counterparts (/z/ and /v/) are similar, but with much more low-frequency energy (Delgutte and Kiang, 1984a).

Appropriately aligned at the bottom of Figure 14.5 are the pooled responses of a large group of primary neurons stimulated separately by each of these two syllables. Arranged by the respective characteristic frequencies of the neurons, these response profiles clearly show that, as in the case of vowels, the neurons that responded most vigorously to each sound were the ones tuned most closely to one of its formant frequencies. The consistency of such behavior across neurons and across animals is such that we can tell, with just a glance at the response-rate profiles in the bottom row, which consonant was sounded.

Several important consequences of the high-frequency content of these consonants deserve mention. First, because these formants are in the 5- to 10-kHz range they are in the frequency region most severely compromised in many hearing-impaired listeners (see Chapter 16). Thus such hearing-impaired people have trouble understanding words containing these consonants, although information distinguishing them does exist at lower frequencies (in the structures of the vowel sounds that either immediately precede or follow them). Second, as the frequencies passed through telephone lines are nominally limited to the band between 0.3 and 3.2 kHz, the formant frequencies of neither of these syllables would reach the far end of a telephone line, making it difficult for a normally hearing listener to tell them apart. Is it any wonder that telephone communications are so easily misunderstood?

CLASS OF USEFUL MODELS

Many of the attributes of primary-neuron responses to speech sounds, such as the data in Figures 14.3–14.5, can be accounted for *qualitatively* by the class of models depicted in Figure 14.6. In these models the output of each

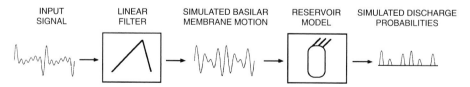

Figure 14.6. Simple two-stage model of cochlear processing useful with low-frequency signals. The first stage filters; and, roughly speaking, the second stage provides automatic gain control. (From Geisler and Greenberg, 1986, with permission.*)

neuron is calculated using basically two stages. The first stage through which the signal passes is a filter stage, one whose filter function is appropriate for the neuron's location (see Chapter 5). The waveform leaving the filter is then passed through a stage that represents the properties of the hair cell–afferent neuron synapse.

After its introduction decades ago (e.g., Weiss, 1966; Siebert, 1968), numerous variations on this basic model have been developed. For the filter stage, models of cochlear partition mechanics are used (see Chapter 9). Some have linear filter functions (e.g., Deng and Geisler, 1987), and others incorporate nonlinear features (e.g., Carney, 1993). Moreover, these filter functions can be set to match physiological frequency tuning data (e.g., Jenison et al., 1991) or perceptual ("psychoacoustic") data (e.g., Patterson et al., 1992). The synapse stage of the model also has many representations (see Chapter 11). Sometimes only one neurotransmitter reservoir is used, though multiple reservoirs are generally superior. Input–output curves of the inner hair cells are also included in some models.

A few models have even been developed to the point where they are available in computer "toolboxes" (Slaney, 1994). Regardless of their complexity, these models are known to be imperfect. First, most cannot generate any longitudinal effects, such as "high-side" suppression (but see Lyon and Mead, 1988). Nevertheless, this class of models usually provides a reasonable first approximation to the responses of a living primary neuron excited by speech. (For a sampling of current modeling efforts, see Ainsworth and Greenberg, in press.)

RESPONSES TO CONSONANT–VOWEL COMBINATIONS (SYLLABLES)

Spectrogram

The responses to speech of a single primary neuron can be plotted as an ordinary (two-dimensional) amplitude–time waveform, as demonstrated by *each* trace included in Figure 14.4A. The frequency components of such waveforms are difficult to determine from such plots (one winds up counting peaks). We could obtain this frequency information by doing a Fourier analysis on each waveform, but then we would wind up with *four* dimensions —amplitude, frequency, initial phase, and time[3]—three if we ignore phase (which is rarely important in speech perception). There are several ways to plot these three dimensions on a two-dimensional page. One with which we are all familiar is used in sheet music. As seen in Figure 14.7A, each written note gives the tonal frequency to be presented and the time (in measures)

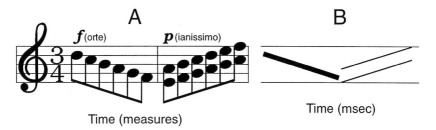

Figure 14.7. Multitonal variable-frequency waveform with standard music notation (*A*) and a spectrogram (*B*). The axes in both *A* and *B* are tonal frequency and time. Strength of tone is denoted either with a symbol (music) or by the darkness of the line (spectrogram).

of its occurrence. The amplitude of the tone is given in written additions: *f* for *forte* (loud), *p* for *pianissimo* (very soft), and so.

A somewhat related display, the *spectrogram*, is traditionally used for hearing and speech research. As with sheet music, the frequency is presented vertically, and time runs horizontally. However, the spectrogram encodes amplitude directly into the plot, as the *darkness* of the traces. Thus the ''forte'' describing the first measure in the sheet music example (Fig. 14.7A) translates into the dark trace in the first half of the spectrogram (Fig. 14.7B), and the ''pianissimo'' becomes the faintness of the two following traces. We regularly encounter this type of three-dimensional plot in other fields. It is used, for instance, in geographical (or weather) maps, where the color, or shading, of an area gives its height (or temperature).

Responses

We have already been introduced to the responses of primary neurons to vowels in Figure 14.4 but were not able to consider accurately the temporal encoding contained in those responses. Equipped with the spectrogram, we are now in a position to do so.

The pressure waveform of the syllable /tu/ is shown in Figure 14.8A. This syllable began with a small pressure pulse caused by the abrupt opening of the totally closed vocal tract. For the first 60 msec following this ''release'' ''unvoiced'' excitation of the vocal tract produced a low-level noisy waveform, after which ''voicing'' commenced and the waveform became much larger and quasirepetitive.

The spectrogram of this syllable (Fig. 14.8B) is shown immediately below the pressure waveform, aligned with it in time. For the first 60 msec, the noisy and high-frequency nature of the syllable's unvoiced segment is reflected in the more intense (darker) but mostly featureless nature of the area

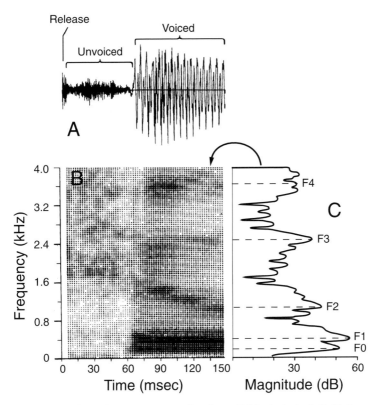

Figure 14.8. Creation of a spectrogram for the syllable /tu/. *A*. Syllable's acoustic waveform; the vowel (voicing) starts at about 70 msec. *C*. Frequency spectrum of a 12.8 msec segment of the syllable centered around the 136 msec mark, with vowel formants labeled. This spectrum is represented by the indicated vertical line in the spectrogram, with the height of the amplitude encoded by the darkness of the line. *B*. Spectrogram. (From Carney and Geisler, 1986, with permission.*)

above 1.6 kHz. When the voicing began at about 70 msec, the picture changed abruptly. Two dark bands suddenly appeared at the bottom of Figure 14.8B, the lowest of which is the "fundamental frequency," F_0. Horizontal striations are also apparent throughout this latter half of the spectrogram, each of which corresponds to one of the higher harmonics of the glottal-pulse train. Four vowel formants are plainly visible, each marked on the spectral "snapshot" pulled out of the spectrogram at the 136-msec point (Fig. 14.8C). Once identified in the vowel segment, the various formants can be easily tracked throughout the whole syllable, the second formant dropping with elapsed time while the third rises.

The responses of three primary neurons to this syllable /tu/ are shown in Figure 14.9A–C in spectrogram form.[4] Each response can be qualitatively

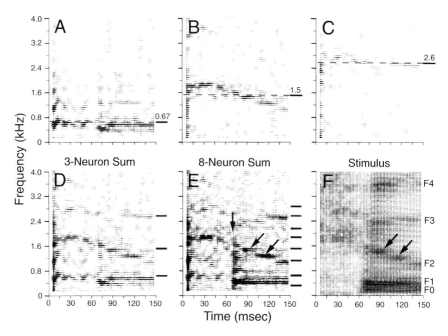

Figure 14.9. Responses of high-spontaneous primary neurons in the cat to the syllable /tu/. $A-C$. Response spectrograms of three individual neurons, with respective characteristic frequencies marked by short bars and dashed lines. Note that the frequency content of each response is largely confined to a narrow band encompassing the characteristic frequency. D. Summed spectrogram of the three neurons in $A-C$. E. Summed response spectrogram of eight primary neurons; their evenly spaced characteristic frequencies are marked by bars on the right ordinate. Note its striking similarity to the stimulus spectrogram (F). (From Carney and Geisler, 1986, with permission.*)

accounted for with the model of Figure 14.6. In particular, the filter stage correctly predicts that each neuron will respond only to frequency components near its characteristic frequency, which is given in each case and marked with a bar and dashed line at the appropriate frequency (height).

In its turn, the synapse (automatic gain control) stage of the model predicts that the amplitude variations of each neural response will be much less than those of the stimulus. Such is the case for all three neurons. Most obviously, the large differences in low-frequency acoustic energy between the unvoiced and voiced segments of the stimulus (Fig. 14.9F) are hardly recognizable in the responses of the 670 Hz neuron (Fig. 14.9A).

To get some idea of the totality of information the central nervous system receives from the periphery in response to this syllable, we need some way to present response spectrograms for the whole set of primary fibers. There is no reasonable way to form such four-dimensional plots, only various abstractions. Here the spectrograms of the various primary neurons are simply added, a process that discards some information (e.g., which neurons encoded which frequency components) but retains overall frequency content. The combination of the three spectrograms (Fig. 14.9A–C) is given in Figure 14.9D, and the sum of eight individual spectrograms (from neurons with evenly spaced characteristic frequencies) is plotted in Figure 14.9E.

Comparisons between the latter neural spectrogram and that of the stimulus (Fig. 14.9F) show that the neurons captured the frequency characteristics of the stimulus in amazing detail, even following the second formant ($F2$) as it dropped from one glottal-pulse harmonic to the next in the ''voiced'' segment (slanted arrows). This ability to follow such abrupt frequency transitions is due to the rapid response capabilities of the primary neurons (see Chapter 13, Responses to Modulated Tones). We can also see that the automatic gain control properties of the neurons were quite effective. The large difference in amplitude between the voiced and unvoiced acoustic segments was mostly reduced to the synchronized ''onset'' responses (Fig. 14.9E, vertical arrow) that were generated at the beginning of the vowel by the neurons with characteristic frequencies below 2 kHz.

Unmentioned so far is the fact that all of the primary neurons featured in Figure 14.9 had high spontaneous rates. The responses of neighboring neurons with lower rates of spontaneous activity behaved differently, as seen in Figure 14.10. Figure 14.10A,B illustrates the fact that some low-spontaneous neurons tended to respond to one segment of the syllable or the other but not to both. These low-spontaneous neurons had lower sensitivities and so responded significantly only when a fair bit of energy fell within their re-

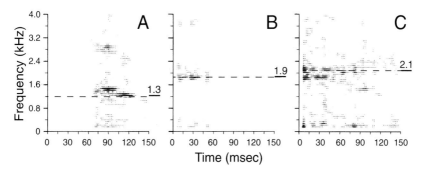

Figure 14.10. Response spectrograms of lower-spontaneous primary neurons stimulated with the syllable /tu/, in the same format as that in Figure 14.9A–C. Note the differential sensitivity to the syllable's two segments. (From Carney and Geisler, 1986, with permission.*)

spective filter passbands. When that energy was present only at the beginning of the syllable, it was registered (as in Fig. 14.10B). If that energy appeared only later, during the vowel, the response also came later (Fig. 14.10A). The net result is that the low-spontaneous neurons tended to segregate the stimulus segments more clearly than did their high-spontaneous companions. The responses of medium-spontaneous neurons, as always, are somewhat intermediate in nature (Fig. 14.10C).

It might be wondered why the simple model of Figure 14.6 is apparently so successful in modeling primary-neuron responses to speech. Part of the answer is that the frequency tuning properties of an apical neuron, such as that of Figure 14.9A, do not vary greatly with stimulus level (e.g. Fig. 13.4) and so are moderately well represented by the model's linear filter.[5] Nevertheless, it has been demonstrated that the level-dependent aspects of their frequency tuning must be included in models of apical neurons if accurate predictions of the response *waveforms* to stimuli of different intensities are desired (Carney and Yin, 1988). What about the effects of the suppressive factors known to be present (see Chapter 13, Responses to Pairs of Tones)? They are there but are inconspicuous in the qualitative comparisons we have been making. For example, the failure of most neurons with characteristic frequencies above 1.5 kHz to reach saturation discharge levels during stimulation with the vowel "eh" presented at a normal speaking intensity (Fig. 14.3D) appears to result from "low-side" suppression exerted by the strong frequency components that occurred in the vicinity of the vowel's first formant (Sachs and Young, 1979). Suppression may also have aided the various formants in dominating the discharge synchrony of neurons in their respective cochlear regions (Fig. 14.4A).

RESPONSES TO SYLLABLES IN NOISE

Speech seldom occurs in quiet. It is almost always just one of many sounds in a person's environment. If these other sounds ("noises") are loud enough, we know from experience that understanding speech becomes impossible. Why? Why do hearing-impaired people, with or without hearing aids, have especially difficult times carrying on conversations in noisy situations? For insights into the physiological causes of these phenomena, the responses of primary neurons to sounds that combine speech and noise are useful.

Some samples of primary-neuron responses to noisy speech are shown in Figure 14.11. The stimulus in this case was again the syllable /tu/, but this time it was presented along with various levels of noise. At the lowest level of noise (when the "signal-to-noise ratio"[6] was 30 dB), the syllable's acoustic waveform was virtually uncontaminated, as seen in its time waveform

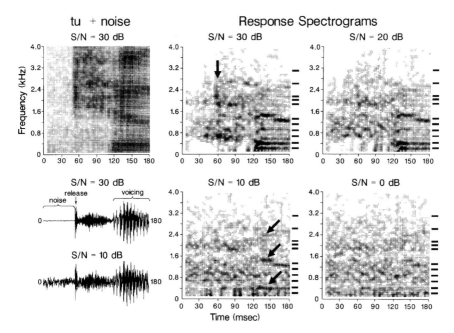

Figure 14.11. Responses of high-spontaneous primary neurons to the syllable /tu/ embedded in various levels of noise having a speech-shaped spectrum. *A.* Spectrogram of the stimulus with a signal-to-noise ratio (S/N) of 30 dB (stimulus waveform is the top trace in *D*). *B.* Summed response spectrogram of 11 high-spontaneous primary neurons to that syllable. The arrow points to their collective ''onset'' responses. Characteristic frequencies are marked by bars on the right ordinate. The other response spectrograms for these neurons (*C, E,* F) are for successively higher noise levels. (From Geisler and Gamble, 1989, with permission.*)

(Fig. 14.11D, top trace) and in its spectrogram (Fig. 14.11A). Yet the summed-response spectrogram of primary neurons with high spontaneous rates (Fig. 14.11B) shows that they responded strongly to the noise—so strongly in fact that the neural spectrogram barely marks the onset of the syllable (arrow). For these high-spontaneous neurons, even that lowest level of noise forced discharge rates toward saturation and almost obliterated (''masked'') the responses to the syllable's unvoiced segment.

As the rest of Figure 14.11 shows, the synchronized response components generated by the syllable became progressively eliminated as the noise level was increased. At a signal-to-noise ratio of 10 dB, the time waveform of the syllable still seemed only mildly affected (Fig. 14.11D, bottom trace). The summed neural response (Fig. 14.11E), however, is dominated by noise, registering only the vowel's formants (arrows). Even the formants are almost completely lost when the noise level is made equal to that of the vowel (Fig. 14.11F). Similar findings were reached in a study using pure vowels as the speech stimuli (Delgutte and Kiang, 1984b).

It is instructive to consider the mechanisms by which the noise captures the discharge synchrony of the primary neurons. Central is the "line busy" effect, due simply to the tendency of an afferent neuron to fire on the positive peaks of its hair cell's receptor potential. Visualize, for instance, the result of a peak in the noise waveform. If it should evoke a spike, the primary neuron would enter a refractory state and so would be unlikely to respond to either noise or syllable for the next few milliseconds. Thus the noise peak would have effectively blanked out a short segment of the syllable for that neuron. The greater the noise intensity, the more often would noise peaks determine the moments of discharge and the ensuing blanking periods. In short, the primary neurons tend to be "peak pickers," allowing relatively weak signals to be completely masked by stronger noise (see Fig. 11.7). Suppression, the other known factor in the power struggle between two competing waveforms (Delgutte, 1990), probably plays a secondary role in this case.

As might be expected from their wider dynamic ranges, primary neurons with lower spontaneous rates are more tolerant of the noise. Roughly speaking, they can take about 10 dB more noise than the high-spontaneous neurons before showing comparable degrees of syllable "masking" at normal voice levels (Silkes and Geisler, 1991). Those figures indicate that some syllable information (primarily about vowel formants) is successfully transmitted by these less-sensitive neurons even when the noise is of the same intensity as the vowel.

Taking these responses of cat primary neurons to reflect at least qualitatively what is going on in human ears, we would predict that consonant syllables of this type would be perceived correctly in noise of all levels up to and perhaps including that of equality with the vowels. Unfortunately, it is difficult to compare this prediction with perceptual performances because varying noise spectra were generally employed in the relevant studies. For instance, in the classic psychoacoustic study that presented consonant–vowel syllables in noise, correct identifications were made about 45% of the time when a signal-to-noise ratio of 0 dB was used (Wang and Bilger, 1973). The agreement of results in the two studies is pleasingly close, yet differences in the noise spectra[6] used suggest caution. Reassuringly, about that same performance level was reached in the study of Plomp and Mimpen (1979), who presented a group of young adult subjects with everyday Dutch sentences embedded in a noise whose spectrum was similar to that of the physiological study. The 50%-correct level in that study lay at a noise level about equal to that of the vowels.

SUMMARY

The inner ear of mammals has the ability to encode, in a robust fashion, the aspects of speech that are important to human perception (Delgutte, 1997). Syllable onsets are clearly marked (sometimes by low-spontaneous neurons if not by the high-spontaneous neurons); formants are accurately tracked (even through rapid transitions); glottal-pulse periods are recorded in particularly robust fashion; and the spectral profiles of both consonants and vowels are faithfully reproduced.

Whether in quiet or in noise, even in whispers (Voight et al., 1982), the encoding of the identifying features of speech by primary auditory neurons remains strong. The mammalian ear, it seems, is well attuned to speech sounds.

NOTES

1. Useful as it is when accounting for the general aspects of speech signals, the acoustic theory of speech production is known to overlook significant nonlinear processes (Teager and Teager, 1990).

2. We follow the widespread custom of referring, somewhat inaccurately, to the major peaks in the spectral profile of a vowel as its "formants." A formant, by definition, however, characterizes the vocal tract. Thus a vowel's spectral peak occurs exactly at a formant frequency *only* when one of the harmonic components of the glottal-pulse waveform happens to fall there (e.g., the fifth harmonic of a glottal-pulse waveform would coincide exactly with a formant frequency of 500 Hz only if its fundamental frequency were 100 Hz, not 90 or 110 Hz). For our purposes, this distinction is insignificant.

3. In its formal definitions, Fourier analysis applies to infinitely long waveforms. Although "windowing" procedures for the treatment of shorter records have been developed, what does one do with waveforms such as speech, whose basic tonality varies with time? There are several methods available. One is to use "short-time" Fourier analysis, applied in a manner not unlike the making of a motion picture. That is, the waveform is chopped up into a sequence of short segments, or "windows," and Fourier analysis is then applied sequentially to each segment as if *its* particular frequency content were unvarying (resulting in spectra such as that of Fig. 14.8C). When the resulting spectra are displayed together in their temporal sequence, as in Fig. 14.8B, a display of frequency change with time is achieved.

4. The procedure for forming these neural spectrograms is identical to that used for making stimulus spectrograms, except that a *linear* amplitude-to-darkness scale is used with poststimulus time histograms instead of the *logarithmic* scale used with acoustic stimuli.

5. Recall that one attribute of linear filters is their complete indifference to stimulus intensity: their frequency tuning is the same for all signals, no matter what the magnitudes are.

6. The signal-to-noise ratio in the study of Figure 14.11 was defined as the ratio (expressed in decibels) of the root mean square sound pressure level of the syllable's vowel divided by that of the noise. Because of the properties of logarithms, this ratio is also simply the *difference* in the sound pressure levels of the vowel and the noise, each expressed in decibels. The physiological data of Figure 14.11 and the psychoacoustic data of Plomp and Mimpen (1979) were obtained with noises having the same average amplitude spectrum as speech; Wang and Bilger (1973) used "white noise."

15

FEEDBACK FROM THE CENTRAL NERVOUS SYSTEM

We have followed the acoustic signal step by step through the auditory periphery, from pinna to primary afferent neuron. We have considered enough of the myriad mechanisms involved to enable us to predict with some accuracy the neural responses to many types of acoustic stimuli. Regardless, the story is still incomplete, as the ear, though serving as the portal through which auditory information enters the brain, does not operate rigidly. Adaptable, the ear modifies itself in response to signals *from* the brain as well as sending information into it.

We have already considered one of the feedback systems, that of the middle ear muscles (see Chapter 4). From what we know, their function is mostly protective. They attenuate intense sounds, both externally and internally generated, on their way into the cochlea. Such protection is important, as intense sounds are known to cause temporary reductions in sensitivity as well as permanent damage if the intensities are high enough (see Chapter 16). The neural circuitry involved in this neuromuscular feedback system is still largely unknown, but a good start has been made with the identification of the motoneurons involved (Guinan et al., 1989).

The cochlea itself is also innervated by the central nervous system. Although the existence of this neural feedback has been known for more than 50 years (Rasmussen, 1946), an understanding of its functions has proved elusive. Although the evidence is still fragmentary, the picture coming into focus is that one of the principal missions of these cochlear efferent systems is to provide the primary afferent neurons with yet another form of gain control. Other roles are also suggested.

ANATOMY

Medial Olivocochlear System

As was indicated in Figure 11.2, the terminals of the efferent neurons are known to contact outer hair cells and afferent terminals directly. There is overwhelming evidence that the axons providing these terminals come from the auditory brain stem, in particular the superior olivary complex (for a review see Warr, 1992). The two distinct efferent systems known to serve each cochlea are shown in Figure 15.1, a cross-sectional (coronal) sketch of the brain stem. One of these systems arises from large cell bodies scattered near the bases of the bilateral brain stem nuclei known as the *medial superior olives*. Located on both sides of the midline, the neurons of the medial olivocochlear (MOC) system send their axons dorsally toward the fourth

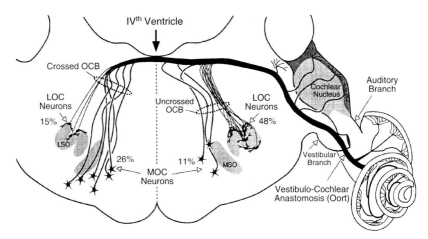

Figure 15.1. Origins and course of the olivocochlear bundle (OCB) innervating each cat cochlea, with respective percentages provided by the efferent groups given. The lateral olivocochlear (LOC) neurons have unmyelinated axons; the medial olivocochlear (MOC) neurons have myelinated axons. The efferent axons exit the brain stem in the vestibular branch of the VIII cranial nerve, cross to the auditory branch via the anastomosis of Oort, and enter the cochlea. The floor of the fourth ventricle (arrow) provides a convenient location for stimulating or recording from the crossed OCB. (From Warr, 1992, with permission.*)

ventricle where they join the *olivocochlear bundle* and head for one or the other of the two cochleas (or both). Most of these axons, all of which are myelinated, cross the midline and enter the vestibular branch of the VIII cranial nerve, finally arriving at the "contralateral" (opposite side) cochlea via a small branch (*anastomosis*) connecting the vestibular and auditory sections of the nerve.

Once inside the cochlea, the MOC axons synapse directly with the outer hair cells (see Fig. 11.5). As the number of these neurons (ca. 400–500 on each side in the cat) is so much smaller than the number of outer hair cells, extensive terminal branching is entailed. Even so, the axon terminations of any one MOC neuron innervate only a restricted cluster of outer hair cells, those located on a short sector of the cochlear partition whose length averages about 1.6 mm in the cat (Liberman and Brown, 1986). Recall that this span of the basal cochlear partition separates locations that differ in characteristic frequency by about half an octave (see Fig. 12.9). As shown on the left side of Figure 15.2, this terminal field of an MOC neuron tends to lie just basal to the origin of the primary afferent axons that drive (via several synapses) that particular MOC neuron (see below).

Lateral Olivocochlear System

The other set of cochlear efferent neurons, which in the cat number nearly twice as many as the MOC group, are located on the upper fringes of the nearby *lateral superior olives* (Fig. 15.1). Recent evidence indicates that the lateral olivocochlear (LOC) system is composed of two distinct groups of neurons, differing both in sites of origin and lengths of terminal arbor (Warr et al., 1997). One group is composed of small "intrinsic" neurons located within the lateral superior olive proper. The axon of each intrinsic neuron appears to terminate within a very small segment of the cochlea, providing a dense patch of synaptic connections, presumably with primary afferent axons (Fig. 15.2, right side). The other LOC group is made up of large "Shell" neurons which border the lateral superior olive. Typically the axon of each Shell neuron bifurcates within the cochlea, each branch joining the spiral axon bundle running under the inner hair cells (see Fig. 11.2) and innervating diffusely with numerous *en passant* synapses. Both types of LOC neurons have *un*myelinated axons.

The extent to which efferent axons (presumably of LOC neurons) also synapse *directly* with the inner hair cells is unclear. Most reports indicate that such axosomatic synapses are rare or nonexistent (e.g., Spoendlin, 1973; Kimura, 1975). Liberman (1980a) found only one such synapse in his serial electron micrographs of the cat cochlea. Nevertheless, one study of the guinea pig cochlea reported an average of seven to nine efferent synapses

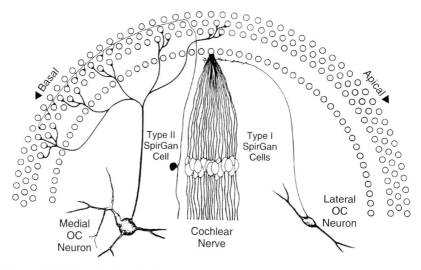

Figure 15.2. Hypothetical depiction of the afferent and efferent innervation related to a single mid-cochlear segment. Two types of afferent neurons (SpirGan) and two types of efferent neurons (OC) are tuned to the segment's frequency. Note the partial spatial overlap of the MOC efferent and type II afferent innervation patterns in the region immediately basal to the segment. The LOC neuron shown is of the ''intrinsic'' type. (From Warr, 1992, with permission.*)

on each inner hair cell (Hashimoto et al., 1990). Moreover, electron microscopic studies of cochleas obtained from young mice (12 days old) show a bewildering variety of efferent synapses, including ''triadic'' and ''reciprocal'' ones, which involve both the afferent axons and the inner hair cells (Sobkowicz et al., 1997). Thus at present the extent to which inner hair cells are under direct efferent control appears to be a function of species, perhaps even of age.

Functional Organization

The cat cochlea's complete afferent–efferent feedback system, displaying its truly bilateral nature, is sketched in Figure 15.3. The loops begin with the primary afferent neurons, which send their axons into the brain stem's *cochlear nucleus*, where they terminate in obligatory synapses. In the next link of the chain, cochlear nucleus neurons send their output into the bilateral superior olivary complexes. Finally, each cochlea receives at least some innervation from all four of the olivocochlear centers. At minimum, therefore, each feedback loop is composed of three neurons. The complete feedback system is no doubt much more complicated than this, as the superior

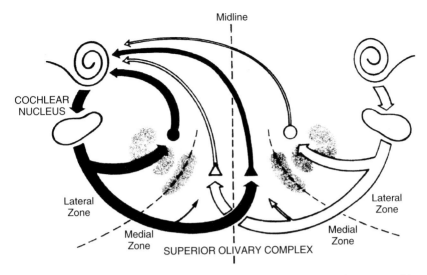

Figure 15.3. Binaural organization of the efferent system innervating one cochlea. Solid arrows and symbols represent pathways driven by acoustic stimulation of the ipsilateral cochlea. Open arrows and symbols represent the smaller pathways driven by the contralateral ear. A convergence of inputs from the two ears occurs in the medial zone. (From Warr, 1992, with permission.*)

olivary complex is known to receive descending innervation from higher brain stem centers such as the inferior colliculus (Vetter et al., 1993).

RESPONSES OF SINGLE EFFERENT NEURONS

By placing microelectrodes appropriately, the discharges of individual efferent neurons can be monitored at the point where their axons enter the cochlea (e.g., Liberman and Brown, 1986). Such axons, when labeled with tracer molecules, always have had their cell bodies in the MOC region. The conclusion is that all microelectrode recordings in the olivocochlear bundles have been from MOC axons. Because these axons are myelinated, like those of the type I primary afferent neurons, it follows that the responses of the *un*myelinated members of the feedback loops, the LOC efferent neurons and the type II primary afferent neurons (see Chapter 11), remain unmeasured. Their roles thus remain a mystery.

Electrophysiological experiments have shown that the MOC neurons are driven by acoustic stimuli, some nearly as readily as the primary afferent neurons, but in a somewhat complementary manner. Whereas first-order neurons discharge at random intervals (see Fig. 11.6), MOC neurons fire with almost clock-like regularity (Liberman and Brown, 1986). Moreover, whilst the response ranges of some primary afferent neurons are limited, sometimes only 20 dB in magnitude (see Chapter 12), MOC neurons respond over wide dynamic ranges. Typical are the rate-level curves of Figure 15.4. For the efferent neurons that had characteristic frequencies above 2 kHz (Fig. 15.4A), the curves generally did not show signs of saturation within the sound levels used. Those neurons with lower characteristic frequencies also had wide dynamic ranges, but with rates that typically saturated (Fig. 15.4B).

It seems worth mentioning that this particular combination of MOC attributes is ideally suited for the rapid, accurate signaling of stimulus intensity. In a sequence of regularly spaced spikes such as these neurons generate, a single interspike interval (e.g., of 25 msec) allows an estimate of sound level to be made (55 dB SPL for the neuron of Fig. 15.4A: follow the dashed line).

The term "characteristic frequency" used above with MOC neurons is appropriate, as they are indeed individually tuned to particular frequencies, with about half the frequency selectivity of comparable primary afferent neurons. Examples of MOC threshold tuning curves are shown in Figure 15.5 for two characteristic-frequency groups. The efferent neurons tuned to 10 kHz (Fig. 15.5B) even displayed the same type of "tail" region exhibited by basally located primary neurons (see Fig. 12.7D). The similarities be-

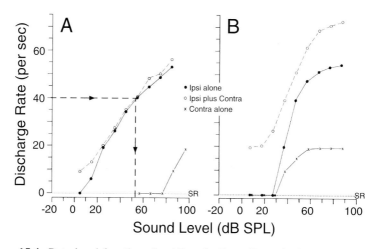

Figure 15.4. Rate-level functions for (*A*) an ipsilaterally excited MOC efferent neuron and (*B*) a binaurally excited one for tonal excitation at their respective characteristic frequencies. In the binaural case, only the level of the ipsilateral tone was varied. A discharge rate of 40 spikes/sec in *A* corresponds to a stimulating level of about 55 dB SPL (follow the dashed line). (From Liberman and Brown, 1986, with permission.*)

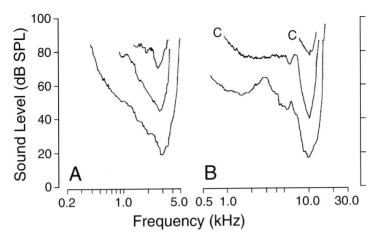

Figure 15.5. Frequency tuning curves of cat MOC efferent neurons from several animals grouped according to characteristic frequency. The curves marked with a C resulted from acoustic stimulation of the contralateral ear. Note the similarity to the corresponding curves of afferent neurons (see Fig. 12.7C,D). (From Liberman and Brown, 1986, with permission.*)

tween the afferent and efferent tuning curves imply that each MOC neuron traces its major excitation back to a highly restricted group of inner hair cells. Moreover, the terminal field of that MOC neuron tends to lie just basal to that small cluster of inner hair cells, the region believed to amplify the tones to which they are tuned (see Chapter 9).

In keeping with the bilateral anatomy of the MOC system, several of the curves in Figure 15.5 were produced with contralateral stimuli. Only about 30% of MOC neurons are driven monaurally by contralateral stimuli; most (about 60%) are driven monaurally only by ipsilateral sound. The remainder (ca. 10%) respond to monaural stimulation of either ear. Regardless of whether they are driven monaurally by contralateral stimuli, most MOC neurons have their responses to ipsilateral stimuli *enhanced* by the simultaneous presentation of sound to the other ear (Liberman, 1988). With binaural stimuli, discharge rates as high as 150 spikes/sec have been recorded (though most were less than 100 spikes/sec); rates only half that high were provoked with ipsilateral stimuli.

The MOC feedback system depicted in Figure 15.3, perhaps involving only a three-neuron loop of myelinated axons in a small region, seems built for speed. In fact, at high intensities the response latency of the MOC neurons can be less than 10 msec (Liberman and Brown, 1986). Brief as that is, it is much longer than the near-instantaneous onset of two-tone suppression exhibited by the primary afferent neurons (see Chapter 13), thereby eliminating the efferent system as a major factor in the early stages of that form of suppression. At most stimulus levels, MOC neuron latencies to acoustic stimulation are measured in tens of milliseconds.

COCHLEAR RESPONSES TO EFFERENT SYSTEM ACTIVATION

Effects of Electrical Stimulation

On Hair Cells

The portion of the olivocochlear bundle that crosses the midline in the floor of the fourth ventricle on its way to the contralateral cochlea provides investigators with a convenient site for intervention (Fig. 15.1, arrow). One experimental technique is to place electrodes on the ventricle floor directly over the bundle and stimulate it electrically. As crossing MOC axons make up the bulk of the bundle at that point, we expect the principal effects of such stimulation to be exerted on outer hair cells, known targets of the MOC efferent system. Unfortunately, intracellular recordings from these hair cells have not yet been obtained during deliberate efferent bundle stimulation.

Successful intracellular recordings *have* been made from acousticolateralis hair cells of several other vertebrates during stimulation of their efferent systems: in the fish lateral line (Flock and Russell, 1976), in the turtle cochlea (Art et al., 1984), and in the frog sacculus (Ashmore and Russell, 1982). In each case hyperpolarizing synaptic potentials were observed in the hair cells. There is a great deal of indirect evidence indicating that stimulation of the mammalian MOC system also produces hyperpolarizing potentials in outer hair cells.

Supporting this hypothesis are the intracellular recordings obtained from *inner* hair cells during electrical stimulation of the crossing efferent bundle (Fig. 15.6A). Few *direct* effects were observed, only small DC potentials, which seem to be field potentials generated by the outer hair cells (see below). Specifically, the DC potentials recorded just outside the inner hair cells (+0.5 to 2.0 mV) were generally larger than those obtained within those hair cells (0 to +1.5 mV), and there were no accompanying changes in their membrane resistances (Brown and Nuttall, 1984). These negative results are consistent with the known anatomy of the MOC efferent system, which does not include synapses with inner hair cells. Any existing axosomatic synapses of the unmyelinated LOC system on these inner hair cells either were unexcited by the electrical stimulation (unmyelinated axons have much higher thresholds for such stimulation than myelinated ones) (Fitzgerald and Woolf, 1981) or their effects were subtle.

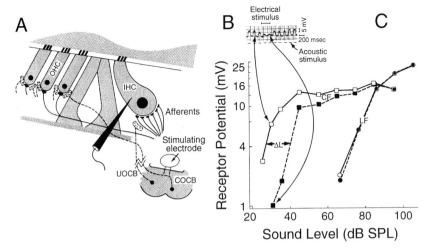

Figure 15.6. Suppression of an inner hair cell's (IHC) receptor potential by the efferent system. *A.* Simplified diagram of the cochlea and of the experimental setup. Crossed olivocochlear bundle (COCB) was electrically stimulated while the intra-cochlear potential of a single inner hair cell was monitored. OHC, outer hair cell; UOCB, uncrossed olivocochlear bundle. *B.* Intracochlear potential generated by repeated tone bursts at the hair cell's characteristic frequency (20 kHz). The COCB was stimulated in the middle of the record, as indicated. *C.* Hair cell's level-response curve for tonal stimulation was shifted to the right (Δ*L*) during efferent stimulation when a characteristic frequency (CF) tone was employed but not when a lower frequency (LF) of 12.4 kHz was used. (From Brown et al., 1983, with permission.*)

What the inner hair cell recordings did show was the selective attenuation of receptor potentials. One example is given in Figure 15.6B, the results of an experiment in which pure tones were presented simultaneously with the efferent stimulation. When the tone was presented at the characteristic frequency of the hair cell (20 kHz), the cell's receptor potential was strongly reduced by the efferent stimulation in a manner reminiscent of two-tone suppression; that is, the entire stimulus-response curve was shifted rightward to higher intensities, by an amount Δ*L* (Fig. 15.6C, CF curves). On the other hand, when acoustic stimulation of a lower frequency (12.4 kHz) was used, no change in receptor potentials was observed (Fig. 15.6C, LF curves). This differential sensitivity to efferent stimulation, combined with the failure to observe intracellular synaptic potentials, provides strong evidence for the conclusion that this type of efferent stimulation does not directly affect the inner hair cells.

On the contrary, the similarities between the efferent suppression of inner hair cells and their two-tone suppressions suggest a common mechanism: namely, loss of "gain" by the cochlear amplifier due to reductions in the transducer potentials of the *outer* hair cells. A similar hypothesis had been offered earlier to account for yet another effect of efferent stimulation, the modification of otoacoustic emissions (Mountain; 1980). At that time, before the motility of the outer hair cells had been discovered, the demonstration of a connection between efferent stimulation and emissions provided important support for the fledgling idea that the outer hair cells were somehow involved in cochlear mechanics.

On Primary Afferent Neurons

Demonstrated even earlier were the effects of efferent bundle stimulation on the responses of the cochlea's primary afferent neurons (Wiederhold and Kiang, 1970). Results of more recent versions of those early auditory nerve experiments are shown in Figure 15.7. In a manner that closely mimics the receptor potential suppressions seen in inner hair cells (Fig. 15.6C), the responses of primary afferent neurons to characteristic-frequency tones were reduced by the efferent stimulation (Fig. 15.7A). The familiar rightward "level shift" of the whole rate-level curve occurred (labeled ΔL in Fig. 15.7A) as well as a reduction (ΔR_M) in the neuron's maximum discharge rate. Some, but not all, of the latter reduction appears due to the long-term suppression effects mentioned in Chapter 13 (Responses to Pairs of Tones).

Particularly interesting is the dependence of the magnitude of suppression on the characteristic frequency of the neuron. As shown in Figure 15.7B,

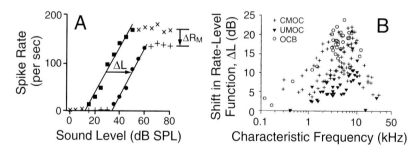

Figure 15.7. Suppression of the discharge rate of primary auditory neurons by the efferent system. *A.* Rate-level function for a single primary neuron with (+) and without (x) electrical stimulation of the MOC efferent system. Points on the rising phases of the curves, indicated by filled symbols, have been fitted with regression lines. The level shift ΔL was measured between those lines. The change in maximum rate ΔR_M is also indicated. *B.* Efferent-induced level shift ΔL displayed by a sample of 161 primary neurons, plotted as a function of their respective characteristic frequencies. Site of MOC stimulation is indicated by symbols: near cell bodies of crossed MOC system (CMOC), near cell bodies of uncrossed MOC system (UMOC), and at the midline of the fourth ventricle (OCB). (From Guinan and Guifford, 1988a, with permission.*)

neurons tuned to frequencies in the 4- to 7-kHz range showed the most suppression (level shift), up to 25 dB. Neurons tuned to either higher or lower frequencies exhibited less suppression; those innervating the extreme apex and base showed almost none. It is worth noting that to obtain these suppression magnitudes the electrical exciting pulses had to be presented at rates of 200/sec, well above the discharge rates evoked by even binaural acoustic stimuli in this same species (when anesthetized).

This spatial dependence of efferent suppression is illustrated in Figure 15.8, which shows the (threshold-level) frequency tuning curves for selected groups of primary afferent neurons, obtained with and without simultaneous efferent stimulation. The maximum suppressive effect was always obtained at or near the respective neuron's characteristic frequency. For basal neurons (i.e., those tuned to high frequencies) the suppression was largely confined to the tip region (Fig. 15.8, right columns), whereas for apical neurons similar magnitudes of suppression seemed to occur at all frequencies (Fig. 15.8, left columns). This pattern of efferent suppressions is similar to that of two-

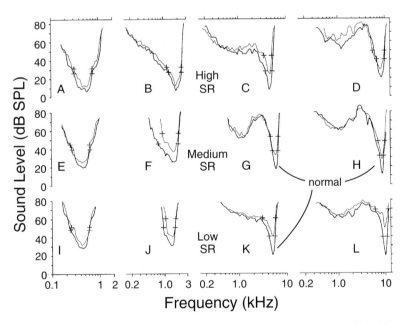

Figure 15.8. Examples of primary-neuron frequency tuning curves, with (thin top traces) and without (thick bottom traces) efferent activity. Data are segregated according to spontaneous rate (row) and characteristic frequency (column). Efferent activation was by electrical stimulation of the crossed olivocochlear bundle at the midline of the fourth ventricle. Points marked with "+" were used to make frequency selectivity (Q_{20}) measurements. (From Guinan and Gifford, 1988c, with permission.*)

tone suppressions (see Chapter 13), both types presumably dependent on the cochlear amplifier.

A line joining the average values of the threshold reductions caused by efferent suppression, normalized to the maximum level, is shown in Figure 15.9 (filled circles). That line has nearly the same shape as normalized curves showing the amount of MOC efferent innervation that exists at various points along the cochlea (Fig. 15.9, open circles), as judged by the total areas of the efferent synapses on all three rows of outer hair cells. This close agreement between the relative magnitudes of efferent suppression and the density of efferent synapses on the outer hair cells lends further strength to the reigning theory of cochlear mechanics, that outer hair cells are the engines of the cochlear amplifier (see Chapter 9).

As suggested by the data in Figure 15.8 (different rows were used for different spontaneous-rate classes), not all primary afferent neurons were equally affected by efferent stimulation. The quantitative comparisons of Figure 15.10 show that the neurons with the lowest spontaneous-discharge rates were the most strongly suppressed (Fig. 15.10, triangles). Not only were their suppressions largest in magnitude, they were the least affected by location within the cochlea. In addition, only members of the low-spontaneous class suffered large reductions in their maximum discharge rates

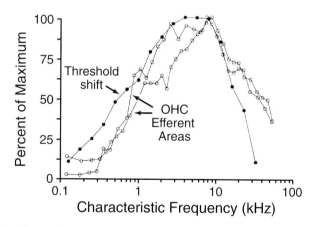

Figure 15.9. Comparison between the anatomical concentration and physiological effects of MOC efferents, in the cat. Plotted, as percent of maximum, are the average threshold shifts that occurred at characteristic frequency during maximum efferent stimulation displayed by a large sample of primary neurons (closed circles) and the total area of efferent terminals found below the cell nucleus on all three rows of outer hair cells in two ears (open circles). The data are plotted as functions of characteristic frequency, inferred for the anatomical data from the characteristic frequency/space map of the cat cochlea (see Fig. 12.9). (From Liberman et al., 1990, with permission.*)

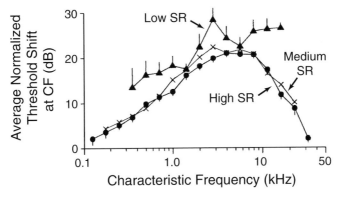

Figure 15.10. Average efferent-induced threshold shifts at characteristic frequency for a sample of 406 primary auditory neurons. Each point shows the average over an octave band of characteristic frequencies (adjacent points have half-octave overlaps). Data for neurons in each class of spontaneous rate (SR) are plotted separately, as indicated (error bars are shown for low-spontaneous and high-spontaneous neurons only). Note the extraordinary suppressibility of low-spontaneous neurons. Data were normalized to account for variations among animals. (From Guinan and Gifford, 1988c, with permission.*)

($\Delta R_m > 20\%$). As primary afferent neurons of all spontaneous-rate classes receive their innervation from the same inner hair cells, suppressive factors beyond those affecting the receptor potentials of these hair cells *must* have been at work on the low-spontaneous neurons (or their synapses). Recall that a similar conclusion was reached when considering two-tone suppression data (see Chapter 13).

In addition to the rapidly acting effects of efferent stimulation described above, much slower inhibitory effects with time constants lasting tens of seconds have been reported (Sridhar et al., 1995). These "slow" effects, which may be due to the build-up of Ca^{2+} ions within the outer hair cells (see below), seem to share the basic electrical and pharmacological characteristics of the fast effects.

As indicated in Chapter 14 (see Fig. 14.11), the presence of added noise can "mask" a primary neuron's responsiveness to a simultaneously occurring signal. Such masking occurs because the noise by itself causes a considerable discharge, about 130 spikes/sec in the example of Figure 15.11A (solid arrow), and reduces the primary neurons' maximum discharge rate down to about 280 spikes/sec, the latter probably through adaptation to the increased spike rate caused by the continuous stimulation. The combination of these two effects squeezes the neuron's remaining range of possible responses to the tone pip down to about 150 spikes/sec (i.e., to between 130 and 280 spikes/sec).

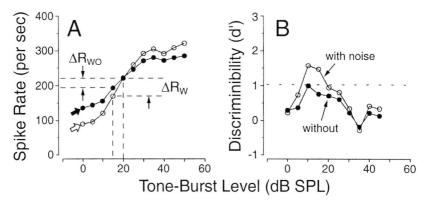

Figure 15.11. Effects of contralateral noise on the response of a single primary neuron to ipsilateral stimuli consisting of tone bursts of various levels and continuous ("masking") noise of a fixed intensity. *A.* Discharge rates measured during the tone burst, plotted as functions of tone burst level, with contralateral noise (open circles) and without it (closed circles). Note the increased dynamic range provided by the contralateral noise. A change in tone-burst level from 15 to 20 dB SPL would produce a larger rate change with the presence of contralateral noise (ΔR_{w}) than without it (ΔR_{wo}). *B.* Discriminability of 5 dB increments in tone-burst level, for the data in *A.* The dashed line indicates a d' value of 1 (i.e., high probability of correctly detecting increment). (From Kawase et al., 1993, with permission.*)

When the crossed efferent system is also activated during such noisy conditions, by either electrical stimulation of the crossed olivocochlear bundle (Winslow and Sachs, 1987) or the presentation of noise to the opposite ear (Kawase et al., 1993), the masking effects of the noise are partially compensated. In Figure 15.11A, from the latter study, the cross-ear efferent stimulation reduced the neuron's responsiveness, allowing its response to the noise alone to drop below 100 spikes/sec (open arrow). In turn, less excitation by the noise resulted in restoration of the maximum rate to a level above 300 spikes/sec. Under these conditions the neuron had rate changes of more than 200 spikes/sec with which to respond to the added tonal signals.

This increased dynamic range is presumed to allow better amplitude discriminations by the central nervous system. For example, a 5 dB change in the level of the masked tone of Figure 15.11A (from 15 to 20 dB SPL) caused a change of about 50 spikes/sec (ΔR_{w}) in the neuron's response rate with cross-ear efferent activation, but only about half that much (ΔR_{wo}) without it. Considering the inherent randomness of primary-neuron discharges (see Fig. 11.6), any estimator of average rates would have an easier time detecting a change in the average spike rate if it were 50 spikes/sec (ΔR_{w}) than if it were 25 spikes/sec (ΔR_{wo}).

To obtain an idea of what improvement in detectability might have resulted from this efferent stimulation, these investigators employed a common statistical technique used to detect signals in noise. The output of this technique is a single number, called d' (read "d prime"), whose magnitude is indicative of the confidence with which one can say that a signal occurred (Green and Swets, 1966). As shown in Figure 15.11B, without the presence of the crossed-ear efferent stimulation (filled circles) the d' measure for detecting a 5 dB difference in stimulus level never reached 1.0 (a value indicating, with good probability, that a difference occurred). With efferent stimulation, on the other hand, d' exceeded unity at two of the lowest tone levels (10 and 15 dB SPL). It appears therefore that efferent system activity should improve central nervous system detection of changes in the amplitudes of noise-embedded signals. If so, the question remains as to why efferent stimulation is not equally effective across all primary afferent neurons, instead of being concentrated in the 1- to 20-kHz region of the cochlea, as was documented in Figure 15.9.

Effects of Bilateral Acoustic Stimulation

The bilateral nature of the cochlear efferent systems suggests that sound presented to one ear could cause suppression in the other cochlea. Such cross-ear suppression does indeed occur, causing shifts of the rate-level curves that are indistinguishable from those produced by electrical stimulation of the olivocochlear bundle (Warren and Liberman, 1989). Such suppression was abolished when the entire olivocochlear bundle was cut but remained largely intact if only the crossed bundle was severed. Referral back to the functional anatomy of the efferent innervation (Fig. 15.3) indicates that the MOC group must have been the principal efferent system involved in this cross-ear acoustic suppression, in agreement with our previous interpretation of the electrical stimulation results.

Suppressive effects of acoustically stimulating the cross-ear efferent system have also been demonstrated in *awake* animals (Hensen et al., 1995). In these experiments brief tone pips at 61 kHz were presented to one ear of the animal (a mustache bat), sometimes with and sometimes without the simultaneous presentation of noise to the other ear. In either case termination of the tone pip produced a "ringing" offset response (damped oscillations) in the cochlear microphonic potential of the animal's ear, which is *very* sharply tuned to that frequency. With simultaneous noise presented to the other ear, these pip-evoked oscillations became shorter (i.e., more highly damped) in an orderly manner: the greater the contralateral noise, the shorter the oscillations. There reductions reflect reduced tuning of the basilar membrane (see Fig. 13.1) exactly what we would expect from stimulation of the MOC system (Fig. 15.8).

Acoustic stimulation on one cochlea can also affect otoacoustic emissions generated in the opposite ear (Puel and Rebillard, 1990). Such cross-ear acoustic effects have proved to be useful noninvasive probes of cochlear function (e.g., Kujawa et al., 1994).

NEUROTRANSMITTERS OF THE EFFERENT SYSTEMS

Many lines of evidence indicate that the major neurotransmitter released by the MOC efferent system is acetylcholine (ACh) (for reviews see Eybalin, 1993; Sewell, 1996). Not only is ACh released during stimulation of the olivocochlear bundle, its synthesizing and degrading enzymes, choline acetyltransferase (ChAT) and acetylcholinesterase (AChE), are present at the axon terminal level. Perfusion of the cochlea with a dilute solution of ACh reduced otoacoustic emissions from those ears, as did electrical stimulation of MOC neurons (see Cochlear Responses to Efferent System Activation, above). Moreover, these reductions due to ACh perfusion vanished when known antagonists (blockers) of olivocochlear efferent activity (curare and strychnine) were added to the perfusate (Kujawa et al., 1992).

Pharmacologically, it appears that the outer hair cells' ACh receptors are nicotinic in nature but in an uncommon class that does not respond well to nicotine (Erostegui et al., 1994). More specifically, there is good evidence that these ACh receptors contain the newly discovered $\alpha9$-subunit (Elgoyhen et al., 1994).

The ionic mechanisms presumably activated by stimulation of the MOC efferent system have been illuminated by the direct application of ACh to isolated outer hair cells (Housley and Ashmore, 1991). Hyperpolarizations as great as 10 mV occurred owing to the outward flow of K^+ ions. Similar hyperpolarizations due to ACh-induced K^+ currents have also been seen in turtle and chick auditory hair cells (Art et al., 1984; Fuchs and Murrow, 1992).

It might seem strange that ACh, the excitatory transmitter at neuromuscular junctions, acts in an inhibitory manner when applied to outer hair cells. Experiments with ''short'' hair cells of the chick cochlea have provided the clearest picture of this role reversal (Fuchs and Morrow, 1992). In these particular hair cells, somewhat analogous to mammalian outer hair cells, exposure to ACh results in a small, transient inward current followed by a much larger, longer-lasting outward current that is dependent on the presence of free intracellular Ca^{2+} ions. Experimental manipulations led to the conclusion that the ACh receptor itself is a nonspecific cation channel, which upon opening allows some Ca^{2+} ions to enter the hair cell. These incoming Ca^{2+} ions are then recruited to open nearby Ca^{2+}-activated K^+ channels, initiating the dominant efflux of K^+ ions (Fuchs, 1996). The system may be more complicated than this simple picture, as there is pharmacological evidence that "second messengers" are involved (Kakehata et al., 1993). Whatever the mechanism(s), the ACh-initiated K^+ flows seem to be of a different nature than the potassium currents associated with the voltage-activated calcium channels described in Chapter 7 (Nenov et al., 1996).

In addition to ACh, associated with both efferent systems, other neurotransmitters are also involved in the feedback loops of the mammalian cochlea (Eybalin, 1993). Most prominent among these is γ-aminobutyric acid (GABA), which has been identified immunologically with one of the two subdivisions of the LOC system (Vetter et al., 1991). The other LOC subdivision stains positively with antibodies to calcitonin gene-related peptide. Dopamine and enkephalins are among the other neurotransmitters that have been identified in cochlear tissue. Little is known about the functions of these other transmitters, although hypotheses have sprung from experiments in which a transmitter is applied through a multibarreled pipette to the region just underneath the inner hair cells of the guinea pig cochlea (e.g., Oestreicher et al., 1997). When so applied, ACh proved to increase the rates of spike activity recorded with the pipette, presumably from the terminal axons of the type I afferent neurons, whereas GABA decreased those rates (Felix and Ehrenberger, 1992). A modulatory role for the LOC system is suggested.

MODEL OF MOC EFFERENT ACTIVITY

Although other explanations exist (see Guinan, 1996), the previous electrical circuit model of the outer hair cell (see Fig. 8.2) can be extended to account for many of the observed effects of MOC system stimulation simply by adding a single branch (Fig. 15.12). This branch, representing ACh-activated K^+ channels, has three elements: a total channel resistance (R_{eff}), a battery equivalent to the net thermal driving force on K^+ ions due to the differences in their concentration on opposite sides of the cell's basolateral membrane (i.e., the potassium ion Nernst potential, E_k), and an ACh-controlled switch (S_{eff}).

Analysis of the circuit with the efferent system quiescent (switch S_{eff} open) shows that sinusoidal modulation of its apical conductance ($\Delta G \sin \omega t$) results in a receptor potential being developed across the hair cell's basal membrane whose equation is

$$E_{rec}(t) \approx \Delta G \sin(\omega t) * (I_0 R_{bas} R_{ap}^2 / R_{tot}) \tag{15.1}$$

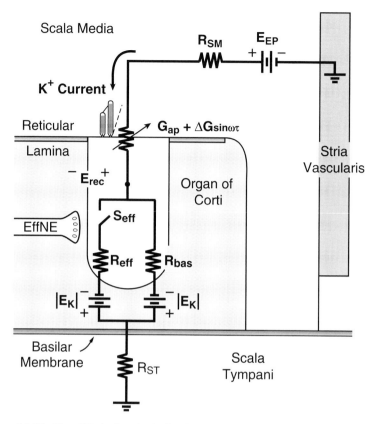

Figure 15.12. Simplified electrical circuit model of a mammalian outer hair cell under efferent control. Added to the general hair cell circuit of Figure 8.2 is an additional branch representing current flow through efferent-activated K^+ channels located in the basal membrane. Efferent activation (closing switch S_{eff} in the left branch) can be thought of as "shunting" current away from the standard basolateral ion channels (right branch), thereby reducing receptor potentials (and changing extracellular potentials). The efferent branch includes R_{eff}, the total resistance of all efferent-activated channels when conducting, and E_K, the Nernst potential for potassium ions at the basolateral surface.

where R_{tot} is the sum of all the fixed resistances, $R_{SM} + R_{ap} + R_{bas} + R_{ST}$, and I_0 is equal to the total DC driving voltage, $(E_{EP} + |E_K|)$, divided by R_{tot} (see Eq. 8.1).

When the efferent synapse is activated (switch S_{Eff} closed), this equation for transmembrane voltage undergoes only one change: R_{bas} is replaced with a resistance of lower value (the parallel combination of R_{bas} and R_{eff}). Because the numerator of Eq. 15.1 is reduced more than the denominator (of which R_{bas} is only a minor part), the receptor potential is also reduced.

According to prevailing theory (see Chapter 9), this reduction in outer hair cell receptor potential results in reduced cochlear amplifier "gain" in tip region frequencies and consequently in reductions of the discharge activity of the primary afferent neurons at those frequencies.

Consideration of the currents flowing through the hair cell during efferent activation is also instructive. The equation for the AC portion of the hair cell current in the circuit of Figure 15.12 during synaptic quiescence, is

$$i_{ac}(t) \approx \Delta G \sin(\omega t) * (I_0 R_{ap}^2 / R_{tot}) \qquad (15.2)$$

Because the only term that changes in this equation during efferent activation is a reduction in the effective value of R_{bas}, which now appears only in the denominator of the equation, the magnitude of $i_{ac}(t)$ increases when the efferent synapse is activated. Because $i_{ac}(t)$ flows through R_{ST} (the summed resistances of scala tympani and the organ of Corti), an application of Ohm's law shows that the extracellular AC potential in scala tympani (the "cochlear microphonic") also increases when efferent stimulation occurs. This increase is in fact observed experimentally (Wiederhold and Peake, 1966), providing further support for this model.

The DC portion of the current (I_{DC}) flowing through the hair cell in Figure 15.12 also changes during synaptic activation. When the efferent synapse is quiescent, the equation for that current is

$$I_{DC} = (E_{EP} + |E_K|)/R_{tot} \qquad (15.3)$$

As was true for Eq. 15.2, only R_{bas} (in the denominator of this equation) changes when the efferent synapses are activated. Thus the DC current flowing through the outer hair cell also increases with efferent stimulation. Because this current flows through the summed resistances of scala tympani and the organ of Corti (R_{ST}) on its way to ground, an increase in the magnitude of I_{DC} means that positive extracellular potentials are developed in those locations.

In addition to accounting for the previously mentioned positive extracellular potentials observed in the vicinity of the inner hair cells during electrical stimulation of the crossed olivocochlear bundle (Brown and Nuttall, 1984), this increased extracellular potential may also explain several other aspects of efferent stimulation. Among them is the reduction in primary-neuron spontaneous activity observed during efferent stimulation (Guinan and Gifford, 1988b). Recall that the positive efferent-produced extracellular potentials observed by Brown and Nuttall (1984) were accompanied by smaller positive potentials within the inner hair cells (see Cochlear Responses to Efferent System Activation, above). It follows that the inner hair cells must have been *indirectly* hyperpolarized by the efferent stimulation. A reduction in the rate of release of transmitter would have followed (see Chapter 12), and the spontaneous discharge rates of the primary neurons would have dropped accordingly, as was observed.

By the same reasoning, the nerve terminals of the afferent neurons must have been hyperpolarized by the positive extracellular potentials resulting from the efferent stimulation. If one assumes that the spike-generating mechanisms of the low-spontaneous neurons were particularly sensitive to this hyperpolarization, the exaggerated efferent-induced suppressions displayed by these neurons (Fig. 15.10) would also be accounted for. The same mechanism might also account for the extraordinary susceptibility of these same neurons to two-tone suppression (see Chapter 13).

FUNCTIONS OF THE COCHLEAR EFFERENT SYSTEMS

Our understanding of the major role(s) of the cochlear efferent systems in behaving animals is still immature. Part of the difficulty has been the inaccessibility of the cochlea. No one yet has been able to record its efferent neural activity in the awake animal, let alone correlate that activity with other neural signals or behavior. The relevant experiments that *have* been successfully accomplished provide only indirect evidence. Nevertheless, the picture emerging indicates that a major role of at least the MOC system is to provide centrally determined gain control to the primary afferent neurons. Only hints exist regarding the role(s) of the LOC system.

Perceptions with Deefferented Cochleas

Human Patients

The treatment of human patients with vestibular disorders such as Ménière's disease (see Chapter 16) sometimes involves severing the vestibular branch of the VIII cranial nerve, an operation that leaves the auditory branch intact while presumably disrupting the olivocochlear system completely (but see Giraud et al., 1995). There is a surprising paucity of data concerning the hearing of such patients.

Probably the clearest case reported is that of a young man with debilitating vertigo whose successful treatment involved cutting the vestibular branch on one side only (Scharf et al., 1994). Hearing sensitivity in both ears, both before and after the operation, was within normal limits. After considerable postoperative perceptual testing, the only differences detected in the patient's sensations to sounds presented first to one ear and then to the other were greater "adaptation" (decline of subjective loudness) to weak sounds presented in the deefferented ear and a *displacusis*; that is, a single tone produced slightly different perceptual pitches depending on which ear was stimulated. Unfortunately, because of the dearth of preoperative testing, it is not known if these differences were present in this patient prior to his surgery.

The only clear perceptual difference produced in that patient by the deefferentation was the *improved* detection of "unexpected" tones in noise, a test in which a long sequence of tones is given, half of which have the same frequency as an oft-repeated "cue" tone. Detection of the other (noncue) tones is thought to test for the "selective attention" the subject is paying to tones of the cue frequency. No satisfying explanation for this peculiar postoperative abnormality of the patient exists.

An extension of such measurements to 15 other patients undergoing destruction of the vestibular branch of the VIII nerve on one side has produced similar results. The only consistent change in their hearing was an improved ability to detect tones of unexpected frequencies (Scharf et al., 1997). The otherwise similarity of hearing through each ear of these patients implies that the functional roles of the efferent systems are indeed subtle.

In other contexts, it has been suggested that efferent effects on the cochlea are influenced by the subject's attentive state, but the evidence for that idea is slim. Not only are there few relevant reports, the ones that do exist are not persuasive. In one (Froehlich et al., 1990), for instance, it was reported that attention to visual stimuli depressed the amplitudes of evoked otoacoustic emissions. Although the changes were repeatable, they were small (< 7%) and observed in only 3 of 16 subjects.

Animal Subjects

Behavioral experiments on animals surgically deprived of efferent systems, usually by section of the crossed olivocochlear bundle, have also been characterized by subtle effects. One early study reported that cats subjected to such deefferenting suffered no loss in detection thresholds for tones presented in quiet, but were somewhat poorer at detecting those tones in noise (Trahiotis and Elliot, 1968). Later studies on cats by another group confirmed that such efferent-deprived animals had normal absolute thresholds and found that they could normally detect changes in both frequency and intensity in the absence of noise (Igarashi et al., 1972, 1979a,b).

The most recent behavioral study of such deefferented animals also shows noise-related deficits (May and McQuone, 1995). In this experiment, cats had to detect 3 dB (30%) level changes in tones of 1 kHz or 8 kHz, in both quiet and noise, before and after bilateral brain stem cuts aimed at severing *all* MOC system axons (Fig. 15.1). The only deficit the successfully deefferented animals displayed was impaired detection of changes in the amplitudes of noise-embedded 8 kHz tones. It has been suggested that such reduced ability is related to the loss of the ''unmasking'' effects normally provided for the primary neurons by the efferent systems (Fig. 15.11).

Responses of Deefferented Cochleas

In keeping with the relatively small behavioral deficits it has induced, chronic de-efferentation of the cochlea has produced few abnormalities in the responses of primary afferent neurons. In the key experiments (Liberman, 1990), each animal had all of the efferent innervation to one ear eliminated (LOC as well as MOC axons) by a lateral brain stem cut that left the contralateral efferent system intact to serve as a built-in control (Fig. 15.1). After various periods of postoperative survival (3–30 weeks), the responses of the animals' primary neurons on the operated side were measured. Their threshold levels were normal, as were their frequency tuning curves and rate-level functions.

The only abnormal attribute these primary neurons manifested was in their reduced rates of spontaneous discharge. Almost all spontaneous rates recorded were below the average sported by normal high-spontaneous neurons (ca. 75/sec) and there were relatively more low-spontaneous neurons than usual. Because cochlear mechanics seemed normal in these animals, the destroyed MOC system can hardly be blamed for these losses of spontaneous rate. Perhaps the LOC system, probably also destroyed by the cuts, was responsible (see Guinan, 1996).

Protective action of a peculiar sort has also been demonstrated by cochlear efferents. This protection was shown in a series of experiments in which loud sounds were briefly applied and the extent of the temporary damage to the cochlea determined (reviewed in Rajan, 1992). Monitored in this case were not individual-neuron spikes but the synchronized neural discharges of primary neurons recorded at a distance with remotely placed electrodes (the ''compound action potential''). Without an olivocochlear bundle, the temporary shifts produced by the noise in the detection thresholds of these potentials averaged about 25 dB. With intact efferent systems, the temporary threshold shifts were considerably less, about 15 dB. Extrapolation of this improvement to louder or more sustained sounds suggested that efferent activity would reduce the permanent damage the cochlea can incur from intense sounds.

The initial enthusiasm generated by these reports has been dampened by the demonstration that this protective effect is highly circumscribed (Reiter and Liberman, 1995). It seems to occur only in the 14 kHz region and then only for relatively short exposures (< 1 minutes) to intense sounds (> 100 dB SPL) composed of high frequencies (8–10 kHz). As the effects of the "slow" efferent effects also diminish after 60 seconds of continuous stimulation (see Cochlear Responses to Efferent System Activation), it appears that those previously demonstrated protective effects of the efferent system are due to this slow effect. Broadening this restrictive picture, however, are fresh reports that the cochlea's efferent systems provide overload protection against other types of intense sound (e.g., Zheng et al., 1997a,b).

It may be that the efferent system also plays a role in cochlear development, as suggested by an intriguing preliminary report (Walsh et al., 1997). In that study, olivocochlear bundles were transected in neonatal cats. Upon reaching adulthood, the primary auditory neurons of these animals were found to be abnormal, having elevated thresholds and reduced frequency sensitivities.

ROLES OF EFFERENTS IN OTHER ACOUSTICOLATERALIS SYSTEMS

With few exceptions, all acousticolateralis systems studied to date appear to have efferent innervation. In the lateral-line systems, the efferents appear to be inhibitory in all cases, but the effects of efferent stimulation on the vestibular end-organs are far from uniform (for review see Goldberg et al., in press). In fish and mammals efferent stimulation results in *excitation* of vestibular afferent neurons, whereas in frogs and turtles both excitation and inhibition of these neurons occur. There are even variations in efferent effects among the various classes of afferents.

The location of some of these end-organs, particularly the lateral-line sensors, has allowed recordings to be made from them while the animal was alert and capable of movement. In several of these experiments, changes in efferent activity have been correlated with planned movements of the animal. Perhaps the clearest case was obtained in the free-swimming toadfish, where it appears that efferent activity had a role in changing the sensitivity of the lateral-line sensory system to suit the fish's immediate situation (Tricas and Highstein, 1990). In particular, arousal in these fish, even by simply showing them their natural prey (killifish), decreased the discharge rates of primary afferent neurons of those end-organs (Tricas and Highstein, 1990). Controls indicated that these reductions were due to efferent activity, known to be inhibitory in this system. Presumably, this reduction of sensitivity would reduce the rate of discharges evoked by the vigorous swimming motions involved in any attack, possibly preventing overstimulation.

"Volitional" efferent-system modulation of the sensitivity of some primary afferent neurons of the turtle's semicircular canals has also been suggested (Brichta and Goldberg, 1996).

SYNOPSIS

Despite major advances, our understanding of the major functions of the efferent systems in the mammalian cochlea is still limited. Although roles in neutralizing unwanted background noise, protecting from loud sounds, and maintaining homeostatic balances have been demonstrated, it is not entirely clear which of those (if any) are the major responsibilities of these feedback systems. There are increasingly strong indications that dynamic control of cochlear sensitivity may be the principal role of the MOC system. Such control might be involuntary, triggered by acoustic stimulation, or it might involve ''volitional'' anticipation of planned behavior, or both.

In support of this budding theory are demonstrations that the efferent systems of at least some acousticolateralis end-organs adjust afferent neuron sensitivity to suit the animal's needs. Also supportive of the concept of central control of sensory input is the suggestion that the cerebellum is involved in the active adjustment of tactile receptors in the fingers (Gao et al., 1996).

IV

DAMAGE AND TREATMENT

16

DAMAGE TO THE EAR AND HEARING IMPAIRMENT

THREATS TO THE SENSE OF HEARING

The ear does an exquisite job of transforming acoustic signals, varying enormously in amplitude and waveform, into a regimented neural code. The hearing that normally results is one of our greatest gifts. With it we monitor our environment in all directions, communicate with one other, and listen to the music of instruments and babbling children. The loss of this treasure can bring severe behavioral deficits (Gravel and Ruben, 1996) as well as untold personal agony. A poignant example is provided in a moving letter from the 31-year-old Beethoven to his brothers, in which he attempts to describe his misery due to a progressive hearing loss. Not only was he unable to appreciate performances of his music, he found it difficult to communicate with other people and became a virtual recluse. He even contemplated suicide (van Beethoven, 1802).

Unfortunately, many processes can damage the ear and rob one of hearing, among which are aging, noise, certain "ototoxic" drugs (Garetz and Schacht, 1996), inherited defects (Steel and Kimberling, 1996), infections (Woolf, 1996), trauma, tumors, and disorders of the vascular, neural, skeletal, and immune systems. In the midst of so many hazards, it is a tribute to the robustness of the ear that we retain our hearing as well as we do.

For most of us, aging is the chief cause of hearing loss. With *presbycusis* (loss of hearing due to aging), hearing is impaired gradually and probably does not become a problem until sometime during one's retirement. The data in Figure 16.1 show the pattern of hearing loss during "normal aging." Given in the form of an *audiogram*,[1] these data indicate that hearing loss typically begins in the high frequencies at a surprisingly young age and increases steadily in severity and frequency range as the years go by. By the time one is 90 years old, much of normal speech, particularly the high-frequency consonants (see Chapter 14), is likely inaudible.

Some appreciation for the difficulties imposed by hearing deficits on the understanding of speech and the appreciation of music can be obtained by listening to the auditory simulations available on the lower half of the World Wide Web page containing our visual animations (See Fig. 1.1).

Based on the correlation between the hearing abilities of aged patients and the damage identified in their cochleas postmortem, four types of cochlear pathology associated with aging have been clinically recognized: sensory (hair cells), neural, strial, and general (Schuknecht, 1967; Schuknecht

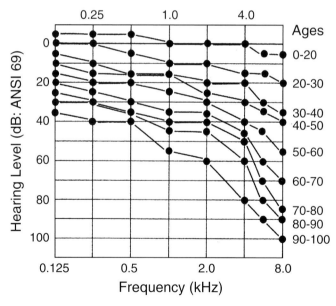

Figure 16.1. Pure-tone audiograms illustrating the patterns of "normal aging" that occur in patients of various ages, as encountered in urban medical practice. Each passing decade brings with it progressive hearing losses, particularly at high frequencies. (From Goodhill, 1979, with permission.*)

and Gacek, 1993). *Sensory* loss is correlated with a loss in high-frequency sensitivity, *strial* atrophy with a loss of sensitivity at all frequencies, and *neural* loss with diminished word recognition. No consistent pathological correlates have been found for hearing losses that gradually increase with frequency, so those cases are placed in the *general* category.

Although hearing losses are certainly not limited to the aged, Schuknecht's categories of presbycusic pathology are employed here as the framework for a more general consideration of cochlear malfunction. Damage to the external and middle ears is also considered. Intended as a non-technical introduction, this chapter covers just a few of the most common impairments. Those interested in delving further are referred to standard medical texts (e.g., Goodhill, 1979; Schuknecht, 1993). More information is also available from the American Speech–Language–Hearing Association.[2]

DEFECTS IN THE EXTERNAL AND MIDDLE EARS ("CONDUCTIVE" HEARING LOSSES)

Types of Defects

The sound-funneling role of the external ear is clearly compromised if the ear canal becomes partially or totally blocked. Such blocking can occur through the natural accumulation of "ear wax" (*cerumen*) or through introduction of a foreign body, such as a bead. Removal of foreign bodies should be left to qualified professionals, as it requires technical skill and equipment to extract the obstruction without forcing it farther into the canal, perhaps even rupturing the eardrum and causing middle ear damage.

Such a rupture is illustrated in Figure 16.2, along with several other impairments of the middle ear. From an acoustic point of view, eardrum rupture (or "perforation") defeats much of the middle ear's signal-transmitting functions (see Chapter 4). No longer does all of the impinging acoustic pressure push on the outer face of the eardrum; some sound enters the middle ear cavity and exerts force on the inside face of the eardrum as well. The *net* force on the eardrum is thereby reduced, as in the reptile ear (see Fig. 4.1), and eardrum vibrations are accordingly attenuated.

In addition, the sound pressures leaking into the middle ear cavity tend to be exerted nearly equally on the oval and round windows. As these two windows must move "out of phase" with each other for normal inner ear function (see Fig. 5.1), this "in phase" pressure exerted on the two windows reduces effective stimulation of the cochlea. The larger the rupture, the greater are these various effects. The resulting reductions in hearing sensi-

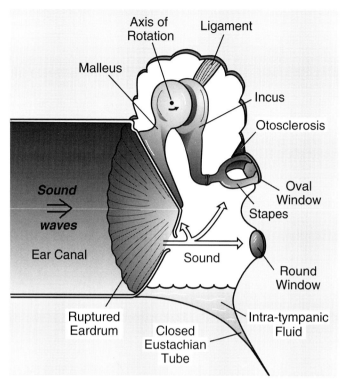

Figure 16.2. Cross section through the human middle ear, depicting three middle ear impairments: ruptured eardrum, otitis media (causing intratympanic fluid and a closed Eustachian tube), and otosclerosis. All three conditions impede motion of the stapes, thereby producing "conductive" hearing losses.

tivity, appropriately labeled "conductive" losses, can generally be treated with hearing aids or surgery (see Chapter 17).

A much more common impairment, particularly in young children, is the accumulation of fluid within the middle ear due to infection (*otitis media*). From an acoustic point of view, this "intratympanic" fluid disrupts normal middle ear function. The simple reduction of air volume in the middle ear cavity increases the effective stiffness of the eardrum (see Chapter 4). Moreover, should the fluid come to lie directly against the eardrum or to engulf the ossicles, middle ear vibrations would be even more sharply reduced. Depending on the volume and viscosity of the fluid, the hearing losses that ensue may range from 5 to 50 dB, with primary involvement of the low frequencies (Goodhill, 1979). If antibiotic treatment does not clear up this condition (which because of possible complications should not be neglected), a tiny ventilating ''tube'' may need to be temporarily placed in the eardrum surgically. When the tube is removed, the eardrum usually heals itself.

The final defect illustrated in Figure 16.2 is *otosclerosis* (literally ''hardening of the ear''), which is abnormal outgrowth from the bone surrounding the oval window. This condition is not rare, being observed histologically in the preserved cochleas of about 8% of people in the United States (Soifer et al., 1970). Only occasionally affecting young children, otosclerosis usually begins during early or middle adulthood (Goodhill, 1979). The disease progressively immobilizes the stapes, resulting in increasingly severe ''conductive'' hearing losses. Surgical procedures are the standard treatment for this condition.

Diagnostic Tools

There are two valuable tools for the differential detection of conductive hearing losses. The first is *tympanometry*, the measurement of eardrum mobility (the inverse of stiffness). In the normal ear the eardrum is optimally positioned within its moorings for maximum mobility. Almost anything that changes the ability of the middle ear to transmit sound changes this mobility.

For example, the air pressures within the ear canal and middle ear are normally equal (i.e., the *net* pressure on the eardrum is zero). When the two pressures become unequal a net force is exerted on the eardrum, and it bulges outward or inward, depending on whether middle ear pressure is greater or less than the canal pressure. This bulging, in *either* direction, increases eardrum stiffness and thus causes an increase in sound reflection from the eardrum. As passengers in an aircraft that is changing altitude, we often become aware of such bulging (sometimes painfully) and of the loss in hearing sensitivity that accompanies it. In the laboratory the tympanometer supplies the varying air pressures and compares stiffness and stiffness changes with normal templates. Various middle ear impairments cause signature departures from those templates.

The other diagnostic tool is based on the fact that acoustic vibrations within the cochlea (and thus hearing) can be generated by touching a vibrating device to the head, effectively bypassing the middle ear. Indeed, that is the principle behind one type of hearing aid (see Chapter 17). In the diagnostic situation, the thresholds for these ''bone-conducted'' tones are compared with those for conventional air-conducted tones. As middle ear defects principally affect the latter, abnormal differences are created between these two groups of thresholds. These differences (called ''air–bone gaps'') have diagnostic significance.

DEFECTS IN THE INNER EAR ("SENSORY" AND "STRIAL" LOSSES)

Damage to Hair Cells

Damage to any element within the inner ear can potentially affect hearing. Pivotal, of course, are the hair cells. Without them (or their electronic substitutes), we cannot hear. As discussed in preceding chapters, the prevailing evidence from studies of normal ears is that the inner hair cells are the principal translators of sound information (see Chapters 12–14), and the outer hair cells mediate collection of that information at low intensities (see Chapter 9). It is known that both types of hair cell can be damaged by ototoxic drugs and acoustic overstimulation (for reviews see Willott, 1991; Garetz and Schacht, 1996). Such impairing effects are to be avoided in normal daily life, but in the laboratory they provide opportunities to unravel the complex processes involved in acoustic transduction.

Damage Produced by Acoustic Overstimulation and Ototoxic Drugs in Animals

One of the primary lines of evidence to support the distinctions just made between hair cell types comes from investigations of damaged cochleas. A classic example is shown in Figure 16.3, which presents data from an ear exposed to a narrow band of intense noise centered at 9 kHz for several hours. Almost all of the hair cells in that cochlea were still physically present a month later (Fig. 16.3A), with appreciable losses[3] confined to a narrow region.

At a finer level of damage assessment[4] the degree of damage to the stereocilia of the hair cells remaining in this cochlea was determined, as shown in Figure 16.3B. Damage to inner hair cell cilia was spread over more than 3.5 mm (the length of the cat's cochlea having characteristic frequencies ranging over the octave from 10 to 20 kHz). Damage to outer hair cell cilia, though almost equally widespread, was not so severe.

Frequency tuning curves obtained from three spiral ganglion neurons positively localized within that cochlea by intracellular labeling, are shown in Figure 16.3C–E. Shown for comparison are frequency tuning curves for normal neurons of those cochlear locations. Neuron 77, at the apical (left) edge of the lesion, showed little abnormality (Fig. 16.3C). By contrast, neuron 34, located only 2 mm away but at the epicenter of the damage, suffered more than a 40 dB (100-fold) loss of sensitivity in its "tip" region (Fig. 16.3D). Accompanying that loss was a slight *increase* of low-frequency ("tail") sensitivity. Neuron 101, originating near the basal (right) edge of outer hair cell ciliary abnormalities, sustained tip-region desensitization (Fig. 16.3E) almost equal to that of neuron 34.

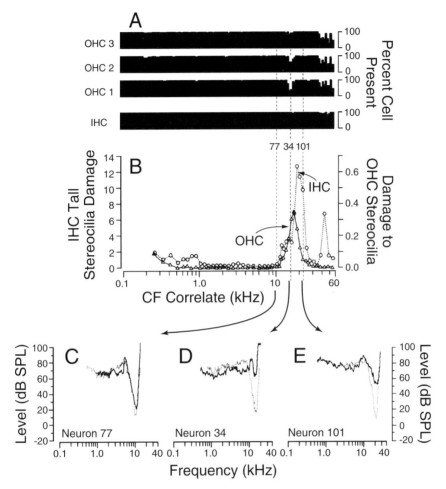

Figure 16.3. Comparison of cochlear pathology with single-neuron frequency tuning curves for one acoustically traumatized cat ear. *A.* The ear's "cytocochleogram," showing (in black) the percentage of hair cells *remaining* in each of the four hair cell rows, regardless of their condition. Few hair cells are missing. *B.* Damage of the cilia of the inner hair cells (IHC) and outer hair cells (OHC) is shown as circles and triangles, respectively. For both hair cell types, the scale expresses the average damage per hair cell, as averaged over roughly 0.6 mm of the organ of Corti. The characteristic-frequency (CF) correlate was inferred from the characteristic-frequency/location map of the cat cochlea (see Fig. 12.9). *C–E.* Frequency tuning curves for each of three labeled primary neurons in this ear (solid curves), the cochlear locations of which are indicated by the dotted lines in *B.* For comparison, corresponding frequency tuning curves from normal ears are shown (dotted curves). (From Liberman and Dodds, 1984, with permission.*)

The spatial pattern of sensitivity damage displayed in Figure 16.3 is especially significant. Whenever damage occurred to the outer hair cells located at and immediately basal to a neuron's location, deficits in tip sensitivity occurred. This basic pattern, seen in numerous other studies, is consistent with the present hydromechanical theory of the basal cochlea (see Chapter 9), which locates a tone's amplification region just basal to its characteristic place. Unexplained by that theory, however, is the large loss in sensitivity suffered by neuron 101, as the outer hair cells located immediately basal to its innervation point on the cochlear partition appeared to be essentially normal. The longitudinal extent of the amplification region for high-frequency tones is still a matter of debate. Some direct data suggest it may be narrower than 0.5 mm in the base of the guinea pig cochlea (Cody, 1992), although more indirect findings imply larger amplification zones in the cat (see Fig. 13.11).

The other noteworthy aspect of the data in Figure 16.3 is the stability of low-frequency sensitivities in the same neurons that suffered massive tip frequency losses. The maintenance of the tail region thresholds in these basal neurons is also expected from the cochlear amplifier theory, which specifies that only tones within the tip region enjoy amplification, and hence only they are adversely affected by damage to the outer hair cells. Thus so long as the inner hair cells are undamaged, the low-frequency thresholds should be unchanged. That theory can account even for the improvement of neuron 34's low-frequency thresholds, if it can be further assumed that the loss of outer hair cells at that neuron's location (Fig. 16.3A) reduced the cochlear partition's stiffness below normal. It follows, according to the equation for a spring ($x = p/k$), that the lower the stiffness (k), the less is the pressure (p) needed to produce a threshold level of displacement (x).

The general findings of this study, which examined a number of cochleas damaged by acoustic overstimulation or the ototoxic antibiotic kanamycin, are shown in Figure 16.4. Broadly speaking, if inner hair cells remained undamaged (Fig. 16.4B,D), low-frequency (tail) thresholds were undiminished, or even sensitized if outer hair cells at that location were lost. Disarray or loss of the inner hair cell cilia reduced overall sensitivity, sometimes precipitously (Fig. 16.4A,C). Finally, to the extent that outer hair cells were damaged, thresholds in the tip region deteriorated. Numerous other studies support this basic pattern of impairment (e.g., Patuzzi et al., 1989), indicating that ''sensory'' pathology must be subdivided into two categories, one for each type of hair cell.

Acoustic overstimulation is not confined to the laboratory. In a sobering case, some chinchillas were taken to a rock concert, where they spent several hours in front of a loudspeaker (Bohne et al., 1976). Histological examination of eight cochleas (from four exposed animals) preserved a few hours

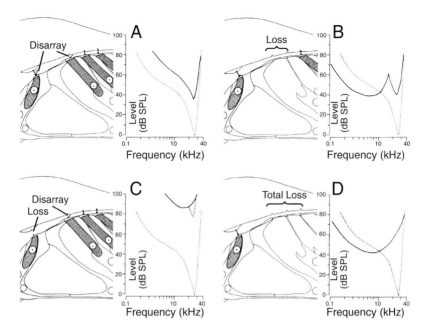

Figure 16.4. Organ of Corti in four states of damage. Each damaged state is shown with the frequency tuning curve typically seen to occur in primary neurons whose peripheral axons innervate such a region (solid curves). For comparison, a normal frequency tuning curve is shown in each panel (dotted curves). (From Liberman and Dodds, 1984, with permission.*)

after the sound exposure, indicated appreciable loss of outer hair cells in both ears of one of these animals (such variability in susceptibility to damage between animals is typical). In the cochleas of two animals allowed a month of recovery after the concert, outer hair cell loss was not appreciably more than normal, but there were severely degenerated sections of the stria vascularis in each animal (see Loss of Endocochlear Potential: Strial Damage, below).

Possible Noise-Related Hair Cell Losses Suffered by Humans

For obvious reasons, it is difficult to determine the degree of damage inflicted by noises or drugs on human cochleas. When the pattern of loss in a human cochlea looks similar to that sustained in controlled animal experiments, a reasonable supposition is that similar effects caused the damage in both human and beast. Consider, for example, the case of a man with impaired hearing who died at age 57 (Schuknecht, 1993). Figure 16.5A shows the pattern of his hair cell pathology: Extensive hair cell loss is ap-

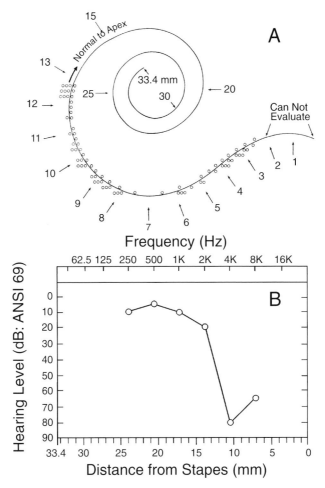

Figure 16.5. Comparison of cochlear pathology with the audiogram of a human patient. *A.* Patient's cytocochleogram, showing in pictorial form the hair cells (circles) remaining in each of the four rows of hair cells, regardless of their condition, plotted as a function of distance from the stapes. Note the extensive hair cell loss in the most basal 12 mm. *B.* Patient's audiogram, showing a profound hearing loss above 2 kHz (top scale of abscissa). The apical border of the extensive hair cell loss corresponds well with the 3 kHz place on the characteristic-frequency/location map for primary auditory neurons in humans (bottom scale of abscissa). (From Schuknect, 1993, with permission.*)

parent throughout the basal region, particularly centered at the 7- and 12-mm locations, where virtually all outer hair cells are missing. The most apical 20 mm of his cochlea appeared normal.

This man's last audiogram (Fig. 16.5B), obtained 2 years before his death, shows a catastrophic loss in sensitivity for frequencies above 2 kHz but only mild losses below that level. Comparison of Figure 16.5A and 16.5B shows good agreement between the characteristic frequencies of the apparently normal cochlear region (from 13 mm to the apex) and the frequencies at which the man had nearly normally hearing. Although the acoustic history of this individual is not known, his selective pattern of impairment, much more severe than that expected from aging alone (Fig. 16.1), is suggestive of appreciable exposure to intense high-frequency noise.

Useful as light microscopy is, it takes electron microscopy to reveal damage at the ultrastructural level.[4] Nadol (1988a), for example, studied the cochleas of three patients who had suffered from neural presbycusis, Ménière's disease (a combined hearing–vestibular disorder), and Usher's syndrome (a genetic disorder that produces hearing loss), respectively. Although light microscopy showed evidence of some neuronal degeneration in each case, it greatly underestimated the degree of ultrastructural degeneration occurring among the remaining processes of the primary afferent fibers.

Diagnostic Devices

Until recently it has been practically impossible to distinguish "sensory" damage from "neural" damage in living humans. The usual diagnosis for nonconductive hearing disorders was a "sensorineural" impairment. Now, with devices to measure cochlear emissions, differential diagnoses become possible (Gorga et al., 1996).

A case in point is shown in Figure 16.6. This patient, a 28-year-old man who regularly used recreational firearms, had severe high-frequency losses in each ear, as indicated by the two audiograms of Figure 16.6A,B. Distortion-product emissions from both ears of this individual fall within the normal range of amplitudes (shaded) at low frequencies but virtually disappear above 3–4 kHz (Fig. 16.6C). The match between hearing loss and emission loss is striking. Even the improvement in the 8 kHz range for the right ear is reflected in the small emissions in that frequency range evoked from that ear. It seems clear that outer hair cells had been damaged in the basal region of each cochlea.

If, by contrast, otoacoustic emissions were to be generated in a frequency region of marked hearing loss, inner hair cell or neural pathology would be suspected (e.g., Prieve et al., 1991).

Effects of Aging

On Humans

Given the differences in our individual histories, it is almost impossible to distinguish the effects of aging in human subjects from environmental

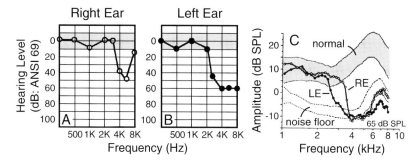

Figure 16.6. Distortion-product otoacoustic emissions of a 28-year-old man who regularly used recreational firearms. *A.* Pure-tone audiogram for the patient's right ear, characterized by a 50 dB loss near 6 kHz. *B.* Audiogram for the patient's left ear, showing a precipitous drop for frequencies above 2 kHz. *C.* Distortion-product emissions measured in the patient's left ear (LE) and right ear (RE), plotted as a function of the geometric mean frequency of the two primary tones (see Fig. 10.10B). The emissions fall within the "normal" range up to a mean frequency of 2 kHz. For both ears the 3- to 4-kHz boundary of severe audiogram loss correlates well with the frequency at which the emissions vanish. (From Martin et al., 1990b, with permission.*)

effects such as noise exposure. For those of us living in industrialized societies, there is no known way of accounting for the effects of the cacophony constantly inflicted on us by our machines. There are, however, groups of people who live far from cities and industrial noises. The hearing abilities of individuals within several of these groups have been tested (Rosen et al., 1962, 1964; Goycoolea et al., 1986). Presumably for these isolated people, the effects of noise exposure are minimal.

Perhaps the most useful of these studies (Goycoolea et al., 1986) was conducted with residents of Easter Island, a small nonindustrialized island belonging to Chile. It is far off the coast and is famous for its huge prehistoric statues. Thresholds for three age groups of residents who had never left the island are shown in Figure 16.7A. Like their industrialized counterparts, the hearing sensitivity of these islanders decreased with age, although their losses were not as great as those in Figure 16.1. For example, the average hearing loss at 8 kHz was about 50 dB for Easter islanders over 65 years of age. For a "typical" urban dweller in that age range, the loss at that frequency was more than 70 dB (Fig. 16.1). It could be argued that these perceptual differences do not prove noise damage but might be the results of differences in genetic makeup, nutrition, and so on.

More secure comparisons, therefore, are those made among the islanders themselves. Shown in Figure 16.7B are the average frequency thresholds of three distinct groups of Easter Islanders: those who had never left the island,

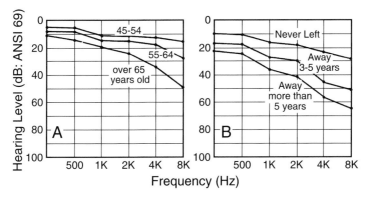

Figure 16.7. *A.* Pure-tone audiograms of Easter Islanders who had always lived on the island, segregated into three age groups. Increasing age was associated with increasing hearing losses but not as severe as those generally encountered in an urban setting (Fig. 16.1). *B.* Audiograms of Easter Islanders having an average age of about 60 years, segregated into groups according to the amount of time spent on the mainland, as indicated. Those who had been on the mainland longest had the greatest losses. (From Goycoolea et al., 1986, with permission.*)

those who had been away on the continent for 3 to 5 years, and those who had been away for more than 5 years. It is clear from these data that, on average, the longer the absence from the island, the greater was the hearing deficit. The obvious inference is that the deleterious effects of aging and noise on hearing must be additive, a conclusion supported by several other studies (for a review see Humes, 1984).

It is interesting that the average audiograms of the mixed-gender group who had never left Easter Island are similar to age-matched audiograms reported in 1984 for a random sample of women in the United States (Ward, 1984). It appears that many women over the age of 45 living in the United States at *that* time had not been appreciably exposed to ear-damaging noise.

In view of the harmful effects of acoustic overload, common sense dictates that we try to limit our exposure to loud sounds as much as is practical. Admittedly, it is difficult to do so in a society of rock concerts and lawn mowers, aircraft engines and electric saws. However, the deliberate choice of quieter pastimes and the judicious use of sound-attenuating earplugs or earmuffs would moderate the most damaging acoustic forces tugging at our hair cells.

On Animals

Animal studies indicate exactly the same trends. In one investigation (Schmiedt et al., 1990) Mongolian gerbils either lived their entire lives in quiet or, for long periods of time, in continuous noise presented at a moderately high sound level (average about 85 dB SPL). When studied during adulthood (24–43 months), neural data from the two groups of animals differed significantly. For those raised in quiet, the frequency tuning curves of typical individual primary neurons were mildly abnormal at all frequencies but showed thresholds as low as 20 dB SPL at 4 kHz (Fig. 16.8A). By contrast, primary neurons of the gerbils who lived their lives in constant noise exhibited considerably elevated neural thresholds in the band of frequencies (0.5–4.0 kHz) contained within the noise (Fig. 16.8B). Moreover, few of the latter neurons exhibited two-tone suppression, implying that cochlear amplifiers in the noise-exposed ears were largely inoperative (see Chapter 10).

The sensitivity reductions of these few individual primary neurons are reflected in the more global measure of summed ganglion cell responses to tones obtained from a remote electrode (the ''compound action potential''). For six gerbils raised in quiet, the profile of their compound action potential thresholds showed appreciable losses at the higher frequencies but only mild losses below 2 kHz (Fig. 16.9A). For five compatriots subjected to long-term noise, further large reductions in these thresholds marked the 2- to 8-kHz range (Fig. 16.9B). In all five of those animals, the band-limited noise caused a restricted sensitivity loss (or ''notch''). Such notches are reminiscent of those suffered by people in particular occupations: the ''aviator's notch'' inflicted on flyers during World War II by reciprocating aircraft en-

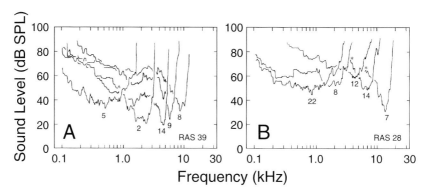

Figure 16.8. *A*. Frequency tuning curves obtained from five primary auditory neurons in a aged gerbil (RAS39) who had lived its entire 38 months of life in quiet. When compared to the sensitivities of young gerbils (e.g., 6 months old), there is a threshold shift of about 20 dB at all frequencies. *B*. Frequency tuning curves for five primary neurons in a gerbil aged 24 months (RAS28) who had lived in a noise field for 1 year. Tails of the curves marked with an asterisk are omitted for clarity. As shown, a severe threshold shift, not attributable to age, occurred in the 1- to 8-kHz region. (From Schmiedt et al., 1990, with permission.*)

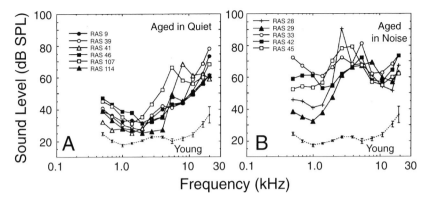

Figure 16.9. Thresholds for the remotely recorded cochlear "compound action potential" in two groups of aged gerbils: those who lived all of their lives in quiet (*A*) and those who had lived in a continuous noise field since the age of about 8 months (*B*). For comparison, the average thresholds for a group of young animals are shown (dotted lines). The sensitivity losses seen here for the ensemble responses of primary neurons appear similar to those seen for the single-neuron data of Figure 16.8. Note the much larger mid-frequency losses in the noise-exposed animals. (From Schmiedt et al., 1990, with permission.*)

gines, and the 3- to 6-kHz notch exhibited by many professional violinists, particularly in their left ears (Royster et al., 1991).

Before proceeding, it is worth pointing out that the age-related losses demonstrated by aged gerbils (Fig. 16.9A) are similar to those of normally aged humans (Fig. 16.1), despite the 25-fold difference in their typical lifespans. As pet owners know, aged cats and dogs also suffer frequently from hearing loss. Evidently, the ear ages at different rates in different mammals, seemingly at about the same rate generally operative in its species.

Loss of Endocochlear Potential (Strial Damage)

As discussed in Chapter 8, the endocochlear potential is important to normal cochlear function. Damage to its source, the stria vascularis, is therefore likely to be an important cause of hearing impairment. Such damage can occur through noise exposure (see Damage Produced by Acoustic Overstimulation and Ototoxic Drugs in Animals, above) as well as through the normal aging process (for summary see Willott, 1991). The losses seen in Figures 16.8A and 16.9A, for instance, are largely attributable to the marked decline in the endocochlear potential that occurs in gerbils as they age (Schmiedt, 1996).

To investigate some of the consequences of reduced strial function in the laboratory, application of the diuretic drug furosemide has been found useful.

Within seconds of its systemic injection the endocochlear potential starts to fall, dropping to just a few millivolts within a minute or so and then slowly recovering to normal values (Evans and Klinke, 1982; Sewell, 1984a). In the latter study, this voltage was measured simultaneously with the frequency tuning curves of individual spiral ganglion neurons, several examples of which are shown in Figure 16.10.

For each of these neurons, sensitivity was impaired at all frequencies. This reaction was expected, as the endocochlear potential provides approximately half of the total voltage drive for the K^+ transduction current flowing through both types of hair cell (see Fig. 8.2). For neurons tuned to low frequencies, the loss in sensitivity was more or less uniform (ca. 20 dB) across the entire range of their frequency sensitivities (Fig. 16.10A), whereas for higher-frequency neurons the loss of sensitivity in their tip regions was much more severe than that in the tails (Fig. 16.10B,C).

This latter pattern is as expected from current theory. Because the cochlear amplifier in basal regions has been demonstrated to be principally effective at frequencies characterizing the local resonance, reducing the magnitude of the transduction current of the outer hair cells theoretically should destroy the tip frequency sensitivity of basal neurons while having negligible effect on their responses to low frequencies. This theory suggests a way of distinguishing the relative contributions to the neural losses of the inner hair cells and the cochlear amplifier. Presumably the latter does not affect the tail sensitivities of high-frequency neurons, so the low-frequency reductions that *did* occur (10–15 dB in Fig. 16.10B,C) can be assigned theoretically to

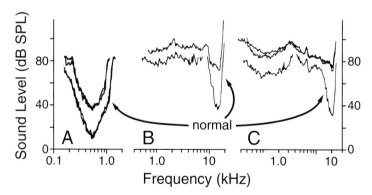

Figure 16.10. Representative examples of the changes in the frequency tuning curves of primary auditory neurons following intravenous administration of furosemide. In all cases the tuning curve obtained before the injection has the lowest threshold. The basally located neurons demonstrated severe losses of threshold near characteristic frequency (*B, C*), whereas apically located neurons encountered more uniform losses of lesser extent (*A*). (From Sewell, 1984a, with permission.*)

inner hair cell effects alone. Hence any losses more than 10–15 dB are assignable to impairment of the cochlear amplifier. The results of that mental arithmetic imply that the cochlear amplifier is powerful and frequency-focused in the base but weak and frequency-indifferent in the apex. Exactly that same conclusion was reached by direct measurements of cochlear partition vibrations (see Chapter 5).

It can therefore be conjectured that strial damage in human patients should have relatively mild effects on their low-frequency hearing (perhaps 20 dB) but should reduce high-frequency sensitivities by larger amounts. Somewhat that same pattern of hearing loss is indeed reflected in four cases of strial atrophy reported by Schuknect and Gacek (1993), when the general effects of aging are also taken into account (the patients were all in their seventies at death).

DEFECTS OF PRIMARY AUDITORY NEURONS (NEURAL PATHOLOGY)

Loss of Neurons

Loss of primary auditory neurons is the most consistent form of pathology in the aged human ear (Schuknecht and Gacek, 1993). Otte et al. (1978) documented an average loss of about 1200 primary neurons per decade of life; and severe reductions in spiral ganglion populations, even in the presence of abundant hair cells, have been reported in other studies (Schuknecht and Gacek, 1993; Felder and Schrott-Fischer, 1995).

Based on the large number of primary neurons operative in the normal ear, it is tempting to hypothesize that *thresholds* should not be greatly affected by moderate neural losses, as the remaining neurons should be able to transmit adequately something so simple as the mere presence of a stimulus. However, because of the complexity of speech, we would expect that there is some relation between the number of primary neurons remaining in an impaired human cochlea and the owner's speech-recognition abilities.

Consistant with these expectations, Otte et al. (1978) deduced that approximately 10,000 spiral ganglion neurons are necessary for some understanding of speech. A later study from the same group (Pauler et al., 1986) found that speech discrimination was correlated with the cochlea's innervation density in the region tuned to frequencies between 1 and 3 kHz, the same frequency range that encompasses most of the second formants of English-language vowels (see Chapter 14).

Such results must be interpreted with caution. Because the understanding of speech is certainly dependent on central structures, it is risky to assume that all losses in speech perception are due to peripheral impairments alone. Indeed, a recent study comparing the speech recognition of young and elderly subjects concludes that both peripheral and central auditory dysfunctions are involved in presbycusis (Frisina and Frisina, 1997).

Tumors

When action potentials generated on the axons on primary auditory neurons cannot complete their journeys into the brain, hearing is impaired even though cochlear transducing functions are normal. This neural pulse traffic can be disrupted, for example, by tumors such as the ''acoustic neuroma'' (though it is neither a neuroma nor restricted to the auditory branch of the VIII nerve). Although benign, when this type of tumor grows large enough it compresses the auditory nerve, producing symptoms that may include tinnitus on the affected side, hearing loss (designated ''retrocochlear''), and imbalance. Treatment of the tumor is surgical removal if it is not contraindicated (Goodhill, 1979).

TINNITUS

Tinnitus—variously described as the sensation of sound in the absence of acoustic stimulation, phantom sounds, or ''ringing in the ears''—is suffered by a surprisingly large number of people. Estimates are that about 17% of people in the United States and Europe are affected, among whom nearly half seek help. Almost 2 million Americans have tinnitus of such severity that normal life is impossible (Jastreboff and Sasaki, 1994).

With the discovery of spontaneous otoacoustic emissions almost 20 years ago (see Chapter 10), it was hoped that the physical basis for these sensations had been discovered. Investigations since then have shown that there is a clear connection between spontaneous emissions and tinnitus in fewer than 5% of such cases (Penner and Jastreboff, 1996).

There are several ways to demonstrate such a cause-and-effect relation between emissions and tinnitus. One could, for example, record someone's emissions and then play the recording back to the subject, asking if the pitch of the recorded emissions matched the pitch of the tinnitus. That test has indeed been used, but it is not definitive: It does not measure how good the ''matches'' were. It is far better to have the subject adjust the frequency of an independent tone so its pitch matches as closely as possible the pitch of the tinnitus. The degree and consistency of agreement between the frequencies of the matching tone and the emission are then indicators of the closeness of their relationship. Another method of comparison is to sound tones that suppress the spontaneous emissions (see Chapter 10) and determine if the tinnitus then vanishes. Based on such tests, it is concluded that spontaneous emissions are causative in only about 4.5% of tinnitus cases (Penner, 1990).

This conclusion is not surprising in light of the fact that spontaneous emissions in humans usually come only from normal ears (see Chapter 10) whereas tinnitus is often associated with hearing loss in the frequency region of the phantom sensations (e.g., Fowler, 1944). Moreover, striking differences usually exist between the perceptions of tinnitus and those produced by externally applied tones (Wilson, 1986; Penner and Jastreboff, 1996). For example, perception of a pure tone can always be eliminated (masked) by stronger tones at neighboring frequencies, whereas tinnitus, when maskable at all, may be masked by tones covering unpredictable ranges of frequency and intensity.

Although the root causes of tinnitus are still unknown, damage to the ear seems ultimately responsible for most cases. Not only is tinnitus highly correlated with ear disorders (Fowler, 1944; McFadden, 1982), but large doses of aspirin, a drug known to reduce cochlear sensitivity (see Chapter 9), can produce temporary tinnitus in human subjects. Indeed, such aspirin doses administered to laboratory animals produced behavioral responses that suggested they too were experiencing tinnitus (Jastreboff, 1990; Penner and Jastreboff, 1996). Hopefully, investigations with this animal ''model'' will produce deeper understanding and better treatment of this debilitating disorder.

The mechanisms within the brain that produce the sensations of tinnitus are completely unknown. Among the many causes suggested are disruptions of the randomness that ordinarily characterizes the spontaneous discharges of primary afferent neurons (Eggermont, 1990). Another possibility is spotty damage to the cochlea (recall that spotty irregularities are thought to produce spontaneous emissions) (see Chapter 10). Primary neurons on the opposing sides of a boundary between regions of damage and normalcy would then be responding differently to acoustic stimuli, creating a problem for processors in the central nervous system. That is, do the persistent differences that exist between the responses of the primary neurons located on the two sides of that boundary indicate the continuous presence of acoustic stimulation *at* the boundary? Central adjustments to that pesky anomaly might then create tinnitus.

Whether that conjecture is right or wrong, the central nervous system is deeply involved in most cases of tinnitus, as indicated by the fact that noise sounded in either ear can often mask it. Most convincingly, the drastic measure of surgically cutting the auditory nerve has rarely eliminated tinnitus (Goodhill, 1979). Thus, regardless of whether a particular case of tinnitus has its origin in cochlear malfunction, it is to the central nervous system that relief efforts are usually directed (see Chapter 17).

SUMMARY

Damage to the auditory system can occur anywhere along the long line of processes involved in hearing: the external and middle ears (''conductive'' losses); the cochlea's vibration sensors (''sensory'' pathology) and vascular supply (''strial'' atrophy); and the generation and transmission of ensuing nerve discharges (''retrocochlear'' losses), which may involve either the primary auditory neurons (''neural'' pathology) or the brain itself. Despite advances in treatment (see Chapter 17), the efficacy with which modern medicine and technology relieve the misery and handicaps imposed by those disorders declines in roughly that same order.

NOTES

1. An ''audiogram'' plots increasing hearing loss *downward*. Such losses, obtained at selected frequencies, are usually judged relative to the ANSI 1969 standard (*A*merican *N*ational *S*tandards *I*nstitute). A loss of less than 20 dB is usually considered to lie within the range of ''normal'' hearing.

2. Information on hearing disorders can be obtained from the American Speech–Language–Hearing Association, 10801 Rockville Pike, Rockville, MD 20852-3279. Phone: 800-638-8255.

3. When outer hair cells degenerate, the apical tips of the phalangeal processes of the Deiters' cells enlarge to fill completely the holes left in the reticular lamina (Bohne and Rabbitt, 1983). This remarkable process evidently reestablishes the rings of tight junctions that completely encircle all reticular lamina elements, thereby preventing the mixing of endolymph and perilymph, a happenstance that would render any remaining hair cells totally inoperative and unable to maintain a sustained K^+ current (see Fig. 6.10).

4. Histological examination of the cochlea can be conducted at several levels. Using light microscopy, the presence or absence of hair cells is readily ascertained. Assessing the degree of damage to the cilia and other parts of *intact* hair cells with light microscopy is much more demanding because that method's limit of resolution is close to the width of a stereocilium. Electron microscopy is needed to evaluate still smaller elements, such as nerve terminals and synapses.

17

TREATMENTS FOR DAMAGED EARS

Appropriately, this last chapter concerns the relief currently available for people with various forms of hearing impairment. It is good to celebrate the improvement in their lives brought about by present treatments and hearing aids. It is also important to pay tribute to the army of workers—scientists, clinicians, technicians, manufacturers—who have labored long and hard to understand and alleviate the disabilities and distress of hearing impairment. Moreover, clinical treatments and aids to hearing comprise a sort of final examination, providing practical tests of the depth with which we understand the workings of the ear. It is such understanding that largely determines the methods used for treating ailing elements within the ear and finding substitutes or assistive devices for missing or defective stages. The treatments achieved remain subject, of course, to the limitations imposed by the present state of science as a whole and by available technology.

As we shall see, treatments for impaired ears have improved considerably since the mid-1980s. In fact, some who were essentially totally deaf[1] now hear well enough to use the telephone. Although there are many dimensions to the treatment of ear disorders (e.g., metabolic, surgical, antibiotic, psychological), it is to the area of physical aids and substitutes that we direct most of our attention (for a review see Working Group, 1991). The course of this chapter follows the general outline of the book and in a sense recapitulates its main themes. After a short section on the treatment of middle ear problems, the bulk of the chapter deals with aids of several types that improve the hearing of people suffering from cochlear impairment. Treatments for tinnitus, presumably a neural problem, are then briefly discussed. Finally, as a glimpse of possible things to come, we end on the note of self-repairing cochleas.

PROCEDURES AND PROSTHESES FOR TREATING MIDDLE EAR DISORDERS

For many conductive hearing losses correction is possible with surgery, sometimes on an outpatient basis. For instance, many specialists would recommend surgical repair of a large eardrum perforation (as in Fig. 16.2). Surgical treatment may also be indicated when the movements of the ossicles are greatly impaired by such conditions as advanced otosclerosis (Goodhill, 1979). Should it be the stapes that is immobilized, it can be freed sometimes by cracking or removing parts of the abnormal bone growth ("stapes mobilization"). In other cases the stapes must be removed entirely and replaced by a tiny artificial strut.

Hearing aids (preferably called "hearing instruments") can also be effective in the treatment of middle ear disorders. For instance, if the ossicular motion of a patient were only 1% of normal, a hearing instrument (aid) that amplifies its input 100-fold would nominally restore normal vibrations to the oval window. In reality, normal hearing is never completely restored by these instruments, as the impairments inevitably have affected the mass, stiffness, or damping of the ossicles, thereby changing the frequency response of the middle ear (see Chapter 4).

In some severe cases of middle ear impairment, the hearing instrument of choice delivers a mechanical vibration instead of sound. When placed against the scalp just behind the ear, these "bone-conducting" hearing instruments produce vibrations in the underlying bone that are transmitted to the cochlea within, where *normal* acoustic traveling waves are produced, and hearing is therefore restored. It might be puzzling that simply vibrating the head generates normal traveling waves within the cochlea, as the usual input port (the oval window) is apparently not used. In fact, normally traveling acoustic waves can be generated in a hydromechanical model of the cochlea when it is driven from its *apex* (von Békésy, 1960, p. 510ff). Although difficult to visualize, the origin of these "paradoxical" waves can be accounted for theoretically (Siebert, 1974). Basically, two oppositely directed traveling waves are produced by *any* source, no matter where it is located along the cochlear partition; but the wave traveling in the base-to-apex direction is by far the dominant one (see Fig. 10.11).

In the few cases of middle ear malfunction that cannot be treated by surgery or with normal hearing instruments, the entire ossicular chain may have to be removed. In its place a semiimplantable middle ear prosthesis might be substituted, perhaps of the type shown in Figure 17.1 (Heide et al., 1988). This device consists of a small capsule placed deep within the ear canal that picks up incoming sound, amplifies it, and then applies it to an encased electromagnetic coil. The magnetic field produced in the coil vibrates an implanted magnetic prosthesis attached directly between the eardrum and the oval window. Electrical currents in the coil are thereby translated directly into motions of the oval window, functionally replacing the ossicles. Other variations exist, some implanted partially and some totally (Suzuki et al., 1988).

AIDS FOR TREATING INNER EAR DISORDERS

At the present time there are no medical treatments for hearing impairments that involve the loss of cochlear hair cells or of primary auditory neurons. For such patients, hearing instruments and other assistive devices (e.g., pocket amplifiers, telephone amplifiers, wireless headphone systems) are usually of great help.

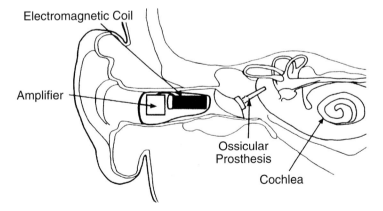

Figure 17.1. Semiimplantable replacement for severely impaired ossicles. The amplifier picks up the sound and translates it into an AC electrical current that energizes the coil. The coil's magnetic field in turn drives the prosthesis and vibrates the oval window. (From Heide et al., 1988, with permission.*)

Functional Attributes of Cochlear Malfunction

If faced with the task of designing a hearing instrument for a particular hearing-impaired person, we would probably start with that person's audiograms, such as the ones in Figure 16.6. For the patient's left ear, the indicated high-frequency loss (Fig. 16.6B) suggests that the instrument would need to amplify frequencies above 2 kHz by about 60 dB (1000-fold). The end result ought to be restoration of normal hearing: a 60 dB loss compensated by a 60 dB amplifier. This type of reasoning, with various modifications, has in fact been the general guide for the design of hearing instruments ever since their first appearance, despite notoriously poor performances in some situations (e.g., noisy restaurants).

The problem is that hearing-impaired people suffer from far more than just the inability to hear soft sounds (i.e., reduced *sensitivity*). They also suffer deficiencies in many other dimensions of sound perception, such as frequency *selectivity* (i.e., the ability to discriminate frequencies) and the detection of brief silent gaps (Ludvigsen, 1985; Glasberg and Moore, 1989). Although reduced sensitivity in various frequency bands is clearly the dominant factor in impaired speech perception, another important yet often overlooked factor concerns the abnormal perceptual loudnesses of the sounds hearing-impaired people *do* hear.

This difficulty can be appreciated by reference to Figure 17.2A, where the case of a typical young adult with normal hearing is shown (Villchur, 1974). The lower solid curve indicates the familiar perception threshold (see Fig. 2.4). The upper solid curve is an "equal-loudness" contour: the connection of points at which tones of various frequencies are judged to be equally loud. In other words, a tone of 1 kHz presented at 74 dB SPL is judged about as loud as a tone of 2 kHz presented at 70 dB SPL (top arrows). The area in the sound–pressure/frequency plane that encompasses normal speech is indicated by the shaded area. As can be seen, the upper boundary of the speech area is remarkably close to the equal-loudness contour.

The corresponding average audiogram and appropriate equal-loudness contour for six severely impaired patients are shown in Figure 17.2B. The threshold curve (bottom solid line) shows average sensitivity losses that grow with increasing stimulus frequency, from about 50 dB at the low frequencies to almost 90 dB at 5 kHz. The equal-loudness contour shown for these patients (top solid line) is that which corresponds most closely to the upper boundary of the sound–pressure/frequency band within which the subjects preferred listening to speech. Note the differences in the *dynamic ranges* of the two panels (i.e., the separations between the upper and lower solid lines). For normally hearing listeners (Fig. 17.2A), there is a 60- to 70-dB difference between the just-audible sounds and those near the upper

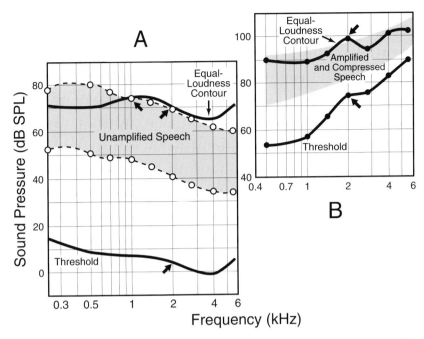

Figure 17.2. *A.* Range of sound pressure levels involved in normal conversational English (shaded band) comfortably fits within the dynamic range of normal hearing. An equal-loudness contour corresponding to a comfortable listening level is also shown (top solid curve): Any two tones on that contour (e.g., top arrows) produced auditory sensations of about the same loudness. *B.* For a small selected group of hearing-impaired listeners, the dynamic range available for speech perception was considerably reduced (e.g., arrows), particularly at high frequencies, because the increase in thresholds (e.g., 50–90 dB) was much greater than the increase in comfortable loudness levels (20–30 dB). Thus the amplitude range of speech must be compressed as well as amplified (shaded band) to fit within the reduced dynamic range. (From Villchur, 1974, with permission.*)

limit of preferred listening. By contrast, the average dynamic range of the hearing-impaired subjects (Fig. 17.2B) was less than 40 dB wide in the low frequencies and diminished so sharply with increasing stimulus frequency that, at 5.5 kHz, barely 10 dB separated the just-audible stimulus level from the upper level preferred for speech reception.

These differences in dynamic range have a significant effect on the loudness perceptions of the two groups. Referring to Figure 17.2A, we see that normally hearing listeners would detect a 2 kHz tone presented at about the 4 dB level (bottom arrow), and that they would feel it comfortably loud at 70 dB SPL (top right arrow). Were the tone to be increased to 110 dB SPL, they would most probably judge it to be uncomfortably loud (not shown).

This gradual increase of perceptual loudness with stimulus level for unimpaired listeners is shown as the left-hand curve in Figure 17.3.

By contrast, the hearing-impaired listeners of Figure 17.2B did not hear a 2 kHz tone until it was increased to about 74 dB SPL (bottom arrow), and they found it comfortably loud at 99 dB SPL, only 25 dB more intense (top arrow). They would probably have tolerated a slightly more intense tone than unimpaired listeners before labeling it uncomfortably loud (Kamm et al., 1978). This steep relation between the sound level of a 2 kHz tone and its perceived loudness by the hearing-impaired listeners is indicated by the right-hand curve in Figure 17.3. Such abnormally rapid growth of perceptual loudness with stimulus level is called ''recruitment,'' a somewhat misleading term as the patients actually suffered from drastic *reductions* in their dynamic ranges (Moore, 1982).

These two loudness curves can be accounted for qualitatively with the mechanical response curves of normal and impaired cochleas, respectively. On one hand, the displacement responses of the normal basilar membrane are compressive in nature (see Fig. 5.8C), akin to the left-hand curve in

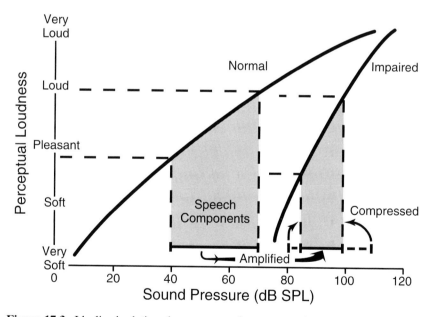

Figure 17.3. Idealized relations between sound pressure and perceptual loudness for subjects with normal hearing (left curve) and those with severely impaired hearing (right curve) for a representative band of frequencies (e.g., around 2 kHz). To produce the same levels of subjective loudness as those experienced by normally hearing listeners, speech for the hearing impaired must be both amplified *and* compressed. (Adapted from Pluvinage, 1994.)

Figure 17.3. On the other hand, when the inner ear's built-in cochlear amplifier is damaged, the responses of the cochlear partition become greatly attenuated at low stimulus intensities but are relatively unaffected at high intensities (see Chapter 10). On the basilar membrane therefore the loss of sensitivity due to impairment of the cochlear amplifier is necessarily accompanied by a loss of compression. Hence the loss of loudness compression suffered by the hearing-impaired listeners appears to be at least partially the result of damage to their internal cochlear amplifiers.

With loudness scales now established, consider how the two groups of listeners respond to the components of the speech waveforms produced by the band of frequencies centered around 2 kHz. For normally hearing listeners, these components range from about 40 to 70 dB SPL in amplitude (Fig. 17.2A). This 30 dB range of sound levels fits well into the middle of the *loudness* range of these subjects, from "pleasant" to "loud" (Fig. 17.3, left shaded area). By contrast, the hearing-impaired listeners have less than a 25 dB range of sound levels between "very soft" (just audible) and "loud" (right-hand curve). The sound-level range separating "soft" and "loud" perceptions for these patients is even smaller than that, probably about 20 dB.

The problem of presenting all of the information contained within the 2 kHz speech band to the patients thus becomes painfully clear. If simply amplified by 40 dB (Fig. 17.3, dashed bar), the soft 2 kHz components would be barely audible, whereas the intense ones would seem very loud. For better and more comfortable perception, it seems that the amplitude variations of the 2 kHz band, which normally span about 30 dB, must be compressed to no more than 15 dB (Fig. 17.3, right shaded area). Moreover, the compressed speech must be amplified just enough to fit snugly within the subjects' narrow perceptual boundaries. Too much amplification, and the more intense sounds would become uncomfortably loud; on the other hand, too little amplification would render the less intense sounds inaudible.

The same calculations can be repeated for each of the frequency bands important for understanding speech.[2] The end result of such considerations suggests that the various frequency bands containing the speech signal should be individually amplified and compressed to fit the speech signal within the narrow strip of the sound–pressure/frequency plane perceptually available to the patient (Fig. 17.2B, shaded area).

Acoustic Hearing Instruments

Analogue Processors

Until recently, almost all hearing instruments had the same basic functional design (Fig. 17.4). The incoming sound is picked up by the micro-

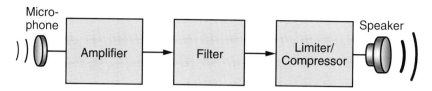

Figure 17.4. Basic elements of an analogue hearing aid. The sound waveform is amplified, filtered, and then limited or compressed in some way. The final waveform is then broadcast into the ear canal by a tiny loudspeaker (or "receiver").

phone and translated into an electrical signal. This signal is first amplified, then filtered, and finally subjected to some sort of amplitude limiting or compression. The resulting electrical waveform is sent to the output speaker, known as the "receiver," which translates the boosted (and filtered) signal back into an acoustic wave. The need for the amplifier is self-evident, as is the need for filtering, because the components at some frequencies must be amplified more than at others. The need for some form of output limiting is also clear, otherwise naturally intense sounds would be amplified well into the danger zone (see Fig. 2.4), causing acute discomfort and possibly damage. Controls and a power supply (not shown) complete the instrument.

The realization of such systems in physical devices parallels the history of electronics (Bergenstoff, 1993). Equipped with vacuum tubes, instruments of the first generation (1940s) were so large containers the size of cigarette packs were needed for the electronics. Worn on the body, these vest-pocket instruments were connected to a large ear mold with a wire (not unlike a Walkman). With the steady shrinking in element size that accompanied the successive revolutions in electronics, the size of the instruments also steadily decreased. Transistors (invented in 1948) allowed the manufacture of instruments small enough to be placed *b*ehind *t*he *e*ar (BTE). When hybrid integrated circuits came along, instruments placed entirely *i*n the pinna of *t*he *e*ar (ITE) became possible. Finally, with the monolithic integrated circuits ("chips") of today, some instruments can now be inserted *c*ompletely with*i*n the ear *c*anal (CIC).

For cosmetic reasons, patients obviously prefer the smallest and least conspicuous instruments. Because the total amount of power (energy) available for amplification is determined by the battery and the total amount of energy stored within a battery is related to its size, the amplification available from a hearing instrument is proportional to its size. Thus although CIC instruments are suitable for treating moderate hearing losses, larger instruments may be needed for severe losses. The size and shape of a patient's ear canal are also important factors in such choices.

Unfortunately, until recently the dramatic reductions in hearing-aid sizes were not accompanied by comparable increases in signal-processing sophistication. A consideration of the limiter/compressor block in the functional diagram (Fig. 17.4) shows one of the impediments to progress.

The easiest way to limit the output of a hearing instrument is to simply include, within its electronics, elements such as diodes that prevent the output from exceeding a certain level (Buerkli-Halevy and Baechler, 1993). This simple limiting process is illustrated in Figure 17.5. When an amplifying device that has a limiter (Fig. 17.5A) is subjected to a waveform that does not reach the limits, the output (Fig. 17.5B, solid curve) is just an amplified copy of the input. However, when the output goes beyond certain set limits, its peaks and troughs are clipped off (Fig. 17.5B, dashed curve). The limiter (or "clipper") is thus successful in preventing excessively large output levels. This protection comes at a high price, as the clipped output

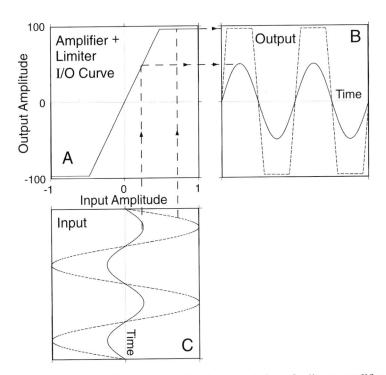

Figure 17.5. Operation of a hearing-aid system consisting of a linear amplifier and a "hard" limiter (A). Sounds of small amplitude (C, solid trace) are amplified linearly (B, solid trace: follow the left dashed line), whereas the amplified versions of intense sounds have their peaks "clipped" off (B, dashed trace) so as not to exceed some preset levels (follow the right dashed line). I/O, input–output.

is badly distorted. From the cochlea's point of view this distortion is composed of higher-harmonic components (see Appendix A), which contaminate the speech components that occur at those higher frequencies, and "intermodulation" components created from the interaction of various frequency components (e.g., quadratic and cubic distortion products). Improvements in performance may be achieved by rounding (or "softening") the abrupt (or "hard") limiter shown in Figure 17.5.

The clipper of Figure 17.5 is a *static* limiting device; it does not change with time. Many hearing instruments presently used obtain compression[3] by exerting *time-varying* control over its amplification. The basic functional diagram for the latter type of instrument, shown in Figure 17.6, is of necessity a feedback circuit. The output is measured, and that measurement is used to control the gain of the amplifier (note the similarity to Fig. 9.5). The simplest form of such a compressor has only two levels of gain. Low-level signals are strongly amplified, and high-level signals are boosted less. This process is indicated in Figure 17.7, with amplifier gains of 200 (46 dB) produced with the "high-gain" setting and 100 (40 dB) with the "low-gain" setting.

The change from one gain to another cannot occur instantaneously. In fact, the time constants of the drop from high gain to low gain (the "attack") and from low gain back to high gain (the "release") are important design parameters (Buerkli-Halevy and Baechler, 1993). Rapid response times (e.g., 1 msec) are used if peak clipping is desired, and slow time constants (e.g., 200 msec attack, 2 second release) are used for slowly varying automatic volume control. Intermediate response times also have their uses, such as

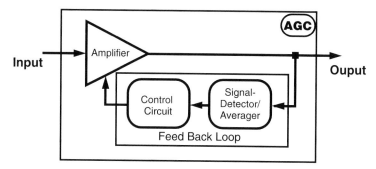

Figure 17.6. Basic elements of an amplifier with automatic gain control (AGC). The output of the amplifier is monitored and its gain continually adjusted to produce output waveforms that vary less in amplitude than the input waveform (see Fig. 17.7). (From Buerkli-Halevy and Baechler, 1993, with permission.*)

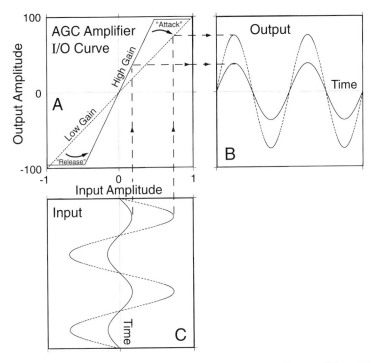

Figure 17.7. Operation of a hearing-aid system consisting of an amplifier with two-level automatic gain control (AGC). Sounds of small amplitude (*C*, solid trace) are strongly amplified (*b*, solid trace: follow the left dashed line), whereas intense sounds (*C*, dashed trace) are more weakly amplified (follow the right dashed line). The time delays involved in switching between amplification gains ("attacks" and "releases") are design factors.

amplifying low-level speech segments (usually consonants) relative to the higher-level segments (typically vowels).

An instrument using the automatic gain control compression of Figure 17.7 would certainly sound better than when using the simple peak clipper of Figure 17.5, but even the performance of the former is not optimal. Sometimes small changes in gain are effective (e.g., to improve the consonant/vowel ratio in speech), and sometimes large differences in gain are needed (e.g., for slowly varying automatic volume control). A number (or continuum) of properly graded gains would be necessary for a hearing instrument to amplify sounds of all intensities appropriately.

Although most hearing instruments commercially available today have the basic functional design depicted in Figure 17.4, the flexibility and quality of the various stages varies enormously. Some instruments have much better quality amplifiers (e.g., lower distortion) than others, an important design feature (Killion, 1993). Some instruments have flexible frequency filters, able to assume a number of configurations (e.g., Westermann, 1994), whereas others have only a few. Some instruments contain continuously variable compression circuits (e.g., Killion, 1993; Pluvinage, 1994; Stypulkowsky, 1994), but many do not.

Several advances in hearing-aid design are proving useful. Perhaps the most widespread is a semiconductor chip insertable in the instruments of many manufacturers that provides continuously increasing compression as sound intensity increases (Killion, 1993). Another improvement, increasingly available, is the use of digital controls for the various hearing-aid stages: Filter configurations and compression characteristics can be changed with the push of a button.

Even more important is the splitting of the sound signal into two or more frequency bands, each of which is processed separately before being merged at the receiver (e.g., Pluvinage, 1994). Thus the high-frequency bands of speech can be compressed more strongly than the low-frequency bands, as required by the greater hearing losses that typically occur at high frequencies (Fig. 17.2B). Although extensive comparison trials between the various instruments have apparently not been undertaken, informal and formal reports (e.g., Stypulkowski, 1994) indicate that the multiband instruments provide improved hearing for many users.

Digital Hearing Instruments

Probably the most significant long-term improvement is only just now appearing–or rather reappearing (see below)—in the form of *totally* digital hearing instruments. Such instruments are fundamentally different from those discussed above. The latter, even the digitally *controlled* (or ''programmed'') ones, share the common feature that the signal being processed is *analogue* in nature. From microphone to receiver, a continuous electrical waveform (perhaps split into several frequency bands) carries the message. If digital elements are present in such instruments, they serve only to set the characteristics of the various stages processing the analogue signal.

By contrast, a truly digital instrument is basically a computer. The incoming signal is converted to a binary (0 or 1) code by an analogue-to-digital (A/D) converter. The resulting blizzard of *numbers* is manipulated within the central processing unit. The result is converted back into a continuous electrical waveform by some sort of digital-to-analogue (D/A) converter and applied to the receiver. The transformations possible with such an instrument are limited only by the power of the computer and the imaginations of the designers.

The first of such digital hearing instruments, the *Phoenix* (Cummins and Hecox, 1987), was introduced in 1988, but its manufacture was discontinued after a few years. A number of reasons have been given for the demise of the Phoenix (Heide, 1994), one of which was psychological resistance to the size of the instrument, which because digital processing units at the time were too bulky to be put into a head-worn instrument had to be worn in a shirt-pocket case, like the original vacuum tube instruments. Such is the pace of modern computer development, that in the few years between the fall of the Phoenix and the present rebirth of digital instruments, digital processors have shrunk much further in size. Now it is possible to put the whole instrument within the ear canal. Because the digital processing in such instruments can do almost any signal manipulation asked for, it is now up to auditory and speech scientists to provide manufacturers with the information needed to find optimum processing. Prospects for restoring good hearing to many of the hearing-impaired have never seemed brighter.

Impediments to the Use of Hearing Instruments

A number of factors limit the use of hearing instruments. One of the more troublesome is feedback: not the deliberate feedback used in compression instruments but the unavoidable feedback that occurs between the output and the input of the instrument. No matter how well sealed the instrument is within the ear canal, *some* of the output signal in the ear canal leaks back out to the input. That returning signal, already amplified once, is then re-amplified, producing more leakage and even more reamplification, and so on. If this feedback leakage is great enough, oscillations at a particular frequency may occur, creating high-pitched squeals that are annoying to by-standers and to the instrument wearer (if it falls within his or her range of hearing). Because of this acoustic feedback, it is seldom possible to achieve more than 60 dB of usable gain from a traditional instrument, although feedback reduction algorithms are now beginning to appear in the new digital instruments. Physically separating microphone and speaker also permits higher gains (Boothroyd, 1993).

As hearing instruments have gotten more sophisticated and smaller, they have also gotten more expensive. It is not unusual to pay several thousand dollars for one of the more advanced instruments. As many types of insurance do not pay for any type of hearing instrument, let alone the more expensive ones, this high cost puts the more advanced instruments beyond the means of many hearing-impaired persons. Some cannot afford even the simplest hearing instruments, although limited funding is available in many states through agency programs. For those concerned, the nonprofit organization *Hear Now*[4] provides used hearing instruments, or the money to buy new ones, to those who need but cannot afford them.

Other Types of Aids: Cochlear Implants

Basic Principles

Not all who are hearing-impaired can use traditional hearing instruments. Most notable are individuals who have extreme losses (> 90 dB); they often do not receive appreciable benefit from even the most powerful acoustic instruments. For such patients there are several remaining options, such as one of the few tactile (skin vibration) aids available (Summers, 1992) or a cochlear implant.

The latter devices pick up the incoming acoustic waves, translate them into electrical waveforms, and apply these electrical signals directly to the afferent nerve axons, bypassing the entire stimulus-encoding machinery of the inner ear. (For reviews, see Clark et al., 1990; Miller and Spelman, 1990). Provided they have sufficient numbers of surviving afferent fibers, patients who suffer "profound" (essentially complete) hearing loss can hear again with such devices. In almost all cases this direct stimulation of the spiral ganglion neurons is accomplished by inserting a flexible bundle of tiny wires (called "electrodes") through the round window of the cochlea and threading it gently into scala tympani. As illustrated in Figure 17.8, the coiling of the cochlea limits the extent to which the wire bundle can be inserted to about one full turn. When enough electrical current is passed between various pairs of the electrodes, spiral ganglion neurons located within the vicinity are stimulated and generate action potentials in cadence with the current waveform (Javel et al., 1987; van den Hornert and Stypulkowski, 1987b).

It was hoped that the neural spike activity so produced would restore something approaching normal hearing. Although hearing *is* restored in this manner, according to the users the sensations that result are nothing like normal (e.g., Heath, 1991).

One reason for this badly distorted restoration of hearing is that the precision with which the individual neurons are stimulated by the implants is orders of magnitude less exact than that which occurs normally. In the case of the normal ear, the geometrical organization is accurate down to the single hair cell level: even closely spaced points on the basilar membrane (e.g., 100 µm apart) are tuned to different frequencies in an orderly manner (Cooper and Rhode, 1992). With the existing implants, however, currents passed between neighboring electrodes produce nearly equal voltages along whole millimeters of the fluid-filled scala tympani. This wide spread of the electrical signals plus the appreciable physical distances that usually separate the electrodes from the neurons results in large numbers of neurons being stimulated by each electrode pair (van den Hornert and Stypulkowski, 1987a).

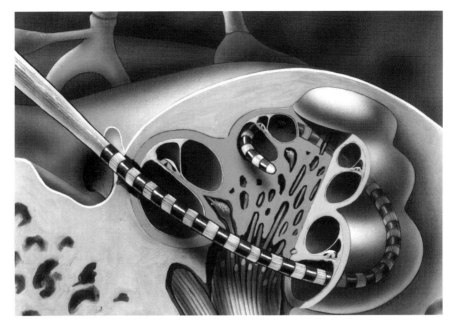

Figure 17.8. Human cochlea showing the apical, middle, and basal turns, with the banded electrode array of a cochlear implant threaded through scala tympani of the basal turn. Some of the electrical currents flowing between various pairs of electrodes pass through the organ of Corti and the modiolus and excite various groups of remaining afferent neurons. (Courtesy of the Cochlear Corporation, USA.)

A further contributor to distorted hearing for individual implant users may be greatly diminished numbers of primary afferent neurons, a condition that often occurs in those with profound hearing losses. With these and other limitations, it is not surprising that the auditory perceptions of cochlear-implant users are not normal. The wonder is that they hear as well as they do.

Practical Results of Cochlear Implants

Cochlear implants are now widely recognized as effective restorative aids for many people suffering from profound hearing impairment. As of the spring of 1995, more than 12,000 people had become users worldwide (National Institutes of Health, 1995). An appreciable fraction of these people have become so skilled in the use of their implants that they can carry on conversations unaided by visual cues, as when using the telephone (Dorman, 1993).

For most users the implants act as aids, providing important supplements to their visual lip-reading (or "speech-reading"). Because of the important roles the lips and teeth play in the production of consonants, "reading" the lips can extract a great deal of the information contained in speech (as much of the information in many languages, including English, is carried by the consonants). What lip-reading does not give is much information about vowels or the pitch or intonation of the voice; those particular attributes of speech are largely established by the tongue and larynx, both functioning out of sight. Combining the partial information about speech obtained visually with the complementary information they extract auditorially allows many implant users to carry on normal conversations, something impossible for them to do with either one of those senses alone. The implants also provide essential environmental sounds that normally hearing people take for granted (e.g., the doorbell or car horn).

Because of the critical importance of a person's early years in speech development, cochlear implants are now being implanted in children who have profound hearing losses when they are as young as 2 years of age. Initial reports with small numbers of these children suggest that the cochlear implants, in conjunction with training, do in fact aid in the acquisition of oral language (National Institutes of Health, 1995). That is good news, as it appears from the few reports available that adult implant users who were deprived of their hearing before learning oral language ("prelingually") usually acquire little benefit from the implants in terms of understanding speech (Dorman, 1993).

Design Strategies

One of the surprising things about cochlear implants is that although the number of companies making them is small, the variety in both hardware and signal-processing schemes is large. The first wearable implants used a single electrode (House and Urban, 1973), whereas more recent ones contain a number of wires, allowing various numbers of independently excitable channels. Although there is no consensus on the optimum number of these channels, it seems that at least four to six are called for. A recent *Nucleus* implant has 21.

Even more varied are the differences in signal-processing strategies (Tyler and Tye-Murray, 1991). for instance, the *Ineraid* device filters the acoustic signal into four frequency bands and applies the output of each band (an *analogue* signal) to a separate electrode channel. By contrast, the $F_0F_1F_2$ version of the *Nucleus* aid extracts the first two speech formants (F1 and F2), as well as the fundamental glottal-pulse frequency (F0). The formant frequencies are encoded by place (i.e., by which electrode channels are stimulated), using *pulse* stimuli whose rates are set by F0 (for unvoiced sounds, aperiodic pulse rates near 100/sec are used). What is truly remarkable is that the "star" users of either aid had comparable performances in word recognition, the best ones approaching 100% correct. Evidently the human brain, given proper training, can make sense out of a wide array of auditory signals.

Electrode location is also a design variable. Although almost all implants are inserted into scala tympani, as in Figure 17.8, a few devices place their electrodes outside the cochlea, on or near the round window (Mecklenburg and Lehnhardt, 1991). Direct insertion of electrodes into the auditory nerve has also been accomplished on an experimental basis (Simmons, 1966). The advantages of using these other electrode locations have not been established.

Finally, it should be mentioned that direct electrical stimulation of the brain stem's cochlear nucleus has provided useful hearing in cases of total deafness resulting from bilateral removal of auditory nerve tumors (Otto and Staller, 1995). In 11 of 12 patients, surface arrays of eight electrodes have provided considerable ability to discriminate speech and environmental sounds.

TREATMENTS FOR TINNITUS[5]

Because the etiologies of tinnitus are varied and its precise neurophysiological mechanisms are unknown (see Chapter 16), many treatments for it have been attempted. Among them are biofeedback, hypnosis, acupuncture, electrical stimulation, changes in ambient air pressure, surgery, drugs, and the addition of acoustic ''masking'' noises (for review see McFadden, 1982). Relief for some patients has been obtained with a number of these treatments, of which drugs and masking noise appear to be the most useful. However, in all but the rare case, those treatments are only partially effective.

Masking Phantom Sounds with Physical Sounds

Suggested by studies going back hundreds of years, supplying acoustic sounds to ''mask'' tinnitus is by far its most common treatment. During the modern era this treatment was pioneered by Vernon (1977), who replaced the microphone in a hearing instrument with a noise-generating circuit. The subsequent melding of hearing instruments and noise maskers into a single combination instrument has made it possible to provide masking noises to almost all tinnitus patients, regardless of whether they have accompanying hearing losses.

Despite early reports by its developers that noise masking was effective in treating tinnitus in many patients, there was considerable skepticism about its widespread applicability. Amid such skepticism a large, comprehensive study carried out in three British hospitals found that noise maskers were indeed effective in helping many of their tinnitus patients (Hazell et al., 1985). Although the noise masking did not change the underlying pathology, it did help to improve the lives of most of the patients. Such help was above and beyond that produced in control groups given only careful diagnostic investigations and counseling (which have proved to be important parts of *any* tinnitus treatment).

Pharmacological Treatments

In a number of studies the drug lidocaine, commonly used as a local anesthetic, has been found effective in reducing or eliminating severe tinnitus (McFadden, 1982). Relief that lasts for minutes, days, and even longer has been reported. Other drugs have also proved capable of helping some tinnitus patients. Because the effective drugs seem to be potent, they can be used only under the direct supervision of physicians able to handle the possible serious side effects. Although most of these drugs are not suitable for chronic management of tinnitus, their successes are promising and provocative. By what mechanisms do they reduce or eliminate tinnitus? Perhaps answers to this question will lead the way to the development of safe, effective drugs for treating this troubling malady.

Electrical Suppression

An unexpected benefit of cochlear implants has been the temporary reduction or elimination or preexisting tinnitus in a number of users, although worsening occurred in a few cases (Hazell, 1991). Not limited to intracochlear stimulation, relief from severe tinnitus has also been obtained with electrodes placed outside the cochlea on the round window. In addition to providing an important avenue for the treatment of disabling cases of tinnitus, such successes provide strong support for the idea that at least some cases of tinnitus are caused by abnormal neural activity that originates within the cochlea. Perhaps the results of this abnormal activity can be lessened by suitable ''conditioning'' of the central nervous system (Penner and Jastreboff, 1996).

REPAIR AND REGROWTH OF THE DAMAGED COCHLEA

All vertebrate organs develop, grow, maintain, and repair themselves and in some instances even regrow after injury. The cochlea is no exception.

Largely ignored, the restorative powers of the cochlea have leaped to center stage with some spectacular demonstrations of repair and regeneration.[6] Fueled by these discoveries, hope is growing that hearing may someday be restored to hearing-impaired patients by promoting the regrowth of missing hair cells and auditory neurons.

Nonmammalian Species

One of the characteristics of many fish and amphibians is that they continue to grow throughout their lives. This continued growth implies continuous expansion of all parts, but it was not until the early 1980s that Corwin (1981, 1985) provided evidence that new hair cells are produced in the acoustico-lateralis systems of some adult vertebrates. In the shark (1981) and the toad (1985) he showed that supporting cells in the inner ear divided at low rates throughout life, continually producing new hair cells and supporting cells. Subsequent studies have confirmed and extended those findings (e.g., Popper and Hoxter, 1990).

Birds, by contrast, do not continue to grow after reaching adulthood and are born with a complete set of cochlear hair cells. It came as a great surprise therefore to learn that the avian cochlea seems to produce new hair cells when recovering from damage imposed by acoustic overstimulation (Cotanche, 1987; Cruz et al., 1987).

The typical sequence of such recovery is shown in Figure 17.9 (Marsh et al., 1990). Before exposure, the hair cells were arranged in a tight matrix, with supporting cells filling in the cracks (Fig. 17.9A). Immediately following a 2-day exposure to a 900 Hz tone presented at 120 dB SPL, extensive hair cell loss occurred, with the apical ends of the supporting cells expanding to close the resulting gaps (Fig. 17.9B). In less than 10 days the damaged cochleas appeared to grow tiny new hair cells (Fig. 17.9C, arrows). The newly appearing hair cells continued to grow, until by 15 days after overstimulation the cochlear surface was beginning to look like its old self (Fig. 17.9D). Even the ciliary orientations were correct; but it was still not a normally equipped cochlea, as cell counts revealed that not all of the lost hair cells had been replaced (Corwin and Warchol, 1991).

Visual evidence can be misleading, and further tests are needed to establish that the newly visible hair cells in Figure 17.9 were in fact newly formed cells and not repaired veterans of the trauma. Because new cells must contain fresh DNA, the incorporation of a DNA marker (radioactive thymidine) applied during the recovery period has been accepted as identifying freshly minted hair cells. The evidence obtained from these radioactive studies is that newly appearing avian hair cells, following both acoustic trauma and

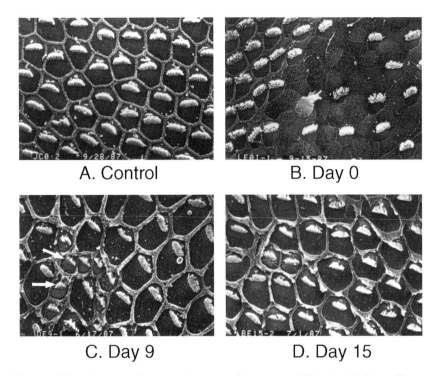

A. Control

B. Day 0

C. Day 9

D. Day 15

Figure 17.9. Electron microscope images of an area within the chick papilla exposed to a 120-dB/900 Hz tone for 48 hours, at various intervals after the exposure. *A.* In the unexposed cochlea the hair cells were uniformly packed, separated by thin wedges of supporting cells. *B.* Immediately after the sound exposure, hair cell surface areas were reduced, supporting cell surfaces were greatly enlarged, and some hair cells had been lost. *C.* By day 9 new hair cells were recognizable (e.g., arrows), although they were much smaller than the surviving hair cells. *D.* On day 15 the papilla had largely recovered its normal appearance, although hair cell size was still variable. (From Marsh et al., 190, with permission.*)

ototoxic poisoning, are indeed newly formed (Corwin and Cotanche, 1988; Lippe et al., 1991).

Of course, replacement of hair cells would have no functional consequence unless the new hair cells were also innervated with operational neurons. There is considerable evidence that at least some of these new hair cells are in fact innervated (Ryals and Westbrook, 1994; Wang and Raphael, 1996).

What about the tectorial membrane, which also suffers loss with acoustic trauma and detachment following ototoxic poisoning? It too eventually recovers in the chick cochlea owing to the secretion of new components (Epstein and Cotanche, 1996).

The picture that emerges is that the avian cochlea is a dynamic organ, one that monitors its own state and repairs itself from serious injuries by replacement of at least some damaged hair cells and regrowth of their attachments.

Hair Cell Regrowth in Mammals

The restorative powers of the mammalian cochlea have long been known from perceptual experiments. After being subjected to intense sounds, human subjects develop a temporary loss of sensitivity, one that gradually recovers over the course of hours or even days (ask any rock-concert fan). Unfortunately, these recoveries do not always succeed in returning hearing to normal, with the result that a permanent loss in sensitivity sometimes occurs. The cellular mechanisms behind such recoveries are only now coming to light.

In contradistinction to the avian cochlea, the mammalian cochlea apparently does not replace severely damaged hair cells; it repairs them instead. Although unambiguously new mammalian hair cells (i.e., incorporating tritiated thymidine) have not yet been reported in damaged mammalian cochleas, some astonishing examples of hair cell repair have been found. An example is shown in Figure 17.10, a microphotograph of a damaged mouse cochlea developing in "culture," where the phalangeal process of a Deiters' cell has enclosed the top of an injured outer hair cell and appears to have directed its microvilli (arrows) toward the hair cell's surviving stereocilia (Sobkowicz et al., 1996). Instances of the regeneration of the kinocilium (which disappears during normal development) and its apparent involvement in the reorganization of a badly damaged cuticular plate have also been observed (Sobkowicz et al., 1995).

The hope of eventual replacement of mammalian cochlear hair cells is not dead, however, as hair cell regeneration does seem to take place in the mammalian *vestibular* system.[6] Why vestibular, not cochlear? Why in the bird but not in the mammal?

CURTAIN

In most of this, the last, chapter we have been reviewing current efforts to redress damage done to the human ear. Although complete "cures" have occurred in only rare instances, at least partial relief from many hearing maladies *has* been obtained. We have progressed far. Yet there is much more to learn before nearly normal hearing can be restored to all of the hearing-impaired.

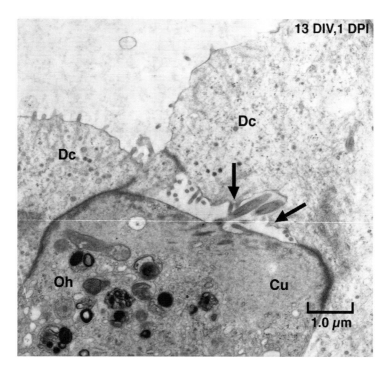

Figure 17.10. Electron microscope image of the apex of an outer hair cell (Oh) in an injured culture of the organ of Corti 1 day after the injury. The phalangeal process of a Deiters' cell (Dc) had wrapped itself around the cuticular plate (Cu) of the injured hair cell and was apparently directing its villi toward some remaining hair cell stereocilia (arrows). The culture, explanted from a newborn mouse, was mechanically injured with the tip of a glass pipette. (From Sobkowicz et al., 1996, with permission.*)

One great difficulty in the job has been the incredibly intricate and ingenious design of the peripheral ear. It has been full of wonderful surprises: on-board amplifiers, dancing hair cells, sound *generation*, feedback of many types, self-repair. What next?

NOTES

1. The word "deaf" is not always used consistently. In some usages it means completely without hearing (as in "stone deaf"), and in others it implies only some degree of hearing impairment. To prevent confusion, the alternate term "hearing-impaired" is used throughout this chapter.

2. The importance of various frequency bands for the recognition of speech has been studied and the results summarized in the "Articulation Index," which assigns

a weight of importance to each of these bands. Interested readers are referred to Humes et al. (1986).

3. The word "compression" can be confusing because it refers to a function (reducing the dynamic range of sounds) rather than to specific types of hearing-aid circuitry. Thus a "compressive" instrument may contain a *static* compressively non-linear input–output characteristic, such as describes cochlear vibrations (see Fig. 5.8C), a *dynamic* automatic gain control system (Fig. 17.6), or a combination of the two (Buerkli-Halevy and Baechler, 1993; Killion, 1996).

4. *Hear Now* is a national nonprofit organization dedicated to providing hearing instruments to low-income children and adults. It is located at 9745 E. Hampden Avenue, Suite 300, Denver, CO 80231-4923. Phone: 1-800-648-HEAR.

5. For those interested in following ongoing developments, there is an organization devoted to furthering the treatment of tinnitus and other auditory impairments, The American Tinnitus Association. The journal it publishes, *Tinnitus Today*, contains nontechnical articles on tinnitus and related topics.

6. For a summary of current work on "Development and Regeneration of the Inner Ear," see Sobkowicz, 1997.

APPENDIX A

FOURIER THEORY: REPRESENTATION OF CONTINUOUS WAVEFORMS WITH SINUSOIDS

SINUSOIDS (SINES AND COSINES)

A sinusoid is a wave shape defined by the familiar sine and cosine terms of elementary trigonometry but with arguments that change continuously with time. Because of the nature of sinusoids they are insensitive to increases in their arguments of 2π or any integer multiple of 2π. For example, cosine $(2\pi + \theta)$ = cosine (θ). Thus as time progresses, the waveform of a sinusoid repeats itself over and over indefinitely with each 2π increase in the argument.

By definition, each sine and cosine term varies between $+1$ and -1. To achieve larger or smaller variations, a sinusoid must be multiplied by a factor, which may be either constant or time-varying. A constant-amplitude sinusoid (our focus) can be described by three values: amplitude, frequency, and initial phase angle. An example is:

$$x(t) = A \cos(2\pi f_0 t + \theta). \tag{A.1}$$

The amplitude (A) is the maximum value the waveform can have. The frequency (f_0) is the number of times the waveform repeats itself per second. Its units were originally given the descriptive name *cycles per second* but have in recent years been relabeled *Hertz* (an eminent German physicist of the nineteenth century). The initial phase angle, (θ) is related to the time at which each sinusoidal period begins.

A convenient, insightful way to think about a sinusoid is as the projection on the horizontal axis of a narrow bar (e.g., a clock arm) A units long rotating counterclockwise at a constant angular velocity about the origin of the coordinate system. The bar completes exactly f_0 revolutions every second. Each rotation sweeps out $360°$ or 2π radians. Thus the bar sweeps out $2\pi f_0$ radians per second. This value, $2\pi f_0$, is the angular (radian) frequency of the bar and is usually represented by the Greek letter omega (ω_0). The tip of the bar goes in a circle (hence the source of another name for these waveforms: circular functions), as shown in Figure A.1. By simple trigonometry it can be seen that the length of the projection of the bar on the horizontal axis is $A \cos(\omega_0 t + \theta)$, where $\omega_0 t + \theta$ is the angle between the bar and the horizontal axis.

The angle θ is just the angle of the bar at $t = 0$: It contributes a time shift of the resulting cosine waveform. How much time? To calculate it, recall that the cosine cycle begins when its argument is zero (e.g., when $\omega_0 t + \theta = 0$). Thus the bar crosses the horizontal axis (and its projection on the horizontal axis is maximum) when $t = -\theta/\omega_0$. Hence when the cosine wave of Eq. A.1 has a positive value of θ, the bar can be thought of as having rotated past the horizontal axis shortly *before* time $t = 0$, arriving at a positive starting angle. The resulting sinusoidal wave shape is said to have a ''phase lead'' over a cosine wave for which θ has the value zero. A ''phase lag''

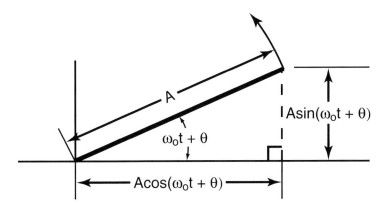

Figure A.1. Representation of $A \sin(\omega_0 t + \theta)$ and $A \cos(\omega_0 t + \theta)$ as the projections on the vertical and horizontal axes, respectively, of a vector (thin rigid bar) of amplitude A rotating counterclockwise with a constant angular speed of ω_0 radians/sec. At $t = 0$, the angle of the bar, relative to the positive horizontal axis, is θ radians.

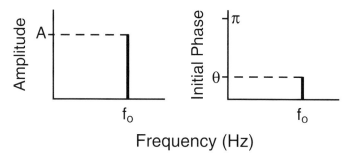

Figure A.2. *Frequency* domain representation of a sinusoid. A sinusoidal waveform is presumed, so only its parameters need be represented: amplitude (A), frequency (f_0), and initial phase angle (θ).

occurs when θ is less than zero (i.e., when the bar rotates past the positive horizontal axis shortly *after t = 0*).

A sinusoidal waveform can be represented in a variety of ways. An examination of its argument (see Eq. A.1) shows that it is a function of both time and frequency, so it can be represented in both the time and frequency "domains." In the time domain it has the familiar hill and valley shape (see Fig. A.3). In the frequency domain it occurs at only one frequency (f_0). At that frequency it has both an amplitude and an initial phase, which must be represented separately. Thus Eq. A.1 can be represented in the frequency domain by the paired graphs shown in Figure A.2.

It is important to stress that Figure A.2 forms a *complete* description of the function described in Eq. A.1. Note how much simpler it is than the time waveform, which from a formal point of view extends to infinity in both directions. This difference is not because the frequency domain is a simpler domain but because we knew that the waveform was a sinusoid *before* we considered Figure A.2. Herein lies one key to the usefulness of the frequency domain. Because we already know the stereotyped shape any sinusoidal wave must have, once we ascertain that a wave is indeed sinusoidal all we need to define it completely are its frequency, amplitude, and initial phase (the three numbers shown in Fig. A.2).

USEFULNESS OF SINUSOIDS

What good does this knowledge do us, as in real life wave shapes are seldom if ever purely sinusoidal? It was shown to us by the great French mathematician Fourier (1768–1830) that a particular combination of sines and cosines can match, with negligible error, virtually any[1] periodic waveform. Why would anybody want to do that?

First, it is often useful from a mathematical point of view to decompose a wave shape into a sum of sinusoids, as in many cases it is much easier to solve the mathematical equations describing events when sinusoids are the stimuli than when arbitrarily shaped waveforms are involved. Thus Fourier sinusoidal methods have become highly advanced, and they have been applied with outstanding success to solving equations dealing with an incredible range of systems, including the ear.

Second, there is the interesting coincidence that sinusoidal vibrations also approximate the natural modes of response for simple flexible systems having little internal friction. For instance, when a bell or a piano string is sharply struck, each "rings" with a waveform closely matching that of a sinusoid whose amplitude is slowly diminishing: so does each sector of the inner ear. More importantly from our perspective, the frequency of this "natural" oscillation marks the approximate frequency of the sinusoidal input to which the flexible system is most sensitive. Each inner ear sector, for instance, responds best (is "tuned") to that restricted group of sinusoidal sound waves whose frequencies nearly match that of its natural oscillations (see Chapter 5).

Finally, there is the curious circumstance that a sinusoidal pressure wave sounds like a "pure" tone to many of us. Indeed, western music is written in terms of sinusoids. The standard note A, for instance, signifies a sinusoidal sound wave having a frequency of 440 Hz.

For these and other reasons, sinusoids and Fourier analysis seem to be peculiarly suited to the vertebrate auditory system; accordingly, they have been heavily utilized to characterize it, particularly the ear. Of necessity therefore we must understand Fourier analysis to appreciate fully those characterizations. It should be kept in mind, however, that the ear is not a Fourier analyzer, although it behaves a bit that way.

HARMONIC RELATIONS

Before proceeding with formal Fourier theory, we must establish the concept of harmonic relations. Starting with one sinusoid of frequency f_0, another sinusoid of frequency nf_0 is said to be harmonically related to the first sinusoid when n is a positive integer. If so, we say that the second sinusoid is the nth harmonic of the first sinusoid.

There is one important property of harmonically related sinusoids: They *all* are periodic with a period of T (= $1/f_0$). To see this, consider the second harmonic of f_0, which repeats itself every $T/2$ seconds. Thus exactly two

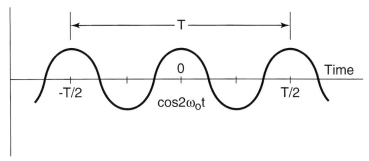

Figure A.3. Short segment of the (infinitely long) *time* domain representation of the sinusoidal function $\cos(2\omega_0 t)$, where ω_0 is equal to $2\pi/T$. The waveform is periodic, with both period $T/2$ and period T.

repetitions of its wave shape require T seconds. Consequently, a waveform segment composed of two periods of a sinusoid with frequency $2f_0$ repeats itself every T seconds (Fig. A.3). Thus the waveform generated by $\cos(2\pi * 2f_0 t)$ is periodic with period T as well as with period $T/2$. Likewise, for a sinusoid of frequency nf_0, the waveform segment composed of n periods of the waveform is exactly T seconds long, and so it too repeats itself every T seconds. Thus $\cos(2\pi * nf_0 t)$ is periodic with period T as well as with period T/n.

FOURIER SERIES

Consider now the sum of a group of harmonically related sinusoids, such as

$$y(t) = \sin(2\pi f_0 t) + \cos(2\pi * 2f_0 t) + \sin(2\pi * 6f_0 t + \pi/2) \quad \text{(A.2)}$$

Because each term is periodic with period T, the whole waveform $y(t)$ must also be periodic with period T. This point can be easily proved mathematically [substitute $(T + t)$ for t in Eq. A.2] but can also be appreciated intuitively. Consider, for example, the hands of a clock. The minute hand revolves exactly 12 times in 12 hours while the hour hand revolves just once. Thus the clock face has a periodic appearance (with $T = 12$ hours) and looks exactly the same 12 hours from now as it does this minute.

This point puts us in a promising position. The sum of a series of harmonically related sinusoids is periodic with period T. Perhaps if we could determine the proper amplitudes and phases (we already know the frequencies) we could represent at least some periodic wave shapes as the sums of sinusoids. That is just what Fourier has given us: a method for determining the composition of these sums. There are essentially no restrictions on the use of the method. It is true that there are several mathematical niceties that must be observed, but they are automatically met by any waveform that could be observed on an oscilloscope (Carslaw, 1950). For practical matters, a sum of sinusoids can always be found that match any given periodic waveform "perfectly."[1]

The general form of the Fourier series includes *all* of the harmonics:

$$x(t) = A_0 + A_1 \cos(\omega_0 t + \theta_1) + A_2 \cos(2\omega_0 t + \theta_2) + \cdots \qquad (A.3)$$

where the A_n terms ($n = 1$ to ∞) are constants. For matters of convenience it is helpful (but not necessary) to split up each of the sinusoids into a cosine and a sine term. Using elementary trigonometric identities, we have

$$x(t) = A_0 + (A_1 \cos \theta_1)\cos(\omega_0 t) + (-A_1 \sin \theta_1)\sin(\omega_0 t)$$

$$+ (A_2 \cos \theta_2)\cos(2\omega_0 t) + (-A_2 \sin \theta_2)\sin(2\omega_0 t) + \cdots \qquad (A.4)$$

Denoting the constant $(A_n\cos\theta_n)$ by a_n, and the constant $(-A_n\sin\theta_n)$ by b_n, we have

$$x(t) = a_0 + \sum_{n=1}^{\infty} [a_n \cos(n\omega_0 t) + b_n \sin(n\omega_0 t)] \qquad (A.5)$$

Now all that remains is to find the a_n and b_n terms. The way we do this is to apply, for each sinusoid, a template of that sinusoid and literally extract from the periodic wave everything that matches the template. The tool for that extraction is the operation of integration.

Consider, for example, the square wave with a period of 2 msec shown in Figure A.4. In order to match the waveform, the sum of sinusoids must repeat every 2 msec, so that must be the basic repetition period (i.e., $T = 2 * 10^{-3}$ sec, so $\omega_0 = 2\pi f_0 = 2\pi/2 * 10^{-3} = \pi * 10^3$). The template for each sinusoid is simply itself. Thus to find the amplitude of b_1 we multiply the periodic waveform $x(t)$ by $\sin(\omega_0 t)$ and integrate over one complete period (taken anywhere along the time axis). Thus

$$b_1 = (2/T) \int_0^T x(t)\sin(\omega_0 t) \, dt$$

$$= (2/T) \int_0^{T/2} (+V)\sin(\omega_0 t) \, dt + (2/T) \int_{T/2}^T (-V)\sin(\omega_0 t) \, dt \qquad (A.6)$$

This equation can be evaluated with elementary calculus to yield $b_1 = 4V/\pi$.

Why does this method work? The answer is related to several factors, one being the combination of the multiplication and area-taking (integration) operations. If a wave shape is positive when the template is positive, their product is positive. If, on the other hand, the wave shape is negative when the template is positive, a negative product results. The integration operation essentially sums all of these products (the $2/T$ in front of the integral sign means that we are really averaging, not summing). Thus the more closely the template tracks the wave shape, the larger is the sum (and average) of all of the products.

Let us apply this reasoning to the waveform of Figure A.4. For the first half-cycle $(0 < t < T/2)$, the waveform $x(t)$ is positive $(+V)$ and so is $\sin(\omega_0 t)$. Thus the product over this entire first half-cycle is positive. For $T/2 < t < T$, both $x(t)$ and $\sin(\omega_0 t)$ are negative, and so their product is positive over the second half-cycle as well. In fact, the product of $x(t)$ and $\sin(\omega_0 t)$ is positive over the entire period, and so its average value is some large positive number ($4V/\pi$, which is larger than V).

Now consider the cosine term having frequency ω_0. During the first quarter-cycle $(0 < t < T/4)$ both terms are positive, and so the product is of course positive. However, over the second quarter-cycle $(T/4 < t < T/2)$ the cosine term is negative, whereas $x(t)$ remains positive; a negative product is produced. Positive and negative products alternate during the last half of the period as well. With part of the period producing positive products and the

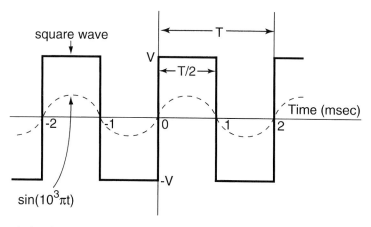

Figure A.4. Time waveform of a periodic square wave having amplitude V and period $T = 2$ msec (solid curve). The waveform of $\sin(2\pi f_0 t)$, the first term in its Fourier expansion, is also shown (dashed curve). Note that the product of the two waveforms is never negative.

other part producing negative products, the average is going to be rather small. In fact, solution of the equation for a_1 can easily be shown to produce a value of zero. *All* of the other a_n values are zero as well.

Solution of the equations for the b_n shows that $b_n = 4V/n\pi$ for odd values of n and zero for even values of n. Thus

$$x(t) = 4V/\pi[\sin(\omega_0 t) + (1/3)\sin(3\omega_0 t) + (1/5)\sin(5\omega_0 t) + \cdots]$$

$$= 4V/\pi \sum_{n=1}^{\infty} (1/n)\sin(n\omega_0 t), \qquad n = \text{odd} \qquad (A.7)$$

Equation A.7 is an enormous achievement. It accomplishes what we started out to do: replace $x(t)$ by a series of sinusoids. But what price victory? We need an infinite number of terms to achieve the equality. How can it be argued that this is a simplification, when all we have done is exchange one complexity (an infinite sequence of $+V$ values and $-V$ values) for another (an infinite number of sinusoids, each of which requires the solution of an integral equation)?

If no further simplifications were possible, the objection would be valid. However, there are many manipulations of the integral equations that can lead to generalizations (Carslaw, 1950). That is, in many cases (as in this one), it may be possible to solve just one general equation for all of the b_n or for all of the a_n. If so, only a few integral equations need be solved, not an infinite number of them. In practice, some simplifications are usually possible.

Furthermore, an infinite number of harmonics is never needed for our purposes. Fourier-series decomposition has the fortunate attribute that the approximation it provides with only a finite sum of terms (i.e., a truncated series) improves with each term added. That is, if the root mean square (rms) error between the original waveform and the sum of the first ten Fourier terms is 2%, for example, the error would be smaller if the 11th term were to be added, still smaller with the 12th, and so on. Thus an arbitrarily good match[1] to a periodic signal can be achieved with a finite Fourier-series representation, simply by adding more and more terms to that series.

FAST FOURIER TRANSFORM

The solution of Fourier integrals (e.g., Eq. A.6) is seldom practiced these days, as the Fourier-series decomposition of the most complicated waveform can be performed on any modern computer in microseconds using a computational process called the *fast Fourier transform* or *FFT* (Ramirez, 1985). However, because all digital computers have finite memories and can deal only with discrete numbers, FFT processing is not exactly the same as the Fourier-series process described by Eq. A.5.

Differences between the two are instructive. First, finite computer memories mean that the FFT can be calculated only for a signal of finite length, not the infinitely extended periodic waveforms implicit in Eq. A.5. This distinction is inconsequential for us, as the FFT processing treats the finite-length waveform as if it were one period of an infinitely long periodic signal. That is, if the waveform analyzed is a measurement of eardrum motion lasting 100 msec, the FFT analysis treats that 100-msec signal as if it were one cycle of a periodic wave having a fundamental frequency of 10 Hertz (Hz). This implicit periodicity produces troublesome artifacts if the value of the last sample taken from the signal is not nearly equal to the first because then the assumed periodic waveform contains discontinuities between successive periods. Various ''windowing'' techniques are used to moderate these artifacts.

A second difference is due to the fact that FFT analysis includes only a finite number of sinusoids in its series, not the infinite number summed in Eq. A.5. However, this finite number of harmonics is not a problem, as it is well known that their sum perfectly matches the necessarily finite sequence of numbers (samples) with which the computer represents the waveform being analyzed (Oppenheim et al., 1983). So long as those samples are taken ''rapidly enough'' (i.e., satisfy the well known ''Nyquist criterion''), FFT analysis can be treated essentially like Fourier-series analysis of the original analogue signal.

APERIODIC SIGNALS

So far, we have considered only periodic signals. What about signals that do not repeat, such as a twig snap? These nonrepeating (or *a*periodic) signals can be handled by an extension of Fourier theory called the Fourier *Transform* (distinct from both the Fourier Series and the FFT). We need not go into the mathematics of the Fourier Transform but simply note that it decomposes any aperiodic signal (so long as it is drawable and finite in area) into a continuum of sinusoids, rather than a series of them. The transient response of a simple flexible system, for example, is decomposed by the Fourier Transform into a continuous band of sinusoids whose frequencies are grouped around that of the single sinusoid that most resembles the response.

The Fourier analysis of transient signals therefore produces continuous *bands* of sinusoids, in contrast to the *series* of sinusoids used to represent periodic signals. For our purposes, however, this distinction is largely academic. Owing to universal use of computers (which can sum but not integrate), almost all transient signals to which we refer were analyzed by FFT methods (i.e., treated as being simply one period of a periodic signal).

OTHER ANALYSIS TECHNIQUES

Fourier methods, valuable as they have proved, are not well suited to handling certain types of signal. For instance, analogue signals containing discontinuities (e.g., square waves) are troublesome, requiring large numbers of harmonics to be included when representing them accurately[1] with a truncated Fourier series (the only practical kind). At a more fundamental level, waveforms emitted by sources that are *not* time-invariant (as in speech production) create conceptual difficulties for Fourier analyses that can be overcome only partially (see Chapter 14).

Consequently, a number of other techniques for analyzing signal waveforms have been developed (see Gade and Gram-Hasen, 1997). Notable among them is *wavelet* analysis, a rising star in recent years, which does an efficient job of representing signals that contain transients or discontinuities (Meyer, 1993; Bruce et al., 1996). That technique is only now beginning to be utilized in auditory science.

NOTE

1. The complete Fourier series (which may have an infinite number of terms) provides, for any periodic time waveform that can be drawn, an *exact* match to those parts of the waveform that are continuous. If the waveform has discontinuities (e.g., square-wave edges) the match is imperfect right *at* the discontinuities. Note, for example, that the Fourier series for the square wave of Figure A.4 has value zero at the wave's discontinuities. However, as these mismatches between waveform and Fourier series exist for only single instants (lasting zero time) during each period, they introduce zero average error into any possible numerical calculations.

APPENDIX B

ACOUSTIC RESONANCES

The basic mechanism of tube resonances can be appreciated by considering the acoustics of a closed rigid tube with a movable piston at one end (Fig. B.1). Assume that at time $t = 0$ the piston instantaneously advances a small amount (d) into the tube (Fig. B.1A). The molecules swept to the right by the piston cause compression of the air directly in front of it (see Fig. 2.1). This thin sheet of compression propagates at the speed of sound (c) to the end of the tube, where it is totally reflected from the immovable terminal wall (see Fig. 3.2C). The reflected compression sheet arrives back at the piston (total round-trip length = $2L$) at time $t = 2L/c$ (Fig. B1.B). At that point it is rereflected from the piston and begins its second trip down the tube.

Let us further assume that as the first reflected compression sheet completes the round trip, the piston instantaneously moves another increment (d) to the right (Fig. B.1C). This movement creates a second compression sheet that begins its own journey down the tube. If this second compression sheet happens to coincide with the twice-reflected first sheet, an even denser compression sheet (producing double pressures) results. This addition of the compression from one cycle of a wave to that of another is what makes up "acoustic resonances."

In the mammalian ear canal (see Fig. 3.5), a resonance occurs because the acoustic impedance of the eardrum (see Appendix C) does not exactly

328

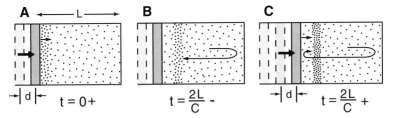

Figure B.1. Phenomenon of acoustic resonance. *A.* The piston in one end of a circular tube moves a small distance *d* (greatly exaggerated here), starting an acoustic compression wave. *B.* The wave is reflected from the far end and heads back to the plate, where it will be re-reflected. *C.* If, at the moment of its arrival back at the plate (*t* = 2*L*/*c*), the old wave is joined by a new wave of compression, the two compression waves superimpose and a traveling sheet of double compression (hence increased pressure) moves down the tube.

match that of the ear canal (see Chapter 4). Thus some of a compression sheet arriving at the eardrum is reflected backward (outward). When it arrives back at the outer end of the ear canal, another impedance mismatch occurs (between air confined in the canal and the free air outside the canal), and some of this once-reflected compression sheet is re-reflected back into the ear canal, although this time it is transformed into a rarefaction sheet (Beranek, 1993). If the doubly reflected sheet, now rarefied and headed back toward the eardrum coincides with the arrival of an incoming rarefaction sheet, the two rarefactions add (e.g., resonance occurs).

Note that timing between cycle arrivals is critical for tonal resonances. The tone's period (e.g., the intervals separating the arrivals of successive cycles) must be such that doubly reflected compressions (transformed to rarefactions by the last reflection) add to incoming rarefactions (''constructive'' interference). If, instead, a doubly reflected compression (transformed to rarefaction by the last reflection) wave coincides with an incoming compression wave, the doubly reflected rarefaction partially cancels the incoming compression, and ''destructive'' interference (or ''antiresonance'') occurs, producing *reduced* pressures.

For the continuously varying pressure waves of pure tones, various degrees of constructive and destructive interference occur, depending on the precise relation between the tone's wavelength and the length of the tube. The principal resonance of the mammalian ear canal, for example, occurs when the length of the ear canal is equal to one-fourth of the stimulating tone's wavelength. As the average adult human ear canal is a little more than 1 inch long (ca. 3 mm), this ''quarter-wavelength resonance'' occurs at about 2.5 kHz (see Fig. 3.7).

APPENDIX C

IMPEDANCE

RESPONSES OF LINEAR (TIME-INVARIANT) SYSTEMS

In a linear time-invariant (unchanging) system, the only possible responses to a sinusoidal input are sinusoids of that same frequency. The validity of this statement can be illustrated by considering the terms in the set of equations describing a linear system. By definition of linearity, *each* of the terms involving any particular system response variable (the particle velocity v, for example) *must* contain v (or *one* of its integrals or derivatives) to the first power only (neither higher nor lower). Suppose, for example, one of the terms in the system equations is

$$v = b * dp/dt \tag{C.1}$$

where the input function is the pressure $p = P_0 * \sin(\omega t)$, and b is a constant. Taking the derivative and using trigonometry, we have

$$v = bP_0\omega * \cos(\omega t) = bP_0\omega * \sin(\omega t + \pi/2) \tag{C.2}$$

In short, for *any* linear acoustic or mechanical system, we know that each time the derivative of the input sinusoid (or any of *its* derivatives) is taken, the result is that same sinusoid with a different amplitude and an added phase angle of $\pi/2$ radians.

The next step is to combine into one all of the various terms involving v in the system equation(s). Suppose, for example, that the (linear) system equation is

$$v = a * p(t) + b * (dp/dt) \tag{C.3}$$

With the help of Eq. C.2, this equation can be rewritten as

$$v = aP_0 * \sin(\omega t) + bP_0\omega * \sin(\omega t + \pi/2) \tag{C.4}$$

Because each of the sinusoidal terms has the same frequency, more trigonometry allows us to combine them all (no matter how many) into a single sinusoidal term. Thus *any* output (velocity in this case) of *any* linear system driven by a pressure at radian frequency ω *must* be of the form $V_0 * \sin(\omega t + \phi)$, where only the amplitude V_0 and the added phase angle ϕ need to be calculated.

IMPEDANCE CALCULATIONS

Comparison of Eqs. C.3 and C.4 is revealing. By introducing the use of a sinusoidal forcing function, the differential equation (Eq. C.3) was transformed into a trigonometric equation (Eq. C.4). As the latter type is usually much easier to solve, it represents a major simplification in the equations. This simplification, coupled with the Fourier methods of decomposing any driving waveform into the sum or integral of sinusoids (see Appendix A), accounts in large part for the great usefulness of Fourier theory.

Acoustic impedance is defined in Chapter 3 as the ratio between driving pressure and the resulting "volume velocity" (velocity times cross-sectional area). We are now in a position to calculate the acoustic impedances of various idealized acoustic elements. Air has mass, so let us start by calculating the acoustic impedance of a thin slab or sheet of air in a cylindrical tube, considering (for the moment) only its mass. To find the acoustic impedance of this thin sheet of air (Fig. C.1A), we must invoke Newton's second law ($\Sigma F = ma$):

$$A * p(t) = m * (d^2x/d^2t) = m * (dv/dt) \tag{C.5}$$

where $p(t)$ represents the pressure acting on the left side of the sheet (for

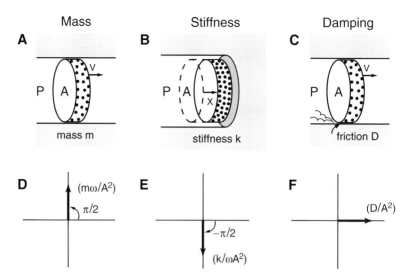

Figure C.1. *A–C.* Three idealized elements often used to model acoustic systems: mass, stiffness, damping. Below each element is a sketch that represents the element's acoustic impedance (i.e., the relation between the sinusoidal pressure acting on the element and its resulting sinusoidal volume velocity). *A.* For a mass, the pressure sinusoid is advanced relative to ("leads") the velocity sinusoid by one-fourth cycle (*D*). *B.* For a stiffness, pressure "lags" velocity by one-fourth cycle (*E*). *C.* For a damping element, pressure and velocity are in phase with each other (*F*).

simplicity of derivation, the pressure on the right side of this sheet is set to zero), and A is cross-sectional area. When the rightward-pushing pressure on the sheet is given as $p(t) = P_0 \sin(\omega t)$, we now know that the velocity of the sheet must be of the form $v(t) = V_0 \sin(\omega t + \phi)$. Thus

$$AP_0 \sin \omega t = (mV_0\omega)\cos(\omega t + \phi) = (mV_0\omega)\sin(\omega t + \phi + \pi/2) \quad (C.6)$$

Equating the respective amplitudes and sine arguments on the two sides of this equation results in the two equalities:

$$P_0 = mV_0\omega/A \quad \text{and} \quad \phi = -\pi/2 \quad (C.7)$$

Thus the velocity of the air slab can be written as

$$v = (P_0A/m\omega) * \sin(\omega t - \pi/2) \quad (C.8)$$

To find the acoustic impedance (Z) of the air sheet, the definition dictates that we form the pressure/volume-velocity ratio. Thus

$$Z = \frac{P_0 * \sin(\omega t)}{A * (P_0 A/m\omega) * \sin(\omega t - \pi/2)} = (m\omega/A^2) * \frac{\sin(\omega t)}{\sin(\omega t - \pi/2)} \quad \text{(C.9)}$$

Unfortunately, this impedance is not a number but, rather, the ratio of two time functions. The pressure magnitude (P_0) appeared in both numerator and denominator and so canceled itself, but the sine terms are in ''quadrature'' phase and cannot be canceled. They would have partially canceled if we had been using exponential notation (Guillemin, 1953), but we do not need that complexity here. Instead, let us adopt a shorthand representation (one consistent with Eq. C.9 expressed in exponential notation).

Returning to Eq. C.8, we see that the volume velocity (Av) has an amplitude $A^2/m\omega$ times the magnitude of the pressure, and the phase of the velocity sinusoid differs from that of the pressure sinusoid by $-\pi/2$. Let us simply use these two relative numbers—magnitude *ratio* and phase *change*—to represent acoustic impedance, with volume velocity being the reference for both comparisons. Thus, the *amplitude* of the acoustic impedance (symbolized by $|Z|$) is ($m\omega/A^2$), and its *phase angle* (symbolized by $\angle Z$) is $+\pi/2$. Therefore the acoustic impedance of the mass of the thin sheet of air can be written in symbols as $|Z| = m\omega/A^2$ and $\angle Z = \pi/2$.

It is worth emphasizing that the acoustic impedance is a *comparison*, giving the pressure (both its amplitude and phase) *relative* to the velocity that pressure produces.

It is a nuisance to carry around two numbers, but there is a convenient way to represent (and manipulate) impedances graphically, as straight lines (vectors) in a two-dimensional plot. The magnitude of an impedance sets the length of the line, and the phase of the impedance determines the line's angle (relative to the positive horizontal axis). In this graphical form, the acoustic impedance of the thin sheet's mass is an upward-pointing vector ($\angle Z = +\pi/2$) of magnitude $|Z| = m\omega/A^2$ (Fig. C.1D). Note, incidentally, that this magnitude grows proportionally with frequency. In other words, the higher the frequency of the mass's oscillations, the more force it takes to maintain a constant magnitude of velocity (just try to lift weights rapidly up and down).

In addition to mass, the thin sheet of air also has springiness (it pushes back if compressed). To picture this, it is convenient to place our sheet of air at the end of the tube (Fig. C.1B). Pressure applied to the tube compresses the air in the sheet, and so the free (left) face of the sheet moves to the right by an amount x. This movement is described by the equation for a spring:

$F = kx$, where k is a measure of the air's compressibility. Thus substituting in the spring equation,

$$A * p(t) = k * x(t) = k * \int (v * dt) \qquad \text{(C.10)}$$

Substituting the known expressions for p and v, we have

$$AP_0 \sin(\omega t) = kV_0 \int \sin(\omega t + \phi) \, dt \qquad \text{(C.11)}$$

Integration and use of simple trigonometric identities produce

$$P_0 \sin(\omega t) = -(kV_0/\omega A)\cos(\omega t + \phi) = (kV_0/\omega A)\sin(\omega t + \phi - \pi/2) \quad \text{(C.12)}$$

Again, separately equating amplitudes and sinusoidal arguments on the two sides of the equation produces two equalities:

$$P_0 = kV_0/\omega A \quad \text{and} \quad \phi = \pi/2 \qquad \text{(C.13)}$$

Finally, using the shorthand notation, we can then say that the acoustic impedance of the sheet's springiness is

$$|Z| = P_0/AV_0 = k/\omega A^2 \quad \text{and} \quad \angle Z = -\phi = -\pi/2 \qquad \text{(C.14)}$$

shown in Figure C.1E as a downward-pointing vector. Notice that the acoustic impedance of springiness increases as frequency *decreases*; that is, the lower the frequency, the more difficult it is to obtain a certain maximum velocity (try moving workout springs at high velocity but low frequency).

The final attribute of the air sheet to be considered is the friction that occurs when the air molecules slide along the surface of the tube (and interact with each other). The simplest equation for representing friction is $F = Dv$, where D is an approximate measure of how rough the surface is (how much friction it can generate). Writing the friction equation for the air sheet (momentarily ignoring its mass and stiffness properties), we have

$$A * p(t) = D * v(t) \qquad \text{(C.15)}$$

Substitution of the known quantities then produces

$$AP_0 \sin(\omega t) = DV_0 \sin(\omega t + \phi) \qquad \text{(C.16)}$$

Finally, equating amplitudes and arguments in this equation, the acoustic impedance presented by the friction properties of the air sheet is calculated to be

$$|Z| = P_0/AV_0 = D/A^2 \quad \text{and} \quad \angle Z = -\phi = 0 \qquad (C.17)$$

This impedance is represented graphically by a horizontal vector of length D/A^2 (Fig. C.1F). Note that this impedance does not vary as a function of frequency.

Having looked separately at each acoustic property of the air sheet, we are now in a position to put them all together and obtain a description of the completely characterized air sheet. It can be done by recognizing that to move the sheet the pressure must accelerate the mass, compress the gas, *and* overcome wall friction simultaneously. The basic equation representing this combination of effects is

$$F(t) = Ap(t) = m(dv/dt) + k \int (v * dt) + Dv \qquad (C.18)$$

Substituting known quantities (see Eqs. C.6, C.12, and C.16), we have

$$AP_0 \sin(\omega t) = mV_0\omega \cos(\omega t + \phi) - (kV_0/\omega)\cos(\omega t + \phi) + DV_0 \sin(\omega t + \phi)$$
$$(C.19)$$

Trigonometric identities can be used to solve this equation for the velocity, but it becomes algebraically messy. Fortunately, it can be shown that judicious use of the graphical representations of the impedances does the job quickly (Fig. C.2). Specifically, if we ''add'' the acoustic impedances produced by each of the three properties (mass, stiffness, damping), we obtain the total acoustic impedance of the sheet. The quotation marks are put around the term *add* to indicate that this addition must be carried on in a specific way (to preserve the phase relations that exist between pressure and velocity for the various elements).

First, the vertically plotted impedances (mass and stiffness) must be *arithmetically* added together, treating the stiffness impedance as negative. Roughly speaking, the physical meaning of this addition (actually subtraction) is that the force needed to oscillate the mass of an object is opposite in phase to the force needed to sinusoidally stretch and compress that same object. Because *total* force drives the unitary mass-spring object, only the difference between the two out-of-phase force components is significant [e.g., $A \sin(\omega t) + B \sin(\omega t + \pi) = (A - B)\sin(\omega t)$]. This difference (drawn

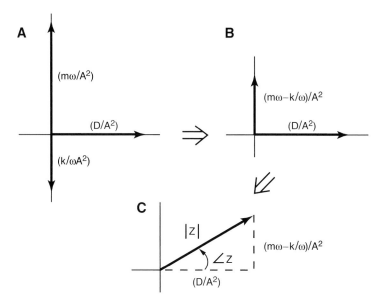

Figure C.2. Graphical determination of the total acoustic impedance of a physical structure having mass, stiffness, and damping. *A.* Impedances of each idealized element of the structure, plotted on the same graph. *B.* Impedance of the stiffness is subtracted from the impedance of the mass to form the "reactive" impedance. *C.* Reactive impedance is added vectorially to the damping ("resistive") impedance to form the total impedance of the structure, *Z*, a term that has both a magnitude $|Z|$ and an angle $\angle Z$.

as the vertical arrow in Fig. C.2B) is termed the "reactive" component of the impedance.

Second, this vertical reactive component must be added *trigonometrically* to the horizontal "resistive" (friction) component (Fig. C.2C). The reason for this trigonometric (vector) addition is that, in essence, we are adding together the three force components needed to oscillate a compressible mass that possesses friction. The net force component needed to oscillate simultaneously the object's mass and compress its springiness (the "reactive" force) is 90° out of phase with the force component that overcomes the friction produced by those oscillations (the "resistive" force). By simple trigonometry on the right triangle thus formed by these quadrature components, we finally obtain the acoustic impedance of the air sheet:

$$|Z| = (1/A^2)\sqrt{[(m\omega - k/\omega)^2 + D^2]} \quad \text{and}$$

$$\angle Z = \tan^{-1}[(m\omega - k/\omega)/D] \tag{C.20}$$

Among the important properties of this total impedance is the form of its reactive component: It can go to zero, which occurs when the mass and stiffness exactly cancel out each other's effects. This "resonance" occurs only when $\omega = \sqrt{(k/m)}$, the "resonant frequency." At frequencies above resonance, the mass dominates the reactive component, whereas at lower frequencies the stiffness predominates.

Although this development has been concerned with *acoustic* impedance, the same development describes *mechanical* impedance. Only the scales are changed. Specifically, mechanical impedance is defined as the ratio of the force acting on an object (the usual driving factor) to object velocity (the response). For the same object (e.g., a thin sheet of air), these impedances differ only by the factor A^2.

REFERENCES

Ainsworth, W., and S. Greenberg (Eds.). *Proceedings of the Workshop on the Auditory Basis of Speech Perception.* New York: Oxford University Press (in preparation).

Allen, J. B. Cochlear micromechanics—a physical model of transduction. *J. Acoust. Soc. Am.* 68:1660–1670, 1980.

Anderson, D. J., J. E. Rose, J. E. Hind, and J. F. Brugge. Temporal position of discharges in single auditory nerve fibers within the cycle of a sine-wave stimulus: frequency and intensity effects. *J. Acoust. Soc. Am.* 49:1131–1139, 1971.

Angelborg, C., and H. Engström. Supporting elements in the organ of Corti. *Acta Otolaryngol. Suppl.* 301:49–60, 1972.

Art, J. J., A. C. Crawford, and R. Fettiplace. Electrical resonance and membrane currents in turtle cochlear hair cells. *Hear. Res.* 22:31–36, 1986.

Art, J. J., R. Fettiplace, and P. A. Fuchs. Synaptic hyperpolarization and inhibition of turtle cochlear hair cells. *J. Physiol. (Lond.)* 356:525–550, 1984.

Arthur, R. M., R. R. Pfeiffer, and N. Suga. Properties of "two-tone inhibition" in primary auditory neurones. *J. Physiol. (Lond.)* 212:593–609, 1971.

Ashmore, J. F. Transducer motor coupling in cochlear outer hair cells. In: *Mechanics of Hearing*, edited by D. Kemp and J. P. Wilson. New York: Plenum, 1989, pp. 107–113.

Ashmore, J. F., and I. J. Russell. Effect of efferent nerve stimulation on hair cells of the frog sacculus. *J. Physiol. (Lond.)* 329:25–26P, 1982.

Ashmore, J. F., F. Mammano, J. E. Gale, and M. J. Tunstall. The pharmacology of the outer hair cell motor. In: *Active Hearing*, edited by Å. Flock, D. Ottoson, and M. Ulfendahl. Tarrytown, NY: Elsevier Science, 1995, pp. 337–348.

Assad, J. A., and D. P. Corey. An active motor model for adaptation by vertebrate hair cells. *J. Neurosci.* 12:3291–3309, 1992.

Assad, J. A., N. Hacohen, and D. P. Corey. Voltage dependence of adaptation and active bundle movement in bullfrog saccular hair cells. *Proc. Natl. Acad. Sci. U.S.A.* 86:2918–2922, 1989.

Assad, J. A., G. M. G. Shepard, and D. P. Corey. Tip-link integrity and mechanical transduction in vertebrate hair cells. *Neuron* 7:985–994, 1991.

Authier, S., and G. A. Manley. A model of frequency tuning in the basilar papilla of the Tokay gecko, *Gekko gecko. Hear. Res.* 82:1–13, 1995.

Bárány E. A contribution to the physiology of bone conduction. *Acta Otolaryngol. Suppl.* 26, 1938.

Beranek, L. L. *Acoustics.* New York: McGraw-Hill, 1954; and Woodbury, NY: Acoustical Society of America, 1993.

Bergenstoff, H. Hearing instruments from past to present. In: *Recent Developments in Hearing Instrument Technology* (*15th Danavox Symposium*), edited by J. Beilin and G. R. Jensen (Scanticon, Denmark), 1993, pp. 13–38.

Bialek, W. Physical limits to sensations and perception. *Annu. Rev. Biophys. Chem.* 16:455–478, 1987.

Bialek, W., and H. P. Wit. Quantum limits to oscillator stability: Theory and experiments on acoustic emissions from the human ear. *Phys. Lett.* 104A:173–178, 1984. (*Copyright owned by Elsevier Science-NL, Sara Burgerhartstraat 25, 1055 KV Amsterdam, The Netherlands.)

Blauert, J. *Spatial Hearing.* Cambridge: M.I.T. Press, 1983.

Bohne, B. A., and K. D. Rabbitt. Holes in the reticular lamina after noise exposure: implication for continuing damage in the organ of Corti. *Hear. Res.* 11:41–53, 1983.

Bohne, B. A., P. H. Ward, and C. Fernández. Irreversible inner ear damage from rock music. *Trans. Am. Acad. Ophthalmol. Otolaryngol.* ORL50–ORL59, 1976.

Boothroyd, A. Profound deafness. In: *Cochlear Implants: Audiological Foundations*, edited by R. S. Tyler. San Diego: Singular Publishing Group, 1993, Chap. 1.

Borg, E., and J-E. Zakrisson. The activity of the stapedius muscle in man during vocalization. *Acta Otolaryngol.* 79:325–333, 1975.

Borg, E., and S. A. Counter. The middle-ear muscles. *Sci. Am.* 260:74–80, 1989.

Borg, E., S. A. Counter, and G. Rösler. Theories of middle-ear muscle function, In: *The Acoustic Reflex*, edited by S. Silman. Orlando, FL: Academic, 1984, Chap. 3.

Brass, D., and Kemp, D. T. Analyses of Mössbauer mechanical measurements indicate that the cochlea is mechanically alive. *J. Acoust. Soc. Am.* 93:1502–1515, 1993.

Brichta, A. M., and J. M. Goldberg. Afferent and efferent responses from morphological fiber classes in the turtle posterior crista. *Ann. N.Y. Acad. Sci.* 781:183–195, 1996.

Brown, A. M., B. McDowell, and A. Forge. Acoustic distortion products can be used to monitor the effects of chronic gentamicin treatment. *Hear. Res.* 42:143–156, 1989.

Brown, M. C., and A. L. Nuttall. Efferent control of cochlear inner hair cell responses in the guinea pig. *J. Physiol.* (*Lond.*) 354:625–646, 1984.

Brown, M. C., A. L. Nuttall, and R. I. Masta. Intracellular recordings from cochlear inner hair cells: effects of stimulation of the crossed olivocochlear efferents.

Science 222:69–71, 1983. (*Copyright owned by the American Association for the Advancement of Science, Washington, DC.)

Brownell, W. E. Observation on a motile response in isolated hair cells. In: *Mechanisms of Hearing*, edited by W. R. Webster and L. M. Aiken. Melbourne: Monash University Press, 1983, pp. 5–10.

Brownell, W. E. Outer hair cell electromotility and otoacoustic emissions. *Ear Hear.* 11:82–92, 1990. (*Copyright owned by Willliams & Wilkins, Baltimore, MD.)

Brownell, W. E., C. R. Bader, D. Bertrand, and Y. de Ribaupierre. Evoked mechanical responses of isolated cochlear hair cells. *Science* 227:194–196, 1985. (*Copyright owned by the American Association for the Advancement of Science, Washington, DC.)

Bruce, A., D. Donoho, and H-Y. Gao. Wavelet analysis. *I.E.E.E. Spectrum* 33(10): 26–35, 1996.

Brugge, J. F., D. J. Anderson, J. E. Hind, and J. E. Rose. Time structure of discharges in single auditory fibers of the squirrel monkey in response to complex periodic sounds. *J. Neurophysiol.* 32:386–401, 1969. (*Copyright owned by The American Physiological Society, Bethesda, MD.)

Buerkli-Halevy, O., and H. Baechler. Digital programmable spectral and temporal properties of AGC circuits allow a wide variety of new applications. In: *Recent Developments in Hearing Instrument Technology* (*15th Danavox Symposium*), edited by J. Beilin and G. R. Jensen (Scanticon, Denmark), 1993, pp. 295–310. (*Copyright owned by The Danavox Jubilee Foundation, Tåstrup, Denmark.)

Butler, R. A., and K. Belendiuk. Spectral cues utilized in the localization of sound in the median sagittal plane. *J. Acoust. Soc. Am.* 61:1264–1269, 1977.

Cai, Y., and C. D. Geisler. Suppression in auditory-nerve fibers of cats using low-side suppressors. II. Effect of spontaneous rates. *Hear. Res.* 96:113–125, 1996. (*Copyright owned by Elsevier Science-NL, Sara Burgerhartstraat 25, 1055 KV Amsterdam, The Netherlands.)

Capranica, R. R. Auditory processing in anurans. *Federation Proc.* 37:2324–2328, 1978.

Carney, L. H. A model for the responses of low-frequency auditory-nerve fibers in cat. *J. Acoust. Soc. Am.* 93:401–417, 1993.

Carney, L. H., and C. D. Geisler. A temporal analysis of auditory-nerve fiber responses to spoken stop consonant-vowel syllables. *J. Acoust. Soc. Am.* 79: 1896–1914, 1986. (*Copyright owned by the American Institute of Physics, Woodbury, NY.)

Carney, L. H., and T. C. T. Yin. Temporal coding of resonances by low-frequency auditory nerve fibers: single-fiber responses and a population model. *J. Neurophysiol.* 60:1653–1677, 1988.

Carslaw, H. L. *Introduction to the Theory of Fourier Series and Integrals.* London: Macmillan, 1930; and New York: Dover, 1950.

Christensen-Dalsgaard, J., and M. B. Jørgensen. One-tone suppression in the frog auditory nerve. *J. Acoust. Soc. Am.* 100:451–457, 1996.

Clark, G. M., Y. C. Tong, and J. F. Patrick (Eds.) *Cochlear Prostheses.* Melbourne, Australia: Churchill Livingstone, 1990.

Clark, W. A., and C. E. Molnar. A description of the LINC. In: *Computers in Biomedical Research*, Vol. II. edited by R. W. Stacy and B. Waxman. Orlando, FL: Academic, 1965, Chap. 2.

Clark, W. W., D. O. Kim, P. M. Zurek, and B. A. Bohne. Spontaneous otoacoustic emission in chinchilla ear canals: correlation with histopathology and suppression by external tones. *Hear. Res.* 16:299–314, 1984.

Cody, A. R. Acoustic lesions in the mammalian cochlea: implications for the spatial distribution of the "active process." *Hear. Res.* 62:166–172, 1992.

Cooper, N. P. Two-tone suppression in cochlear mechanics. *J. Acoust. Soc. Am.* 99: 3087–3098, 1996.

Cooper, N. P., and W. S. Rhode. Basilar membrane tonotopicity in the hook region of the cat cochlea. *Hear. Res.* 63:191–196, 1992.

Cooper, N. P., and W. S. Rhode. Two-tone suppression in apical cochlear mechanics. *Aud. Neurosci.* 3:123–134, 1996. (*Copyright owned by Harwood Academic Publishers, Lausanne, Switzerland.)

Cooper, N. P., and G. K. Yates. Nonlinear input–output functions derived from the responses of guinea-pig cochlear nerve fibres: variations with characteristic frequency. *Hear. Res.* 78:221–234, 1994.

Cooper, N. P., D. Robertson, and G. K. Yates. Cochlear nerve fiber responses to amplitude-modulated stimuli: variations with spontaneous rate and other response characteristics. *J. Neurophysiol.* 70:370–386, 1993.

Corwin, J. T. Postembryonic production and aging of inner ear hair cells in sharks. *J. Comp. Neurol.* 201:541–553, 1981.

Corwin, J. T. Perpetual production of hair cells and maturational changes in hair cell ultrastructure accompany postembryonic growth in an amphibian ear. *Proc. Natl. Acad. Sci. U.S.A.* 82:3911–3915, 1985.

Corwin, J. T., and D. A. Cotanche. Regeneration of sensory hair cells after acoustic trauma. *Science* 240:1772–1774, 1988.

Corwin, J. T., and M. E. Warchol. Auditory hair cells: structure, function, development and regeneration. *Annu. Rev. Neurosci.* 14:310–333, 1991.

Cotanche, D. A. Regeneration of hair cell stereociliary bundles in the chick cochlea following severe acoustic trauma. *Hear. Res.* 30:181–196, 1987.

Crawford, A. C., and R. Fettiplace. The frequency selectivity of auditory nerve fibres and hair cells in the cochlea of the turtle. *J. Physiol. (Lond.)* 306:79–125, 1980.

Crawford, A. C., and R. Fettiplace. The mechanical properties of ciliary bundles of turtle cochlear hair cells. *J. Physiol. (Lond.)* 364:359–379, 1985.

Crawford, A. C., M. G. Evans, and R. Fettiplace. The actions of calcium on the mechanoelectrical transducer current of turtle hair cells. *J. Physiol. (Lond.)* 434: 369–398, 1991. (*Copyright owned by *The Journal of Physiology*, Cambridge, UK.)

Cruz, R. M., P. R. Lambert, and E. W. Rubel. Light microscopic evidence of hair cell regeneration in the chick cochlea after gentamicin ototoxicity. *Arch. Otolaryngol. Head Neck Surg.* 113:1058–1062, 1987.

Cummins, K. L., and K. E. Hecox. Ambulatory testing of digital hearing aid algorithms. Presented at the RESNA 10th Annual Conference, San Jose, CA, 1987.

Dallos, P. Low-frequency auditory characteristics: species dependence. *J. Acoust. Soc. Am.* 48:489–499, 1970.

Dallos, P. *The Auditory Periphery: Biophysics and Physiology.* Orlando, FL: Academic, 1973.

Dallos, P. Neurobiology of cochlear inner and outer hair cells: intracellular recordings. *Hear. Res.* 22:185–198, 1986.

Dallos, P. The active cochlea. *J. Neurosci.* 12:4575–4585, 1992. (*Copyright is owned by the Society for Neuroscience, Washington, DC.)

Dallos, P., B. N. Evans, and R. Hallworth. Nature of the motor element in electro-kinetic shape changes of cochlear outer hair cells. *Nature* 350:155–157, 1991.

Dallos, P., D. Z-z. He, B. N. Evans, and B. Clark. Dynamic characteristics of outer hair cell motility. In: *Biophysics of Hair Cell Sensory Systems*, edited by H. Duifhuis, J. W. Horst, P. van Dijk, and S. M. van Netten. Singapore: World Scientific, 1993, pp. 167–174.

Davis, C. Q., and D. M. Freeman. Direct observations of sound-induced motions of the reticular lamina, tectorial membrane, hair bundles, and individual stereocilia. *Abstr. Assoc. Res. Otolaryngol.* 18:189, 1995.

De Boer, E. Power amplification in an active model of the cochlea: short-wave case: *J. Acoust. Soc. Am.* 73:577–579, 1983.

De Boer, E. On equivalence of locally active models of the cochlea. *J. Acoust. Soc. Am.* 98:1400–1409, 1995a.

De Boer, E. The "inverse problem" solved for a three-dimensional model of the cochlea. II. Application to experimental sets. *J. Acoust. Soc. Am.* 98:904–910, 1995b.

De Boer, E. Mechanics of the cochlea: modeling efforts. In: *The Cochlea*, edited by P. Dallos, A. N. Popper, and R. R. Fay. New York: Springer, 1996, Chapter 5.

De Boer, E., and H. R. de Jongh. On cochlear encoding: potentialities and limitations of the reverse-correlation technique. *J. Acoust. Soc. Am.* 63:115–135, 1978.

Decraemer, W. F., S. M. Khanna, and W. R. J. Funnell. Interferometric measurement of the amplitude and phase of tympanic membrane vibrations in cat. *Hear. Res.* 38:1–18, 1989.

Decraemer, W. F., S. M. Khanna, and W. R. J. Funnell. Malleus vibration mode changes with frequency. *Hear. Res.* 54:305–318, 1991.

Delgutte, B. Some correlates of phonetic distinctions at the level of the auditory nerve. In: *The Representation of Speech in the Peripheral Auditory System*, edited by R. Carlson and B. Granström. Amsterdam: Elsevier Biomedical Press, 1982, pp. 131–149.

Delgutte, B. Peripheral auditory processing of speech information: implications from a physiological study of intensity discrimination. In: *The Psychophysics of Speech Perception*, edited by M. E. H. Schouten. Dordrecht, The Netherlands: Nijhoff, 1987, pp. 333–353.

Delgutte, B. Physiological mechanisms of psychophysical masking: observations from auditory-nerve fibers. *J. Acoust. Soc. Am.* 87:791–809, 1990.

Delgutte, B. Two-tone rate suppression in auditory-nerve fibers: Dependence on suppressor frequency and level. *Hear. Res.* 49:225–246, 1990. (*Copyright owned by Elsevier Science-NL, Sara Burgerhartstraat 25, 1055 KV Amsterdam, The Netherlands.)

Delgutte, B. Auditory neural processing of speech. In: *The Handbook of Phonetic Sciences*, edited by W. J. Hardcastle and J. Laver. Cambridge: Blackwell Publishers, 1997, Chapter 16.

Delgutte, B., and N. Y. S. Kiang. Speech coding in the auditory nerve. III. Voiceless fricative consonants. *J. Acoust. Soc. Am.* 75:887–896, 1984a. (*Copyright owned by the American Institute of Physics, Woodbury, NY.)

Delgutte, B., and N. Y. S. Kiang. Speech coding in the auditory nerve. V. Vowels in background noise. *J. Acoust. Soc. Am.* 75:908–918, 1984b.

Deng, L., and C. D. Geisler. A composite auditory model for processing speech sounds. *J. Acoust. Soc. Am.* 82:2001–2012, 1987.

Denk, W., and W. W. Webb. Forward and reverse transduction at the limit of sensitivity studied by correlating electrical and mechanical fluctuations in frog saccular hair cells. *Hear. Res.* 60:89–102, 1992.

Denk, W., W. W. Webb, and A. J. Hudspeth. Mechanical properties of sensory hair bundles are reflected in their Brownian motion measured with a laser differential interferometer. *Proc. Natl. Acad. Sci. U.S.A.* 86:5371–5375, 1989.

Denk, W., J. R. Holt, G. M. G. Shepard, and D. P. Corey. Calcium imaging of single stereocilia in hair cells: localization of transduction channels at both ends of tip links. *Neuron* 15:1311–1321, 1995.

Diependaal, R. J., E. de Boer, and M. A. Viergever. Cochlear flux as an indicator of mechanical activity. *J. Acoust. Soc. Am.* 82:917–926, 1987.

Dorman, M. F. Speech perception by adults. In: *Cochlear Implants: Audiological Foundations*, edited by R. S. Tyler. San Diego: Singular Publishing Group, 1993, Chap. 4.

Dulon, D., and J. Schacht. Motility of cochlear outer hair cells. *Am. J. Otol.* 13: 108–112, 1992.

Dunn, H. K., and S. D. White. Statistical measurements on conversational speech. *J. Acoust. Soc. Am.* 11:278–288, 1940.

Durlach, N. I., and H. S. Colburn. Binaural phenomena. In: *Handbook of Perception, Vol. 4: Hearing*, edited by E. C. Carterette and M. P. Friedman. Orlando, FL: Academic, 1978, pp. 365–466.

Eatock, R. A., G. A. Manley, and L. Pawson. Auditory nerve fibre activity in the tokay gecko. I. Implications for cochlear processing. *J. Comp. Physiol. A* 142: 203–218, 1981.

Eatock, R. A., M. Saeki, and M. J. Hutzler. Electrical resonance of isolated hair cells does not account for the acoustic tuning in a free-standing region of the alligator lizards cochlea. *J. Neurosci.* 13:1767–1783, 1993.

Eggermont, J. J. On the pathophysiology of tinnitus: a review and a peripheral model. *Hear. Res.* 48:111–124, 1990.

Ehret, G., and R. Romand (Eds.). *The Central Auditory System*. New York: Oxford Univ., 1997.

Elgoyhen, A. B., D. S. Johnson, J. Boulter, D. E. Vetter, and S. Heinemann. α9: An acetylcholine receptor with novel pharmacological properties expressed in rat cochlear hair cells. *Cell* 79:705–715, 1994.

Engström, H., H. W. Ades, and A. Anderson. *Structural Pattern of the Organ of Corti*. Baltimore: Williams & Wilkins, 1966.

Epstein, J. E., and D. A. Contanche. Secretion of a new basal layer of tectorial membrane following gentamicin-induced hair cell loss. *Hear. Res.* 90:31–43, 1995.

Erostegui, C., C. H. Norris, and R. P. Bobbin. In vitro pharmacologic characterization of a cholinergic receptor on outer hair cells. *Hear. Res.* 74:135–147, 1994.

Evans, E. F. Frequency selectivity at high signal levels of single units in cochlear nerve and cochlear nucleus. In: *Psychophysics and Physiology of Hearing*, edited by E. F. Evans and J. P. Wilson. Orlando, FL: Academic, 1977, pp. 185–192. (*Copyright owned by Academic Press, San Diego, CA.)

Evans, E. F. Aspects of the neural coding of time in the mammalian peripheral auditory system relevant to temporal resolution. In: *Time Resolution in Auditory Systems*, edited by A. Michelsen. New York: Springer-Verlag, 1985, pp. 74–95.

Evans, E. F., and R. Klinke. The effects of intracochlear and systemic furosemide on the properties of single cochlear nerve fibers in the cat. *J. Physiol. (Lond.)* 331:409–427, 1982.

Eybalin, M. Neurotransmitters and neuromodulators of the mammalian cochlea. *Physiol. Rev.* 73:309–373, 1993.

Fawcett, D. W. *A Textbook of Histology*, 12 ed. New York: Chapman & Hall, 1994, p. 929. (*Copyright owned by Chapman & Hall, New York, NY.)

Fay, R. R. *Hearing in Vertebrates*: *A Psychophysics Databook*. Winnetka, IL: Hill-Fay Associates, 1988.

Fay, R. R., and A. N. Popper (Eds.). *Comparative Hearing*: *Mammals*. New York: Springer-Verlag, 1994.

Felder, E., and A. Schrott-Fischer. Quantitative evaluation of myelinated nerve fibres and hair cells in cochleae of humans with age-related high-tone hearing loss. *Hear. Res.* 91:19–32, 1995.

Felix, D., and K. Ehrenberger. The efferent modulation of mammalian inner hair cell afferents. *Hear. Res.* 64:1–5, 1992.

Feng, A. S., P. M. Narins, and R. R. Capranica. Three populations of primary auditory fibers in the bullfrog (*Rana catesbeiana*): their peripheral origins and frequency sensitivities. *J. Comp. Physiol.* 100:221–229, 1975.

Fettiplace, R. Electrical tuning of haircells in the inner ear. *TINS* 10:421–425, 1987.

Fettiplace, R. The role of calcium in hair cell transduction. In: *Sensory Transduction*, edited by D. P. Corey and S. D. Roper. New York: Rockefeller University Press, 1992, Chap. 22. (*Copyright owned by The Rockfeller University Press, New York.)

Fettiplace, R., A. C. Crawford, and M. G. Evans. The hair cell's mechanical transducer channel. *Ann. N.Y. Acad. Sci.* 656:1–11, 1992.

Fitzgerald, M., and C. J. Woolf. Effects of cutaneous nerve and intraspinal conditioning on C-fibre efferent terminal excitability in decerebrate spinal rats. *J. Physiol.* (*Lond.*) 318:25–39, 1981.

Flanagan, J. L. *Speech Analysis Synthesis and Perception*, 2nd ed. New York: Springer-Verlag, 1972. (*Copyright owned by Springer-Verlag, New York.)

Flock, Å. Sensory transduction in hair cells. In: *Handbook of Sensory Physiology*, Vol. 1, edited by W. R. Loewenstein. New York: Springer-Verlag, 1971, Chap. 14.

Flock, Å. Physiological properties of relative ion distribution in the inner ear. *Acta Otolaryngol.* 83:239–244, 1977.

Flock, Å., and I. Russell. Inhibition by efferent nerve fibres: action on hair cells and afferent synaptic transmission in the lateral line canal organ of the burbot *Lota lota. J. Physiol.* (*Lond.*) 257:45–62, 1976.

Flock, Å., H. C. Cheung, B. Flock, and G. Utter. Three sets of actin filaments in sensory cells of the inner ear: identification and functional orientation determined by gel electrophoresis, immunofluorescence and electron microscopy. *J. Neurocytol.* 10:133–147, 1981.

Fowler, E. P. Head noises in normal and disordered ears: significance, measurement, differentiation and treatment. *Arch. Otolaryngol.* 39:498–503, 1944.

Freeman, D. M., and T. F. Weiss. The role of fluid inertia in mechanical stimulation of hair cells. *Hear. Res.* 35:201–208, 1988.

Freeman, D. M., and T. F. Weiss. Hydrodynamic forces on hair bundles at low frequencies. *Hear. Res.* 48:17–30, 1990a.

Freeman, D. M., and T. F. Weiss. Hydrodynamic forces on hair bundles at high frequencies. *Hear. Res.* 48:31–36, 1990b.

Freeman, D. M., and T. F. Weiss. Hydrodynamic analysis of a two-dimensional model for micromechanical resonance of free-standing hair bundles. *Hear. Res.* 48:37–68, 1990c.

Freeman, D. M., D. K. Hendrix, D. Shah, L. F. Fan, and T. F. Weiss. Effect of lymph composition on an in vitro preparation of the alligator lizard cochlea. *Hear. Res.* 65:83–98, 1993. (*Copyright owned by Elsevier Science-NL, Sara Burgerhart-straat 25, 1055 KV Amsterdam, The Netherlands.)

Frishkopf, L. S., and D. J. DeRosier. Mechanical tuning of free-standing stereociliary bundles and frequency analysis in the alligator lizard cochlea. *Hear. Res.* 12:393–404, 1983.

Frisina, D. R., and R. D. Frisina. Speech recognition in noise and presbycusis: relations to possible neural mechanisms. *Hear. Res.* 106:95–104, 1997.

Froehlich, P., L. Collet, J. M. Chanal, and A. Morgon. Variability of the influence of a visual task on the active micromechanical properties of the cochlea. *Brain Res.* 508:286–288, 1990.

Fuchs, P. A. Synaptic transmission at vertebrate hair cells. *Curr. Opin. Neurobiol.* 6:514–519, 1996.

Fuchs, P. A., and M. G. Evans. Voltage oscillations and ionic conductances in hair cells isolated from the alligator cochlea. *J. Comp. Physiol. A* 164:151–163, 1988.

Fuchs, P. A., and B. W. Murrow. Cholinergic inhibition of short (outer) hair cells of the chick's cochlea. *J. Neurosci.* 12:800–809, 1992.

Fuchs, P. A., T. Nagai, and M. G. Evans. Electrical tuning in hair cells isolated from the chick cochlea. *J. Neurosci.* 8:2460–2467, 1988.

Fukazawa, T., and Y. Tanaka. Spontaneous otoacoustic emissions in an active feed-forward model of the cochlea. *Hear. Res.* 95:135–143, 1996.

Furness, D. N., C. M. Hackney, and D. J. Benos. The binding site on cochlear stereocilia for antisera raised against renal Na^+ channels is blocked by amiloride and dihydrostreptomycin. *Hear. Res.* 93:136–146, 1996.

Furness, D. N., D. E. Zetes, C. M. Hackney, and C. R. Steele. Kinematic analysis of shear displacement as a means for operating mechanotransduction channels in the contact region between adjacent stereocilia of mammalian cochlea hair cells. *Proc. R. Soc. Lond. B* 264:45–51, 1997.

Furukawa, T., and S. Matsuura. Adaptive rundown of excitatory post-synaptic potentials at synapses between hair cells and eighth nerve fibres in the goldfish. *J. Physiol. (Lond.)* 276:193–209, 1978.

Fuzessery, Z. M. Monaural and binaural spectral cues created by the external ears of the pallid bat. *Hear. Res.* 95:1–17, 1996.

Gade, S., and K. Gram-Hansen. The analysis of nonstationary signals. *Sound and Vibration* 31:40–46, 1997.

Gao, J-H., L. M. Parsons, J. M. Bower, J. Xiong, J. Li, and P. T. Fox. Cerebellum implicated in sensory acquisition and discrimination rather than motor control. *Science* 272:545–547, 1996.

Garetz, S. L., and J. Schacht. Ototoxicity: of mice and men. In: *Clinical Aspects of Hearing*, edited by T. R. Van De Water, A. N. Popper, and R. R. Fay. New York: Springer-Verlag, 1996, Chap. 5.

Geisler, C. D. A model for discharge patterns of primary auditory-nerve fibers. *Brain Res.* 212:198–201, 1981.

Geisler, C. D. Coding of acoustic signals on the auditory nerve. *I.E.E.E. E.M.B. Magazine* June:22–28, 1987. (*Copyright owned by the Institute of Electrical and Electronic Engineers, Piscataway, NJ.)

Geisler, C. D. Two-tone suppression by a saturating feedback model of the cochlear partition. *Hear. Res.* 63:203–211, 1992.

Geisler, C. D. A model of stereociliary tip-link stretches. *Hear. Res.* 65:79–82, 1993.

Geisler, C. D. Further results with the "uniquantal-EPSP" hypothesis. *Hear. Res.* (in press).

Geisler, C. D., and Y. Cai. Relationships between frequency-tuning and spatial-tuning curves in the mammalian cochlea. *J. Acoust. Soc. Am.* 99:1550–1555, 1996.

Geisler, C. D., and T. Gamble. Responses of "high-spontaneous" auditory-nerve fibers to consonant-vowel syllables in noise. *J. Acoust. Soc. Am.* 85:1639–1652, 1989. (*Copyright owned by the American Institute of Physics, Woodbury, NY.)

Geisler, C. D., and J. M. Goldberg. A stochastic model of the repetitive activity of neurons. *Biophys. J.* 6:53–69, 1966.

Geisler, C. D., and S. Greenberg. A two-stage nonlinear cochlear model possesses automatic gain control. *J. Acoust. Soc. Am.* 80:1359–1363, 1986. (*Copyright owned by the American Institute of Physics, Woodbury, NY.)

Geisler, C. D., and A. L. Nuttall. Two-tone "low-side" suppression in responses of basal basilar membrane. In: *Diversity in Auditory Mechanics*, edited by E. R. Lewis, G. R. Long, R. F. Lyon, P. M. Narins, C. R. Steele, and E. Hecht-Poinar. Singapore: World Scientific, 1997a, pp. 305–311. (*Copyright owned by World Scientific Publishing Co., Singapore.)

Geisler, C. D., and A. L. Nuttall. Two-tone suppression on the basilar membrane using a "low-side" suppressor. *J. Acoust. Soc. Am.* 102:430–440, 1997b.

Geisler, C. D., and C. Sang. A cochlear model using feed-forward outer-hair-cell forces. *Hear. Res.* 86:132–146, 1995.

Geisler, C. D., and S. M. Silkes. Responses of "lower-spontaneous-rate" auditory-nerve fibers to speech syllables presented in noise. II. Glottal pulse periodicities. *J. Acoust. Soc. Am.* 90:3140–3148, 1991.

Geisler, C. D., and D. G. Sinex. Responses of primary auditory fibers to combined noise and tonal stimuli. *Hear. Res.* 3:317–334, 1980. (*Copyright owned by Elsevier Science-NL, Sara Burgerhartstraat 25, 1055 KV Amsterdam, The Netherlands.)

Geisler, C. D., W. A. van Bergeijk, and L. S. Frishkopf. The inner ear of the bullfrog. *J. Morphol.* 114:43–58, 1964.

Geisler, C. D., Rhode, W. S., and D. T. Kennedy. Responses to tonal stimuli of single auditory nerve fibers and their relationship to basilar membrane motion in the squirrel monkey. *J. Neurophysiol.* 37:1156–1172, 1974. (*Copyright owned by The American Physiological Society, Bethesda, MD.)

Geisler, C. D., L. Deng, and S. R. Greenberg. Thresholds for primary auditory fibers using statistically defined criteria. *J. Acoust. Soc. Am.* 77:1102–1109, 1985.

Gillespie, P. G. Molecular machinery of auditory and vestibular transduction. *Curr. Opin. Neurobiol.* 5:449–455, 1995. (*Copyright owned by Current Biology, London, UK.)

Giraud, A. L., L. Collet, S. Chéry-Croze, J. Magnan, and A. Chays. Evidence of a medial olivocochlear involvement in contralateral suppression of otoacoustic emissions in humans. *Brain Res.* 705:15–23, 1995.

Glasberg, B. R., and B. C. J. Moore. Psychoacoustic abilities of subjects with unilateral and bilateral cochlear hearing impairments and their relationship to the ability to understand speech. *Scand. Audiology Suppl.* 32:3–25, 1989.

Gleich, O., B. M. Johnstone, and D. Robertson. Effects of L-glutamate on auditory afferent activity in view of its proposed excitatory transmitter role in the mammalian cochlea. *Hear. Res.* 45:295–312, 1990.

Goblick, T. J., and R. R. Pfeiffer. Time-domain measurements of cochlear nonlinearities using combination click stimuli. *J. Acoust. Soc. Am.* 46:924–938, 1969.

Gold, T. Hearing II. The physical basis of the action of the cochlea. *Proc. R. Soc. Edinb. B* 135:492–498, 1948.

Goldberg, J. M., and P. B. Brown. Response of binaural neurons of dog superior olivary complex to dichotic tonal stimuli: some physiological mechanisms of sound localization. *J. Neurophysiol.* 32:613–636, 1969.

Goldberg, J. M., and C. Fernández. Vestibular mechanisms. *Annu. Rev. Physiol.* 37: 1126–162, 1972.

Goldberg, J. M., A. M. Brichta, and P. A. Wackym. Efferent vestibular system: anatomy, physiology and neurochemistry. In: *Neurochemistry of the Vestibular System*, edited by J. H. Anderson, and A. Beitz. Boca Raton, FL: CRC (in press).

Goodhill, V. *Ear Diseases, Deafness, and Dizziness.* New York: Harper & Row, 1979. (*Copyright owned by Lippincott-Raven, Philadelphia, PA.)

Gorga, M. P., L. Stover, and S. T. Neely. The use of cumulative distributions to determine critical values and levels of confidence for clinical distortion product otoacoustic emission measurements. *J. Acoust. Soc. Am.* 100:968–977, 1996.

Goycoolea, M. V., H. G. Goycoolea, C. R. Farfan, L. G. Rodriguez, G. C. Marinez, and R. Vidal. Effect of life in industrialized societies on hearing in natives of Easter Island. *Laryngoscope*, 96:1391–1396, 1986. (*Copyright owned by The Laryngoscope Company, St. Louis, MO.)

Gravel, J. S. and R. J. Ruben. Auditory deprivation and its consequences: from animal models to humans. In: *Clinical Aspects of Hearing*, edited by T. R. Van De Water, A. N. Popper, and R. R. Fay. New York: Springer-Verlag, 1996, Chap. 4.

Green, D. M. *An Introduction to Hearing.* Hillsdale, NJ: Lawrence Erlbaum Associates, 1976.

Green, D. M., and J. A. Swets. *Signal Detection Theory and Psychophysics.* New York: Wiley, 1966.

Greenberg, S. (Ed.). Representation of speech in the auditory periphery. *J. Phonetics* 16(1), 1988.

Guilleman, E. A. *Introductory Circuit Theory.* New York: Wiley, 1953.

Guinan, J. J., Jr. Physiology of olivocochlear efferents. In: *The Cochlea*, edited by P. Dallos, A. N. Popper, and R. R. Fay. New York: Springer-Verlag, 1996, Chap. 8.

Guinan, J. J., Jr., and M. L. Gifford. Effects of electrical stimulation of efferent olivocochlear neurons on cat auditory-nerve fibers. I. Rate-level functions. *Hear. Res.* 33:97–114, 1988a.(*Copyright owned by Elsevier Science-NL, Sara Burgerhartstraat 25, 1055 KV Amsterdam, The Netherlands.)

Guinan, J. J., Jr., and M. L. Gifford. Effects of electrical stimulation of efferent olivocochlear neurons on cat auditory-nerve fibers. II. Spontaneous rate. *Hear. Res.* 33:115–128, 1988b.

Guinan, J. J., Jr., and M. L. Gifford. Effects of electrical stimulation of efferent olivocochlear neurons on cat auditory-nerve fibers. III. Tuning curves and thresholds at CF. *Hear. Res.* 37:29–46, 1988c. (*Copyright owned by Elsevier Science-NL, Sara Burgerhartstraat 25, 1055 KV Amsterdam, The Netherlands.)

Guinan, J. J., and W. T. Peake. Middle-ear characteristics of anesthetized cats. *J. Acoust. Soc. Am.* 41:1237–1261, 1967.

Guinan, J. J., Jr., M. P. Joseph, and B. E. Norris. Brainstem facial-motor pathways from two distinct groups of stapedius motoneurons in the cat. *J. Comp. Neurol.* 287:134–144, 1989.

Gulley, R. L., and T. S. Reese. Intercellular junctions in the reticular lamina of the organ of Corti. *J. Neurocytol.* 5:479–507, 1976.

Gummer, A. W., J. W. T. Smolders, and R. Klinke. Basilar membrane motion in the pigeon measured with the Mössbauer technique. *Hear. Res.* 29:63–92, 1987.

Gummer, A. W., W. Hemmert, and H-P. Zenner. Micromechanics of cellular structures in the mammalian cochlea: auditory and electrical stimulation. In: *Active Hearing*, edited by Å. Flock, D. Ottoson, and M. Ulfendahl. Kidlington, UK: Elsevier Science, 1995, pp. 271–282.

Guth, P. S., A. Aubert, A. J. Ricci, and C. H. Norris. Differential modulation of spontaneous and evoked neurotransmitter release from hair cells: some novel hypotheses. *Hear. Res.* 56:69–78, 1991.

Hackney, C. M., R. Fettiplace, and D. N. Furness. The functional morphology of stereociliary bundles on turtle cochlear hair cells. *Hear. Res.* 69:163–175, 1993.(*Copyright owned by Elsevier Science-NL, Sara Burgerhartstraat 25, 1055 KV Amsterdam, The Netherlands.)

Harris, F. P., B. L. Lonsbury-Martin, B. B. Stagner, A. C. Coats, and G. K. Martin. Acoustic distortion products in humans: systematic changes in amplitude as a function of f2/f1 ratio. *J. Acoust. Soc. Am.* 85:220–229, 1989.

Harris, G. G. Brownian motion in the cochlear partition. *J. Acoust. Soc. Am.* 44: 176–186, 1968.

Harrison, R. V., and I. M. Hunter-Duvar. An anatomical tour of the cochlea. In: *Physiology of the Ear*, edited by A. F. Jahn and J. Santos-Sacchi. New York: Raven, 1988, p. 160. (*Copyright owned by Raven Press, New York, NY.)

Hashimoto, S., R. S. Kimura, and T. Takasaka. Computer-aided three-dimensional reconstruction of the inner hair cells and their nerve endings in the guinea pig cochlea. *Acta Otolaryngol.* 109:228–234, 1990.

Hassan, El-S. A theoretical basis for the high-frequency performance of the outer hair cell's receptor potential. *J. Acoust. Soc. Am.* 101:2129–2134, 1997.

Hazell, J. W. P. Electrical tinnitus suppression. In: *Cochlear Implants: A Practical Guide*, edited by H. Cooper. San Diego: Singular Publishing Group, 1991, Chap. 20.

Hazell, J. W. P., S. M. Wood, H. R. Cooper, S. D. G. Stephens, A. L. Corcoran, R. R. A. Coles, J. L. Baskill, and J. B. Sheldrake. A clinical study of tinnitus maskers. *Br. J. Audiol.* 19:65–146, 1985.

He, N., and R. A. Schmiedt. Fine structure of the $2f_1$-f_2 acoustic distortion product: Effects of primary level and frequency ratios. *J. Acoust. Soc. Am.* 101:3554–3565, 1997.

Heath, A. The experience of being deafened. In: *Cochlear Implants: A Practical Guide*, edited by H. Cooper. San Diego: Singular Publishing Group, 1991, Chap. 21.

Heffner, R. S., and H. E. Heffner. Sound localization, use of binaural cues and the superior olivary complex of pigs. *Brain Behav. Evol.* 33:248–258, 1989.

Heide, J., G. Tatge, T. Sander, T. Gooch, and T. Prescott. Development of a semi-implantable hearing device. *Adv. Audiol.* 4:32–43, 1988. (*Copyright owned by S. Karger, Basel, Switzerland.)

Heide, V. H. Project Phoenix, Inc., 1984–1989: the development of a wearable digital signal processing hearing aid. In: *Understanding Digitally Programmable Hearing Aids*, edited by R. E. Sandlin. Boston: Allyn & Bacon, 1994, Chap. 7.

Hemilä, S., S. Nummela, and T. Reuter. What middle ear parameters tell about impedance matching and high frequency hearing. *Hear. Res.* 85:31–44, 1995.

Henson, M. M., and O. W. Henson Jr. Tension fibroblasts and the connective tissue matrix of the spiral ligament. *Hear. Res.* 35:237–258, 1988.

Henson, O. W., Jr. The activity and function of the middle-ear muscles in echolocating bats. *J. Physiol. (Lond.)* 180:871–887, 1965.

Henson, Jr., O. W., D. H. Xie, A. W. Keating, and M. M. Henson. The effect of contralateral stimulation on cochlear resonance and damping in the mustached bat: the role of the medial efferent system. *Hear. Res.* 86:111–124, 1995.

Hewitt, M. J., and R. Meddis. An evaluation of eight computer models of mammalian inner hair-cell function. *J. Acoust. Soc. Am.* 90:904–917, 1991.

Hill, K. G., G. Strange, A. W. Gummer, and J. Mo. A model proposing synaptic and extra-synaptic influences on the responses of cochlear nerve fibres. *Hear. Res.* 39:75–90, 1989.

Hill, K. G., and C. D. Geisler. Two-tone suppression, excitation and the after effect in rate responses in auditory nerve fibres in the cat. *Hear. Res.* 64:52–60, 1992.

Holley, M. High frequency force generation in outer hair cells from the mammalian ear. *Bioessays* 13:115–120, 1991.

Holley, M. C., and J. F. Ashmore. A cytoskeletal spring in cochlear outer hair cells. *Nature* 335:635–637, 1988a.

Holley, M. C., and J. F. Ashmore. On the mechanism of a high-frequency force generator in outer hair cells isolated from the guinea pig cochlea. *Proc. R. Soc. Lond. B* 232:413–429, 1988b.

Holton, T., and T. F. Weiss. Two-tone rate suppression in lizard cochlear nerve fibres, relation to receptor organ morphology. *Brain Res.* 159:219–222, 1978.

House, W. F., and J. Urban. Long term results of electrode implantation and electronic stimulation of the cochlea in man. *Ann. Otol. Rhinol. Laryngol.* 82:540–514, 1973.

Housley, G. D., and J. F. Ashmore. Direct measurement of the action of acetylcholine on isolated outer hair cells of the guinea pig cochlea. *Proc. R. Soc. Lond. B* 244:161–167, 1991.

Housley, G. D., and J. F. Ashmore. Ionic currents of outer hair cells isolated from the guinea-pig cochlea. *J. Physiol. (Lond.)* 448:73–98, 1992.

Housley, G. D., B. J. Connor, and N. P. Raybould. Purinergic modulation of outer hair cell electromotility. In: *Active Hearing*, edited by Å. Flock, D. Ottoson, and M. Ulfendahl. Kidlington, UK: Elsevier Science, 1995, pp. 221–238.

Huang, A. Y., and B. J. May. Sound orientation behavior in cats. II. Mid-frequency spectral cues for sound localization. *J. Acoust. Soc. Am.* 100:1070–1080, 1996.

Hubbard, A. A traveling-wave amplifier model of the cochlea. *Science* 259:68–71, 1993.

Hubbard, A. E., and D. C. Mountain. Alternating current delivered into the scala media alters sound pressure at the eardrum. *Science* 222:510–512, 1983.

Hubbard, A. E., and D. C. Mountain. Analysis and synthesis of cochlear mechanical function using models. In: *Auditory Computation*, edited by H. L. Hawkins, T. A. McMullen, A. N. Popper, and R. R. Fay. New York: Springer-Verlag, 1996, Chap. 3.

Hubbard, A. E., H. H. Nakajima, E. S. Olson, and D. C. Mountain. Sound induced changes in electrically evoked cochlear emissions. In: *The Mechanics and Biophysics of Hearing*, edited by P. Dallos, C. D. Geisler, J. W. Matthews, M. A. Ruggero, and C. R. Steele. New York: Springer-Verlag, 1990, pp. 186–192.

Hudspeth, A. J. Extracellular current flow and the site of transduction by vertebrate hair cells. *J. Neurosci.* 1:1–10, 1982.

Hudspeth, A. J. How the ear's works work. *Nature* 341:397–404, 1989.

Hudspeth, A. J., and D. P. Corey. Sensitivity, polarity, and conductance change in the response of vertebrate hair cells to controlled mechanical stimuli. *Proc. Natl. Acad. Sci. U.S.A.* 74:2407–2411, 1977.

Hudspeth, A. J., and P. G. Gillespie. Pulling springs to tune transduction: adaptation by hair cells. *Neuron* 12:1–9, 1994.

Hudspeth, A. J., and R. Jacobs. Stereocilia mediate transduction in vertebrate hair cells. *Proc. Natl. Acad. Sci. U.S.A.* 76:1506–1509, 1979.

Hudspeth, A. J., and R. S. Lewis. A model for electrical resonance and frequency tuning in saccular hair cells of the bull-frog, *Rana catesbeiana. J. Physiol. (Lond.)* 400:275–297, 1988.

Humes, L. E. Noise-induced hearing loss as influenced by other agents and by some physical characteristics of the individual. *J. Acoust. Soc. Am.* 76:1318–1329, 1984.

Humes, L. E., D. D. Dirks, T. S. Bell, C. Ahlstrom, and G. E. Kincaid. Application of the articulation index and the speech transmission index to the recognition of speech by normal-hearing and hearing-impaired listeners. *J. Speech Hear. Res.* 29:447–462, 1986.

Igarashi, M., B. R. Alford, Y. Nakai, and W. P. Gordon. Behavioral auditory function after transection of crossed olivo-cochlear bundle in the cat. I. Pure-tone threshold and perceptual signal-to-noise ratio. *Acta Otolaryngol.* 73:455–466, 1972.

Igarashi, M., J. L. Cranford, Y. Nakai, and B. R. Alford. Behavioral auditory function after transection of crossed olivo-cochlear bundle in the cat. IV. Study on pure-tone frequency discrimination. *Acta Otolaryngol.* 87:79–83, 1979a.

Igarashi, M., J. L. Cranford, E. A. Allen, and B. R. Alford. Behavioral auditory function after transection of crossed olivo-cochlear bundle in the cat. V. Pure-tone intensity discrimination. *Acta Otolaryngol.* 87:429–433, 1979b.

Ikeda, K., H. Sunose, and T. Takasaka. Ion transport mechanisms in the outer hair cell of the mammalian cochlea. *Prog. Neurobiol.* 42:703–717, 1994.

International Team for Ear Research (ITER). Cellular vibration and motility in the organ of Corti. *Acta Otolaryngol. Suppl.* 467:151–156, 1989.

Irvine, D. R. F. Physiology of the auditory system, In: *The Mammalian Auditory Pathway: Neurophysiology,* edited by A. N. Popper and R. R. Fay. New York: Springer-Verlag, 1992, pp. 153–231.

Jastreboff, P. J. Phantom auditory perception (tinnitus): mechanisms of generation and perception. *Neurosci. Res.* 8:221–254, 1990.

Jastreboff, P. J., and C. T. Sasaki. An animal model of tinnitus: a decade of development. *Am. J. Otology* 15:19–27, 1994.

Javel, E. Suppression of auditory nerve responses. I. Temporal analysis, intensity effects and suppression contours. *J. Acoust. Soc. Am.* 69:1735–1745, 1981.

Javel, E. Long-term adaptation in cat auditory-nerve fiber responses. *J. Acoust. Soc. Am.* 99:1040–1052, 1996.

Javel, E., C. D. Geisler, and A. Ravindran. Two-tone suppression in auditory nerve of the cat: rate-intensity and temporal analyses. *J. Acoust. Soc. Am.* 63:1093–1104, 1978. (*Copyright owned by the American Institute of Physics, Woodbury, NY.)

Javel, E., Y. C. Tong, R. K. Shepard, and G. M. Clark. Responses of cat auditory nerve fibers to biphasic electrical current pulses. *Ann. Otol. Rhinol. Laryngol.* 96(Suppl.):128:26–30, 1987.

Jen, D. H., and C. R. Steele. Electro-kinetic model of outer hair cell motility. *J. Acoust. Soc. Am.* 82:1667–1678, 1987.

Jenison, R. L., S. Greenberg, K. R. Kluender, and W. S. Rhode. *J. Acoust. Soc. Am.* 90:773–786, 1991.

Jerry, R. A., A. S. Popel, and W. E. Brownell. Outer hair cell length changes in an external electric field. II. The role of electrokinetic forces on the cell surface. *J. Acoust. Soc. Am.* 98:2011–2017, 1995.

Johnson, D. H., and N. Y. S. Kiang. Analysis of discharges recorded simultaneously from pairs of auditory nerve fibers. *Biophys. J.* 16:719–734, 1976.

Johnstone, B. M., and A. J. F. Boyle. Basilar membrane vibration examined with the Mössbauer technique. *Science* 158:390–391, 1967.

Johnstone, B. M., and K. J. Taylor. Physiology of the middle ear transmission system. *J. Otolaryngol. Soc. Aust.* 3:226–228, 1971. (*Copyright owned by Australian Journal of Otolaryngology, St. Leonards, NSW.)

Joris, P. X., and T. C. T. Yin. Responses to amplitude-modulated tones in the auditory nerve of the cat. *J. Acoust. Soc. Am.* 91:215–232, 1992. (*Copyright owned by the American Institute of Physics, Woodbury, NY.)

Joris, P. X., L. H. Carney, P. H. Smith, and T. C. T. Yin. Enhancement of neural synchronization in the anteroventral cochlear nucleus. I. Responses to tones at the characteristic frequency. *J. Neurosci.* 71:1022–1036, 1994. (*Copyright owned by the American Physiological Society, Bethesda, MD.)

Kakehata, S., T. Nakagawa, T. Takasaka, and N. Akaike. Cellular mechanism of acetylcholine-induced response in dissociated outer hair cells of guinea-pig cochlea. *J. Physiol. (Lond.)* 463:227–244, 1993.

Kalinec, F., and B. Kachar. Structure of the electromechanical transduction mechanism in mammalian outer hair cells. In: *Active Hearing*, edited by Å. Flock, D. Ottoson, and M. Ulfendahl. Kidlington, UK: Pergamon, 1995, pp. 181–193. (*Copyright owned by Elsevier Science, Kidlington, UK.)

Kalinec, F., M. C. Holley, K. H. Isawa, D. J. Lim, and B. Kachar. A membrane-based force generation mechanism in auditory sensory cells. *Proc. Natl. Acad. Sci. U.S.A.* 89:8671–8675, 1992.

Kamm, C., D. D. Dirks, and M. R. Mickey. Effect of sensorineural hearing loss on loudness discomfort levels and the most comfortable loudness judgments. *J. Speech Hear. Res.* 21:668–681, 1978.

Kapadia, S., and M. E. Lutman. Are normal hearing thresholds a sufficient condition for click-evoked otoacoustic emissions? *J. Acoust. Soc. Am.* 101:3566–3576, 1997.

Kawase, T., B. Delgutte, and M. C. Liberman. Antimasking effects of the olivo-cochlear reflex. II. Enhancement of auditory-nerve response to masked tones. *J. Neurophysiol.* 70:2533–2549, 1993. (*Copyright owned by The American Physiological Society, Bethesda, MD.)

Kemp, D. T. Stimulated acoustic emissions from within the human auditory system. *J. Acoust. Soc. Am.* 64:1386–1391, 1978.

Kemp, D. T. Evidence of mechanical nonlinearity and frequency selective wave amplification in the cochlea. *Arch. Otorhinolaryngol.* 224:37–45, 1979.

Khanna, S. M., and D. G. B. Leonard. Basilar membrane tuning in the cat cochlea. *Science* 215:305–306, 1982.

Kiang, N. Y. S. Peripheral neural processing of auditory information. In: *Handbook of Physiology, Sensory Processes*, vol. III, edited by I. Darian-Smith, J. M.

Brookhart, and V. B. Mountcastle. Bethesda, MD: American Physiological Society, 1984, p. 640. (*Copyright owned by the American Physiological Society, Bethesda, MD.)

Kiang, N. Y-S., T. Watanabe, E. C. Thomas, and L. F. Clark. *Discharge Patterns of Single Fibers in the Cat's Auditory Nerve.* Cambridge, MA: MIT Press, 1965.

Kiang, N. Y. S., J. M. Rho, C. C. Northrop, M. C. Liberman, and D. K. Ryugo. Hair-cell innervation by spiral ganglion cells in adult cats. *Science* 217:175–177, 1982.

Kiang, N. Y. S., M. C. Liberman, W. F. Sewell, and J. J. Guinan. Single unit clues to cochlear mechanisms. *Hear. Res.* 22:171–182, 1986.

Killion, M. C. The K-AMP$^{T.M.}$ hearing aid: an attempt to present high fidelity for the hearing impaired. In: *Recent Developments in Hearing Instrument Technology (15th Danavox Symposium)*, edited by J. Beilin and G. R. Jensen (Scanticon, Denmark), 1993, pp. 167–229.

Killion, M. C. Compression: distinctions. *Hear. Rev.* 3:29–32, 1996.

Killion, M. C., and P. Dallos. Impedance matching by the combined effects of the outer and middle ear, *J. Acoust. Soc. Am.* 66:599–602, 1979.

Kim, D. O. Cochlear mechanics: implications of electrophysiological and acoustical observations. *Hear. Res.* 2:297–317, 1980.

Kim, D. O., S. T. Neely, C. E. Molnar, and J. W. Matthews. An active cochlear model with negative damping in the cochlear partition: comparison with Rhode's ante- and post-mortem results. In: *Psychological, Physiological and Behavioral Studies in Hearing*, edited by G. van den Brink and F. A. Bilsen. Delft, The Netherlands: Delft University Press, 1980, pp. 7–14.

Kim, P. J., and E. D. Young. Comparative analysis of spectro-temporal receptive fields, reverse correlation functions, and frequency tuning curves of auditory-nerve fibers. *J. Acoust. Soc. Am.* 95:410–422, 1994.

Kimura, R. S. The ultrastructure of the organ of Corti. *Int. Rev. Cytol.* 42:173–222, 1975.

Kirk, D. L., and G. K. Yates. Frequency tuning and acoustic enhancement of electrically evoked otoacoustic emissions in the guinea pig cochlea. *J. Acoust. Soc. Am.* 100:3714–3725, 1996.

Klinke, R., and J. W. Th. Smolders. Performance of the avian inner ear. *Prog. Brain Res.* 97:31–43, 1993.

Knudsen, E. I., and M. Konishi. Mechanisms of sound localization in the barn owl (*Tyto alba*). *J. Comp. Physiol.* 133:13–21, 1979. (*Copyright owned by Springer-Verlag, New York.)

Kobler, J. B., J. J. Guinan Jr., S. R. Vacher, and B. E. Norris. Acoustic reflex frequency selectivity in single stapedius motoneurons of the cat. *J. Neurophysiol.* 68:807–817, 1992. (*Copyright owned by the American Physiological Society, Bethesda, MD.)

Konishi, M. Listening with two ears. *Sci. Am.* 268:66–73, 1993.

Köppl, C. Otoacoustic emissions as an indicator for active cochlear mechanics: a primitive property of vertebrate auditory organs. In: *Advances in Hearing Research*, edited by G. A. Manley, G. M. Klump, C. Köppl, H. Fastl, and H. Oeckinghaus. Singapore: World Scientific, 1995, pp. 207–216.

Köppl, C., and M. Kössl. What is the function of an auditory fovea? *Abstr. Assoc. Res. Otolaryngol.* 20:6, 1997.

Kössl, M. Otoacoustic emissions from the cochlea of the ''constant frequency'' bats, *Pteronotus parnellii* and *Rhinolophus rouxi. Hear. Res.* 72:59–72, 1994.

Kössl, M., and M. Vater. Evoked acoustic emissions and cochlear microphonics in the mustache bat, *Pteronotus parnellii. Hear. Res.* 19:157–170, 1985a.

Kössl, M., and M. Vater. The cochlear frequency map of the mustache bat, *Pteronotus parnellii. J. Comp. Physiol.* 157:687–697, 1985b.

Kringlebotn, M. The equality of volume displacements in the inner ear windows, *J. Acoust. Soc. Am.* 98:192–196, 1995.

Kros, C. J., and A. C. Crawford. Potassium currents in inner hair cells isolated from the guinea-pig cochlea. *J. Physiol. (Lond.)* 421:263–291, 1990.

Kuhn, B., and M. Vater. The postnatal development of F-actin in tension fibroblasts of the spiral ligament of the gerbil cochlea. *Hear. Res.* 108:180–190, 1997.

Kuijpers, W. The origin of the endocochlear resting potential. *Oto. Rhinol. Laryngol. Dig.* Sept:37–42, 1972.

Kujawa, S. G., T. J. Glattke, M. Fallon, and R. P. Bobbin. Intracochlear application of acetylcholine alters sound-induced mechanical events within the cochlear partition. *Hear. Res.* 61:106–116, 1992.

Kujawa, S. G., T. J. Glattke, M. Fallon, and R. P. Bobbin. A nicotinic-like receptor mediates suppression of distortion product otoacoustic emissions by contralateral sound. *Hear. Res.* 74:122–134, 1994.

Liberman, M. C. Auditory-nerve response from cats raised in a low-noise chamber. *J. Acoust. Soc. Am.* 63:442–455, 1978. (*Copyright owned by the American Institute of Physics, Woodbury, NY.)

Liberman, M. C. Efferent synapses in the inner hair cell area of the cat cochlea: an electron microscopic study of serial sections. *Hear. Res.* 3:189–204, 1980a.

Liberman, M. C. Morphological differences among radial afferent fibers in the cat cochlea: an electron-microscopic study of serial sections. *Hear. Res.* 3:45–63, 1980b.

Liberman, M. C. Single-neuron labeling in the cat auditory nerve. *Science* 216:1239–1241, 1982a.

Liberman, M. C. The cochlear frequency map for the cat: labeling auditory-nerve fibers of known characteristic frequency. *J. Acoust. Soc. Am.* 72:1441–1449, 1982b. (*Copyright owned by the American Institute of Physics, Woodbury, NY.)

Liberman, M. C. Response properties of cochlear efferent neurons: monaural vs. binaural stimulation and the effects of noise. *J. Neurophysiol.* 60:1779–1798, 1988.

Liberman, M. C. Effects of chronic cochlear de-efferentation on auditory-nerve response. *Hear. Res.* 49:209–224, 1990.

Liberman, M. C., and M. C. Brown. Physiology and anatomy of single olivocochlear neurons in the cat. *Hear. Res.* 24:17–36, 1986. (*Copyright owned by Elsevier Science-NL, Sara Burgerhartstraat 25, 1055 KV Amsterdam, The Netherlands.)

Liberman, M. C., and L. W. Dodds. Single-neuron labeling and chronic cochlear pathology. III. Stereocilia damage and alternations of threshold tuning curves. *Hear. Res.* 16:55–74, 1984. (*Copyright owned by Elsevier Science-NL, Sara Burgerhartstraat 25, 1055 KV Amsterdam, The Netherlands.)

Liberman, M. C., and M. J. Mulroy. Acute and chronic effects of acoustic trauma: cochlear pathology and auditory nerve pathophysiology. In: *New Perspectives on Noise-Induced Hearing Loss*, edited by R. P. Hamernick, D. Henderson, and R. Salvi. New York: Raven, 1982, pp. 105–135. (*Copyright owned by Raven Press, New York, NY.)

Liberman, M. C., and M. E. Oliver. Morphometry of intracellularly labeled neurons of the auditory nerve: correlations with functional properties. *J. Comp. Neurol.* 223:163–176, 1984. (*Copyright owned by John Wiley & Sons, New York, NY.)

Liberman, M. C., L. W. Dodds, and S. Pierce. Afferent and efferent innervation of the cat cochlea: quantitative analysis with light and electron microscopy. *J. Comp. Neurol.* 301:443–460, 1990. (*Copyright owned by John Wiley & Sons, New York, NY.)

Licklider, J. C. R. Basic correlates of the auditory stimulus. In: *Handbook of Experimental Psychology*, edited by S. S. Stevens. New York: Wiley, 1951, Chap. 25.

Lieberman, P. *Speech Physiology and Acoustic Phonetics*. New York: Macmillan, 1977.

Lim, D. J. Cochlear anatomy related to cochlear micromechanics: A review. *J. Acoust. Soc. Am.* 67:1686–1695, 1980.

Lippe, W. R., E. W. Westbrook, and B. M. Ryals. Hair cell regeneration in the chicken cochlea following aminoglycoside toxicity. *Hear. Res.* 56:302–210, 1991.

Long, G. R., and A. Tubis. Modification of spontaneous and evoked otoacoustic emissions and associated psychoacoustic microstructure by aspirin consumption. *J. Acoust. Soc. Am.* 84:1343–1353, 1988.

Long, G. R., A. Tubis, and K. L. Jones. Modeling synchronization and suppression of spontaneous otoacoustic emissions using Van der Pol oscillators: effects of aspirin administration. *J. Acoust. Soc. Am.* 89:1201–1212, 1991.

Lonsbury-Martin, B. L., and G. K. Martin. The clinical utility of distortion-product otoacoustic emissions. *Ear Hear.* 11:144–154, 1990. (*Copyright owned by Williams & Wilkins, Baltimore, MD.)

Lonsbury-Martin, B. L., G. K. Martin, R. Probst, and A. C. Coats. Spontaneous otoacoustic emissions in a nonhuman primate. II. Cochlear anatomy. *Hear. Res.* 33:69–94, 1988.

Lowen, D. B., and M. C. Teich. Auditory-nerve action potentials form a nonrenewal point process over short as well as long time scales. *J. Acoust. Soc. Am.* 92:803–806, 1992.

Ludvigsen, C. Relations among some psychoacoustic parameters in normal and cochlearly impaired listeners. *J. Acoust. Soc. Am.* 78:1271–1280, 1985.

Lyon, R. F., Automatic gain control in cochlear mechanics. In: *The Mechanics and Biophysics of Hearing*, edited by P. Dallos, C. D. Geisler, J. W. Matthews, M. A. Ruggero, and C. R. Steele. New York: Springer-Verlag, 1990, pp. 395–402.

Lyon, R. F., and C. Mead. An analog electronic cochlea. *I.E.E.E. Trans. Acoust. Speech Sig. Proc.* 36:1119–1134, 1988.

Lyon, R. F., and S. Shamma. Auditory representations of timbre and pitch. In: *Auditory Computation*, edited by H. L. Hawkins, T. A. McMullen, A. N. Popper, and R. R. Fay. New York: Springer-Verlag, 1996, Chap. 6.

Mammano, F., and J. F. Ashmore. Reverse transduction measured in the isolated cochlea by laser Michelson interferometry. *Nature* 365:838–841, 1993. (*Copyright owned by *Nature*, New York, NY.)

Manley, G. A. *Peripheral Hearing Mechanisms in Reptiles and Birds*. Berlin: Springer-Verlag, 1990.

Manley, G. A., G. K. Yates, and C. Köppl. Auditory peripheral tuning: evidence for a simple resonance phenomenon in the lizard *Tiliqua*. *Hear. Res.* 33:181–190,

1988. (*Copyright owned by Elsevier Science-NL, Sara Burgerhartstraat 25, 1055 KV Amsterdam, The Netherlands.)

Marsh, R. R., L. Xu, J. P. Moy, and J. C. Saunders. Recovery of the basilar papilla following intense sound exposure in the chick. *Hear. Res.* 46:229–238, 1990. (*Copyright owned by Elsevier Science-NL, Sara Burgerhartstraat 25, 1055 KV Amsterdam, The Netherlands.)

Martin, G. K., B. L. Lonsbury-Martin, R. Probst, and A. C. Coats. Spontaneous otoacoustic emissions in a nonhuman primate. I. Basic features and relations to other emissions. *Hear. Res.* 33:49–68, 1988.

Martin, G. K., L. A. Ohlms, D. J. Franklin, F. P. Harris, and B. L. Lonsbury-Martin. Distortion product emissions in humans. III. Influence of sensorineural hearing loss. *Ann. Otol. Rhinol. Laryngol.* 99(Suppl. 147):30–42, 1990a.

Martin, G. K., R. Probst, and B. L. Lonsbury-Martin. Otoacoustic emissions in human ears: normative findings. *Ear Hear.* 11:106–120, 1990b. (*Copyright owned by Williams & Wilkins, Baltimore, MD.)

Matthew, G. Synaptic exocytosis and endocytosis: capacitance measurements. *Curr. Opin. Neurobiol.* 6:358–364, 1996.

May, B. J., and S. J. McQuone. Effects of bilateral olivocochlear lesions on pure-tone intensity discrimination in cats. *Auditory Neurosci.* 1:385–400, 1995.

McFadden, D. *Tinnitus: Facts, Theories, and Treatments.* Washington, DC: National Academy Press, 1982.

Mecklenburg, D., and E. Lehnhardt. The development of cochlear implants in Europe, Asia and Australia. In: *Cochlear Implants: A Practical Guide*, edited by H. Cooper. San Diego: Singular Publishing Group, 1991, Chap. 3.

Melnick, W. Hearing loss from noise exposure. In: *Handbook of Acoustical Measurements and Noise Control*, 3rd ed., edited by C. M. Harris. New York: McGraw-Hill, 1991, Chap. 18.

Merchan-Perez, A., and M. C. Liberman. Ultrastructural differences among afferent synapses on cochlear hair cells: correlations with spontaneous discharge rate. *J. Comp. Neurol.* 371:208–221, 1996.

Meyer, Y. *Wavelets: Algorithm and Applications.* Philadelphia: Society of Industrial and Applied Mathematics, 1993.

Middlebrooks, J. C., and D. M. Green. Sound localization by human listeners. *Annu. Rev. Psychol.* 42:135–159, 1991.

Miller, J. M., and F. A. Spelman (Eds.). *Cochlear Implants, Models of the Electrically Stimulated Ear.* New York: Springer-Verlag, 1990.

Miller, J. M., T. Y. Ren, and A. L. Nuttall. Studies of inner ear blood flow in animals and human beings. *Otolaryngol. Head Neck Surg.* 112:101–113, 1995.

Miller, M. I., and M. B. Sachs. Representation of stop consonants in the discharge patterns of auditory-nerve fibers. *J. Acoust. Soc. Am.* 74:502–517, 1983. (*Copyright owned by the American Institute of Physics, Woodbury, NY.)

Miller, M. I., and M. B. Sachs. Representation of voice pitch in discharge patterns of auditory-nerve fibers. *Hear. Res.* 14:257–279, 1984.

Moore, B. C. J. *An Introduction to the Psychology of Hearing*, 2nd ed. Orlando, FL: Academic, 1982.

Mott, J. B., S. J. Norton, S. T. Neely, and W. B. Warr. Changes in spontaneous otoacoustic emissions produced by acoustic stimulation of the contralateral ear. *Hear. Res.* 38:229–242, 1989.

Mountain, D. C. Changes in endolymphatic potential and crossed olivocochlear bundle stimulation alter cochlear mechanics. *Science* 210:71–72, 1980.

Mountain, D. C. Electromechanical properties of hair cells. In: *Neurobiology of Hearing: The Cochlea*, edited by R. A. Altschuler, D. W. Hoffman, and R. P. Bobbin. New York: Raven, 1986, pp. 77–90.

Mountain, D. C., and A. E. Hubbard. Rapid force production in the cochlea. *Hear. Res.* 42:195–202, 1989.

Mountain, D. C., and A. E. Hubbard. A piezoelectric model of outer hair cell function. *J. Acoust. Soc. Am.* 95:350–354, 1994.

Mountain, D. C., and A. E. Hubbard. Computational analysis of hair cell and auditory nerve processes. In: *Auditory Computation*, edited by H. L. Hawkins, T. A. McMullen, A. N. Popper, and R. R. Fay. New York: Springer-Verlag, 1996, Chap. 4.

Mountain, D. C., A. E. Hubbard, and T. A. McMillen. Electromechanical processes in the cochlea. In: *Mechanics of Hearing*, edited by E. de Boer and M. A. Viergever. Delft, The Netherlands: Delft University Press, 1983, pp. 119–126.

Møller, A. An experimental study of the acoustic impedance of the middle ear and its transmission properties. *Acta Otolaryngol.* 59:1–19, 1965.

Møller, A. Neurophysiological basis of the acoustic middle-ear reflex. In: *The Acoustic Reflex*, edited by S. Silman. Orlando, FL, Academic, 1984, Chap. 1.

Müller, M., and D. Robertson. Shapes of rate-versus-level functions of primary auditory nerve fibers: test of the basilar membrane mechanical hypothesis. *Hear. Res.* 57:71–78, 1991.

Müller, M., D. Robertson, and G. K. Yates. Rate-versus-level functions of primary auditory nerve fibres: evidence for square law behaviour of all fibre categories in the guinea pig. *Hear. Res.* 55:50–56, 1991. (*Copyright owned by Elsevier Science-NL, Sara Burgerhartstraat 25, 1055 KV Amsterdam, The Netherlands.)

Musicant, A. D., J. C. K. Chan, and J. E. Hind. Direction-dependent spectral properties of cat external ear: new data and cross-species comparisons. *J. Acoust. Soc. Am.* 87:757–781, 1990. (*Copyright owned by the American Institute of Physics, Woodbury, NY.)

Nadol, J. B. Application of electron microscopy to human otopathology. *Acta Otolaryngol.* 105:411–419, 1988a.

Nadol, Jr., J. B. Comparative anatomy of the cochlea and auditory nerve in mammals. *Hear. Res.* 34:253–266, 1988b.

Naidu, R. C., and D. C. Mountain. Frequency-stiffness relationships in the cochlea: Data vs. models. *Abstr. Assoc. Res. Otolaryngol.* 20:63, 1997.

Narins, P. M. Frog communication. *Sci. Am.* 273:77–83, 1995.

National Institutes of Health. Cochlear implants in adults and children. *NIH Consensus Statement* 13(2), 1995.

Nedzelnitsky, V. Sound pressures in the basal turn of the cat cochlea. *J. Acoust. Soc. Am.* 68:1676–1689, 1980. (*Copyright owned by the American Institute of Physics, Woodbury, NY.)

Neely, S. T., and D. O. Kim. An active cochlear model showing sharp tuning and high sensitivity. *Hear. Res.* 9:123–130, 1983.

Nenov, A. P., C. Norris, and R. P. Bobbin. Acetylcholine response in guinea pig outer hair cells. II. Activation of a small conductance Ca^{2+}-activated K^+ channel. *Hear. Res.* 101:149–172, 1996.

Nummela, S. Scaling of the mammalian middle ear. *Hear. Res.* 85:18–30, 1995. (*Copyright owned by Elseiver Science-NL, Sara Burgerhartstraat 25, 1055 KV Amsterdam, The Netherlands.)

Nuttall, A. L., and D. F. Dolan. Basilar membrane velocity responses to acoustic and intracochlear electric stimuli. In: *Biophysics of Hair Cell Sensory Systems*, edited by H. Duifhuis, J. W. Horst, P. van Dijk, and S. M. van Netten. Singapore: World Scientific, 1993, pp. 288–294.

Nuttall, A. L., and T. Ren. Electromotile hearing: evidence from basilar membrane motion and otoacoustic emissions. *Hear. Res.* 92:170–177, 1995.

Nuttall, A. L., W. J. Kong, T. Y. Ren, and D. F. Dolan. Basilar membrane motion and position changes induced by direct current stimulation. In: *Active Hearing*, edited by Å. Flock, D. Ottoson, and M. Ulfendahl. Kidlington, UK: Elsevier Science, 1995, pp. 283–294. (*Copyright owned by Elsevier Science, the Boulevard, Langford Lane, Kidlington OX5 1GB, UK.)

Oestreicher, E., W. Arnold, K. Ehrenberger, and D. Felix. Dopamine regulates the glutamatergic inner hair cell activity in guinea pigs. *Hear. Res.* 107:46–52, 1997.

Ohmori, H. Afferent synaptic transmission from hair cells. In: *Active Hearing*, edited by Å. Flock, D. Ottoson, and M. Ulfendahl. Kidlington, UK: Elsevier Science, 1995, pp. 53–61.

Ohyama, K., H. Wada, R. Kobayashi, and T. Takasaka. Spontaneous otoacoustic emissions in the guinea pig. *Hear. Res.* 56:111–121, 1991.

Olson, E. S., and D. C. Mountain. Mapping the cochlear partition's stiffness to its cellular architecture. *J. Acoust. Soc. Am.* 95:395–400, 1994.

O'Neill, and A. Bearden. Laser-feedback measurements of turtle basilar membrane motion using direct reflection. *Hear. Res.* 84:125–138, 1995.

Oono, Y., and Y. Sujaku. A model for automatic gain control observed in the firings of primary auditory neurons. *Trans. IECE (Japan)* 58:352–358, 1975.

Oppenheim, A. V., A. S. Willsky, and I. T. Young. *Signals and Systems*. Englewood Cliffs, NJ: Prentice-Hall, 1983.

Otte, J., H. F. Schuknecht, and A. G. Kerr. Ganglion cell populations in normal and pathological human cochleae: implications for cochlear implantation. *Laryngoscope* 88:1231–1246, 1978.

Otto, S., and S. Staller. Multichannel auditory brain stem implant: case studies comparing fitting strategies and results. *Ann. Otol. Rhinol. Laryngol.* 166(Suppl.): 36–39, 1995.

Palmer, A. R., and I. J. Russell. Phase-locking in the cochlear nerve of the guinea-pig and its relation to the receptor potential of inner hair-cells. *Hear. Res.* 24: 1–15, 1986.

Pang, X. D., and W. T. Peake. How do contractions of the stapedius muscle alter the acoustic properties of the middle ear? In: *Peripheral Auditory Mechanisms*, edited by J. B. Allen, J. L. Hall, A. Hubbard, S. T. Neely, and A. Tubis. New York: Springer-Verlag, 1986, pp. 36–43.

Park, J. Y., W. W. Clark, J. M. Coticchia, G. H. Esselman, and J. M. Fredrickson. Distortion product otoacoustic emissions in rhesus (*Macaca mulatta*) monkey ears: normative findings. *Hear. Res.* 86:147–162, 1995.

Parsons, T. D., D. Lenzi, W. Almers, and W. M. Roberts. Calcium-triggered exocytosis and endocytosis in an isolated presynaptic cell: capacitance measurements in saccular hair cells. *Neuron* 13:875–883, 1994.

Patterson, R. D, K. Robinson, J. Holdsworth, D. McKeown, C. Zhang, and M. H. Allerhand. In: *Auditory Physiology and Perception*, edited by Y. Cazals, L. Demany, and K. Horner. Oxford: Pergamon, 1992, pp. 429–446.

Patuzzi, R. Cochlear micromechanics and macromechanics. In: *The Cochlea*, edited by P. Dallos, A. N. Popper, and R. R. Fay. New York: Springer, 1996, Chapter 4.

Patuzzi, R., and P. M. Sellick. A comparison between basilar membrane and inner hair cell receptor potential input-output functions in the guinea pig cochlea. *J. Acoust. Soc. Am.* 74:1734–1741, 1983.

Patuzzi, R., and D. Robertson. Tuning in the mammalian cochlea. *Physiol. Rev.* 68: 1009–1082, 1988.

Patuzzi, R. B., and G. K. Yates. The low-frequency response of inner hair cells in the guinea pig cochlea: implications for fluid coupling and resonance of the stereocilia. *Hear. Res.* 30:83–98, 1987.

Patuzzi, R. B., G. K. Yates, and B. M. Johnstone. Outer hair cell receptor current and sensorineural hearing loss. *Hear. Res.* 42:47–72, 1989.

Pauler, M., H. F. Schuknecht, and A. R. Thornton. Correlative studies of cochlear neuronal loss with speech discrimination and pure-tone thresholds. *Arch. Oto-rhinolaryngol.* 243:200–206, 1986.

Peake, W. T., and A. Ling Jr. Basilar-membrane motion in the alligator lizard: its relation to tonotopic organization and frequency selectivity. *J. Acoust. Soc. Am.* 67:1736–1745, 1980.

Peake, W. T., J. J. Rosowski, and T. J. Lynch III. Middle-ear transmission: acoustic versus ossicular coupling in cat and human. *Hear. Res.* 57:245–268, 1992.

Penner, M. J. An estimate of the prevalence of tinnitus caused by spontaneous otoacoustic emissions. *Arch. Otolaryngol. Head Neck Surg.* 116:418–423, 1990.

Penner, M. J., and Burns, E. M. The dissociation of SOAEs and tinnitus. *J. Speech Hear. Res.* 30:396–403, 1987.

Penner, M. J., and P. J. Jastreboff. Tinnitus: psychophysical observations in humans and an animal model. In: *Clinical Aspects of Hearing*, edited by T. R. Van De Water, A. N. Popper, and R. R. Fay. New York: Springer-Verlag, 1996, Chap. 8.

Penner, M. J., and T. Zhang. Prevalence of spontaneous otoacoustic emissions in adults revisited. *Hear. Res.* 103:28–34, 1997.

Peterson, L. C., and B. P. Bogert. A dynamical theory of the cochlea. *J. Acoust. Soc. Am.* 22:369–381, 1950.

Pfeiffer, R. R. A model for two-tone inhibition of single cochlear-nerve fibers. *J. Acoust. Soc. Am.* 48:1373–1378, 1970.

Pickett, J. M. *The Sounds of Speech Communication*. Baltimore: University Park Press, 1980. (*Copyright owned by Allyn & Bacon.)

Pickles, J. O. A model for the mechanics of the stereociliary bundle on acoustico-lateral hair cells. *Hear. Res.* 68:159–172, 1993.

Pickles, J. O., S. D. Comis, and M. P. Osborne. Cross-links between stereocilia in the guinea pig organ of Corti, and their possible relation to sensory transduction. *Hear. Res.* 15:103–112, 1984.

Pitchford, S., and J. F. Ashmore. An electrical resonance in hair cells of the amphibian papilla of the frog *Rana temporaria*. *Hear. Res.* 29:75–83, 1987.

Plomp, R., and A. M. Mimpen. Speech-reception threshold for sentences as a function of age and noise level. *J. Acoust. Soc. Am.* 66:1333–1342, 1979.

Pluvinage, V. Rationale and development of the ReSound system. In: *Understanding Digitally Programmable Hearing Aids*, edited by R. E. Sandlin. Boston: Allyn & Bacon, 1994, Chap. 2.

Popper, A. N., and B. Hoxter. Growth of a fish ear. II. Locations of newly prolif-erated sensory hair cells in the saccular epithelium of *Astronotus ocellatus. Hear. Res.* 45:33–40, 1990.

Popper, A. N., and R. R. Fay (Eds.) *Hearing by Bats.* New York: Springer-Verlag, 1995.

Preyer, S., W. Hemmert, H-P. Zenner, and A. W. Gummer. Abolition of the receptor potential response of isolated mammalian outer hair cells by hair-bundle treatment with elastase: a test of the tip-link hypothesis. *Hear. Res.* 89:187–193, 1995.

Preyer, S., S. Renz, W. Hemmert, H-P. Zenner, and A. W. Gummer. Receptor po-tential of outer hair cells isolated from base to apex of the adult guinea-pig cochlea: implications for cochlear tuning mechanisms. *Auditory Neurosci.* 2: 145–157, 1996. (*Copyright owned by Harwood Academic Publishers, Lau-sanne, Switzerland.)

Prieve, B. A., M. P. Gorga, and S. T. Neely. Otoacoustic emissions in an adult with severe hearing loss. *Am. Speech Lang. Hear. Assoc.* 34:379–385, 1991.

Probst, R., B. L. Lonsbury-Martin, and G. K. Martin. A review of otoacoustic emis-sions. *J. Acoust. Soc. Am.* 89:2027–2067, 1991.

Probst, R., A. C. Coats, G. K. Martin, and B. L. Lonsbury-Martin. *Hear. Res.* 21: 261–275, 1986. (*Copyright owned by Elsevier Science-NL, Sara Burgerharts-traat 25, 1055 KV Amsterdam, The Netherlands.)

Puel, J-L., and G. Rebillard. Effect of contralateral sound stimulation on the distor-tion product 2F1–F2: Evidence that the medial efferent system is involved. *J. Acoust. Soc. Am.* 87:1630–1635, 1990.

Pujol, R., M. Lenoir, S. Ladrech, F. Tribillac, and G. Rebillard. Correlation between the length of outer hair cells and the frequency coding of the cochlea. In: *Au-ditory Physiology and Perception, Advances in the Biosciences*, vol. 83, edited by Y. Cazals, K. Demany, and K. Horner. New York: Pergamon, 1992, pp. 45– 51.

Puria, S., W. T. Peake, and J. J. Rosowski. Sound-pressure measurements in the cochlear vestibule of human-cadaver ears. *J. Acoust. Soc. Am.* 101:2754–2770, 1997.

Rajan, R. Protective functions of the efferent pathways to the mammalian cochlea: a review. In: *Noise-Induced Hearing Loss*, edited by A. L. Dancer, D. Henderson, R. J. Salvi, and R. P. Hamernik. St. Louis: Mosby, 1992, pp. 429–444.

Ramirez, R. W. *The FFT: Fundamentals and Concepts.* Englewood Cliffs, NJ: Pren-tice-Hall, 1985.

Ranke, O. F. Hydrodynamik der Schneckenflüssigkeit. *Z. Biol.* 103:409–434, 1950.

Raphael, Y., M. Lenoir, R. Wroblewski, and R. Pujol. The sensory epithelium and its innervation in the mole rat cochlea. *J. Comp. Neurol.* 314:367–382, 1991. (*Copyright owned by Wiley-Liss, a subsidiary of John Wiley & Sons, New York, NY.)

Rasmussen, G. L. The olivary peduncle and other fiber projections of the superior olivary complex. *J. Comp. Neurol.* 84:141–219, 1946.

Ravicz, M. E., and J. J. Rosowski. Sound-power collection by the auditory periphery of the Mongolian gerbil *Meriones unguiculatus*: III. Effect of variations in mid-dle-ear volume. *J. Acoust. Soc. Am.* 101:2135–2147, 1997.

Ravicz, M. E., J. J. Rosowski, and H. F. Voight. Sound-power collection by the auditory periphery of the Mongolian gerbil *Meriones unguiculatus*. I. Middle-ear input impedance. *J. Acoust. Soc. Am.* 92:157–177, 1992. (*Copyright owned by the American Institute of Physics, Woodbury, NY.)

Reiter, E. R., and M. C. Liberman. Efferent-mediated protection from acoustic over-exposure: relation to slow effects of olivocochlear stimulation. *J. Neurophysiol.* 73:506–514, 1995.

Relkin, E. M., and J. R. Doucet. Recovery from prior stimulation. I. Relationship to spontaneous firing rates of primary auditory neurons. *Hear. Res.* 55:215–222, 1991.

Reuter, G., A. H. Gitter, U. Thurm, and H-P. Zenner. High frequency radial movements of the reticular lamina induced by outer hair cell motility, *Hear. Res.* 60: 236–246, 1992.

Rhode, W. S. Observations of the vibration of the basilar membrane in squirrel monkeys using the Mössbauer technique. *J. Acoust. Soc. Am.* 49:1218–1231, 1971.

Rhode, W. S. An investigation of post-mortem cochlear mechanics using the Mössbauer effect. In: *Basic Mechanisms in Hearing*, edited by A. R. Møller. Orlando, FL: Academic, 1973, pp. 49–63.

Rhode, W. S. Some observations on two-tone interaction measured with the Mössbauer effect. In: *Psychophysics and Physiology of Hearing*, edited by E. F. Evans and J. P. Wilson. Orlando, FL, Academic, 1977, pp. 27–38.

Rhode, W. S. Some observations on cochlear mechanics. *J. Acoust. Soc. Am.* 64: 158–176, 1978.

Rhode, W. S., and N. P. Cooper. Two-tone suppression and distortion production on the basilar membrane in the hook region of cat and guinea pig cochleae. *Hear. Res.* 66:31–45, 1993. (*Copyright owned by Elsevier Science-NL, Sara Burgerhartstraat 25, 1055 KV Amsterdam, The Netherlands.)

Rhode, W. S., and N. P. Cooper. Nonlinear mechanics in the apical turn of the chinchilla cochlea in vivo. *Auditory Neurosci.* 3:101–121, 1996. (*Copyright owned by Harwood Academic Publishers, Lausanne, Switzerland.)

Rhode, W. S., and P. H. Smith. Characteristics of tone-pip response patterns in relationship to spontaneous rate in cat auditory nerve fibers. *Hear. Res.* 18: 159–168, 1985. (*Copyright owned by Elsevier Science-NL, Sara Burgerhartstraat 25, 1055 KV Amsterdam, The Netherlands.)

Ricci, A. J., and R. Fettiplace. The effects of calcium buffering and cyclic AMP on mechano-electrical transduction in turtle auditory hair cells. *J. Physiol. (Lond.)* 501:111–124, 1997.

Roberts, W. M., R. A. Jacobs, and A. J. Hudspeth. Co-localization of ion channels involved in frequency selectivity and synaptic transmission at presynaptic active zones of hair cells. *J. Neurosci.* 10:3664–3684, 1990.

Robertson, D. Horseradish peroxidase injection of physiologically characterized afferent and efferent neurones in the guinea pig spiral ganglion. *Hear. Res.* 15: 113–122, 1984.

Robertson, D., and G. A. Manley. Manipulation of frequency analysis in the cochlear ganglion of the guinea pig. *J. Comp. Physiol.* 91:363–375, 1974. (*Copyright owned by Springer-Verlag, New York, NY.)

Robles, L., M. A. Ruggero, and N. C. Rich. Nonlinear interactions in the mechanical response of the cochlea to two-tone stimuli. In: *Cochlear Mechanics*, edited by J. P. Wilson and D. T. Kemp. New York: Plenum, 1989, pp. 369–375.

Rose, J. E., J. F. Brugge, D. J. Anderson, and J. E. Hind. Phase-locked response to low-frequency tones in single auditory nerve fibers of the squirrel monkey. *J. Neurophysiol.* 30:769–793, 1967. (*Copyright owned by The American Physiological Society, Bethesda, MD.)

Rosen, S., M. Bergman, D. Plester, A. El-Mofty, and M. H. Satti. Presbycusis study of a relatively noise-free population in the Sudan. *Ann. Otol. Rhinol. Laryngol.* 71:725–743, 1962.

Rosen, S., D. Plester, A. El-Mofty, and H. V. Rosen. High frequency audiometry in presbycusis: a comparative study of the Mabaan tribe in the Sudan with urban populations. *Arch. Otolaryngol.* 79:18–32, 1964.

Rosowski, J. J. The effects of external- and middle-ear filtering on auditory threshold and noise-induced hearing loss. *J. Acoust. Soc. Am.* 90:124–135, 1991. (*Copyright owned by the American Institute of Physics, Woodbury, NY.)

Rosowski, J. J. Models of external- and middle-ear function. In: *Auditory Computation*, edited by H. L. Hawkins, T. A. McMullen, A. N. Popper, and R. R. Fay. New York: Springer-Verlag, 1996, Chap. 2.

Rosowski, J. J., L. H. Carney, and W. T. Peake. The radiation impedance of the external ear of cat: measurements and applications. *J. Acoust. Soc. Am.* 84: 1695–1708, 1988.

Ross, S. A functional model of the hair cell-primary fiber complex. *J. Acoust. Soc. Am.* 99:2221–2238, 1996.

Rossi, M. L., M. Martini, B. Pelucchi, and R. Fesce. Quantal nature of synaptic transmission at the cytoneural junction in the frog labyrinth. *J. Physiol. (Lond.)* 478:17–35, 1994.

Royster, J. D., L. H. Royster, and M. C. Killion. Sound exposures and hearing thresholds of symphony orchestra musicians. *J. Acoust. Soc. Am.* 89:2793–2803, 1991.

Ruggero, M. A. Response to noise of auditory nerve fibers in the squirrel monkey. *J. Neurophysiol.* 36:569–587, 1973.

Ruggero, M. Responses to sound of the basilar membrane of the mammalian cochlea. *Curr. Opin. Neurobiol.* 2:449–456, 1992. (*Copyright owned by Current Medicine, Philadelphia, PA.)

Ruggero, M. A., and N. C. Rich. Application of a commercially-manufactured Doppler-shift laser velocimeter to the measurement of basilar-membrane vibration. *Hear. Res.* 51:215–230, 1991. (*Copyright owned by Elsevier Science-NL, Sara Burgerhartstraat 25, 1055 KV Amsterdam, The Netherlands.)

Ruggero, M. A., N. C. Rich, and R. Freyman. Spontaneous and impulsively evoked otoacoustic emissions: indicators of cochlear pathology? *Hear. Res.* 10:283–300, 1983.

Ruggero, M. A., N. C. Rich, L. Robles, and B. G. Shivapuja. Middle-ear response in the chinchilla and its relationship to mechanics at the base of the cochlea. *J. Acoust. Soc. Am.* 87:1612–1629, 1990.

Ruggero, M. A., L. Robles, and N. C. Rich. Two-tone suppression in the basilar membrane of the cochlea: mechanical basis of auditory-nerve rate suppression. *J. Neurophysiol.* 68:1087–1099, 1992. (*Copyright owned by The American Physiological Society, Bethesda, MD.)

Ruggero, M. A., L. Robles, N. C. Rich, and A. Recio. Basilar membrane responses to two-tone and broadband stimuli. *Phil. Trans. R. Soc. Lond.* B 336:307–315, 1992. (*Copyright owned by The Royal Society, London, England.)

Ruggero, M. A., N. C. Rich, B. G. Shivapuja, and A. N. Temchin. Auditory-nerve responses to low-frequency tones: intensity dependence. *Auditory Neurosci.* 2: 159–185, 1996.

Russell, I. J., and M. Kössl. Modulation of hair cell voltage responses to tones by low-frequency biasing of the basilar membrane in the guinea pig cochlea. *J. Neurosci.* 12:1587–1601, 1992.

Russell, I. J., A. R. Cody, and G. P. Richardson. The responses of inner and outer hair cells in the basal turn of the guinea-pig cochlea and in the mouse cochlea grown in vitro. *Hear. Res.* 22:199–216, 1986. (*Copyright owned by Elsevier Science-NL, Sara Burgerhartstraat 25, 1055 KV Amsterdam, The Netherlands.)

Russell, I. J., and M. Kössl. Measurements of the basilar membrane resonance in the cochlea of the mustached bat. In: *Active Hearing*, edited by Å. Flock, D. Ottoson, and M. Ulfendahl. Kidlington, UK: Elsevier Science, 1995, pp. 295–305.

Russell, I. J., M. Kössl, and E. Murugasu. A comparison between tone-evoked voltage responses of hair cells and basilar membrane displacements recorded in the basal turn of the guinea pig cochlea. In: *Advances in Hearing Research*, edited by G. A. Manley, G. M. Klump, C. Köppl, H. Fastl, and H. Oeckinghaus. Singapore: World Scientific, 1995, pp. 136–144. (*Copyright owned by World Scientific Publishing Company, River Edge, NJ.)

Ryals, B. M., and E. W. Westbrook. TEM analysis of neural terminals on autoradiographically identified regenerated hair cells. *Hear. Res.* 72:81–88, 1994.

Sachs, M. B. Stimulus-response relation for auditory-nerve fibers: two-tone stimuli. *J. Acoust. Soc. Am.* 45:1025–1036, 1969.

Sachs, M. B., and E. D. Young. Encoding of steady-state vowels in the auditory nerve: representation in terms of discharge rate. *J. Acoust. Soc. Am.* 66:470–479, 1979. (*Copyright owned by the American Institute of Physics, Woodbury, NY.)

Santos-Sacchi, J. Reversible inhibition of voltage-dependent outer hair cell motility and capacitance. *J. Neurosci.* 11:3096–3110, 1991.

Santos-Sacchi, J. On the frequency limit and phase of outer hair cell motility: effects of the membrane filter. *J. Neurosci.* 12:1906–1916, 1992. (*Copyright owned by the Society for Neuroscience, Washington, DC.)

Schacht, J., J. D. Fessenden, and G. Zajic. Slow motility of outer hair cells. In: *Active Hearing*, edited by Å. Flock, D. Ottoson, and M. Ulfendahl. Oxford: Pergamon, 1995, pp. 209–220.

Scharf, B., J. Magnan, L. Collet, E. Ulmer, and A. Chays. On the role of the olivocochlear bundle in hearing: a case study. *Hear. Res.* 75:11–26, 1994.

Scharf, B., J. Magnan, and A. Chays. On the role of the olivocochlear bundle in hearing: 16 case studies. *Hear. Res.* 103:101–122, 1997.

Schloth, E., and E. Zwicker. Mechanical and acoustical influences on spontaneous oto-acoustic emissions. *Hear. Res.* 11:285–293, 1983.

Schmiedt, R. A. Effects of aging on potassium homeostasis and the endocochlear potential in the gerbil cochlea. *Hear. Res.* 102:125–132, 1996.

Schmiedt, R. A., J. H. Mills, and J. C. Adams. Tuning and suppression in auditory nerve fibers of aged gerbils raised in quiet or noise. *Hear. Res.* 45:221–236, 1990. (*Copyright owned by Elsevier Science-NL, Sara Burgerhartstraat 25, 1055 KV Amsterdam, The Netherlands.)

Schroeder, M. R., and J. L. Hall. Model for mechanical to neural transduction in the auditory receptor. *J. Acoust. Soc. Am.* 55:1055–1060, 1974.

Schuknecht, H. R. The effect of aging on the cochlea. In: *Sensorineural Hearing Processes and Disorders*. Boston: Little, Brown, 1967, pp. 393–401.

Schuknecht, H. F. *The Pathology of the Ear*, 2nd ed. Malvern, PA: Lea & Febiger, 1993, p. 291. (*Copyright owned by Williams & Wilkins, Baltimore, MD.)

Schuknecht, H. F., and M. R. Gacek. Cochlear pathology in presbycusis. *Ann. Otol. Rhinol. Laryngol.* 102:1–16, 1993.

Sellick, P. M., and B. M. Johnstone. Production and role of inner ear fluid. *Prog. Neurobiol.* 5:337–362, 1975.

Sellick, P. M., R. Patuzzi, and B. M. Johnstone. Measurement of basilar membrane motion in the guinea pig using the Mössbauer technique. *J. Acoust. Soc. Am.* 72:131–141, 1982.

Sewell, W. F. The effects of furosemide on the endocochlear potential and auditory-nerve fiber tuning curves in cats. *Hear. Res.* 14:305–314, 1984a. (*Copyright owned by Elsevier Science-NL, Sara Burgerhartstraat 25, 1055 KV Amsterdam, The Netherlands.)

Sewell, W. F. The relation between the endocochlear potential and spontaneous activity in auditory nerve fibres in the cat. *J. Physiol. (Lond.)* 347:685–696, 1984b.

Sewell, W. F. Synaptic potentials in afferent fibers innervating hair cells of the lateral line organ in *Xenopus laevis. Hear Res.* 44:71–82, 1990.

Sewell, W. F. Neurotransmitters and synaptic transmission. In: *The Cochlea*, edited by P. Dallos, A. N. Popper, and R. R. Fay. New York: Springer-Verlag, 1996, Chap. 9.

Sewell, W. F., and J. A. Evans. Partial identification of a novel neurotransmitter candidate for the hair cell afferent synapse. *Abstr. Assoc. Res. Otolaryngol.* 20: 170, 1997.

Shamma, S. A. Speech processing in the auditory system. I. The representation of speech sounds in the responses of the auditory nerve. *J. Acoust. Soc. Am.* 78: 1612–1621, 1985. (*Copyright owned by the American Institute of Physics, Woodbury, NY.)

Shaw, E. A. G. Transformation of sound pressure level from the free field to the eardrum in the horizontal plane. *J. Acoust. Soc. Am* 56:1848–1861, 1974. (*Copyright owned by the American Institute of Physics, Woodbury, NY.)

Shaw, E. A. G. 1979 Rayleigh medal lecture: the elusive connection, In: *Localization of Sound: Theory and Applications*, edited by R. Gatehouse. Groton, CT: Amphora, 1982, pp. 13–29.

Shaw, E. A. G. External ear response and sound localization. In: *Localization of Sound: Theory and Applications*, edited by R. Gatehouse. Groton, CT: Amphora, 1982b, pp. 30–41.

Siebert, W. M. Stimulus transformations in the peripheral auditory system. In: *Recognizing Patterns*, edited by P. A. Kolers and M. Eden. Cambridge, MA: MIT Press, 1968, pp. 104–133.

Siebert, W. M. Ranke revisited—a simple short-wave cochlear model. *J. Acoust. Soc. Am.* 56:594–600, 1974.

Siegel, J. H. Spontaneous synaptic potentials from afferent terminals in the guinea pig cochlea. *Hear. Res.* 59:85–92, 1992. (*Copyright owned by Elsevier Science-NL, Sara Burgerhartstraat 25, 1055 KV Amsterdam, The Netherlands.)

Siegel, J. H., and E. M. Relkin. Antagonistic effects of perilymphatic calcium and magnesium on the activity of single cochlear afferent neurons. *Hear. Res.* 28: 131–147, 1987.

Silkes, S. M., and C. D. Geisler. Responses of "lower-spontaneous-rate" auditory-nerve fibers to speech syllables presented in noise. I. General characteristics. *J. Acoust. Soc. Am.* 90:3122–3139, 1991.

Simmons, F. B. Electrical stimulation of the auditory nerve in man. *Arch. Otolaryngol.* 84:24–54, 1966.

Simmons, J. A., M. Ferragamo, C. F. Moss, S. B. Stevenson, and R. A. Altes. Discrimination of jittered sonar echoes by the echolocating bat, *Eptesicus fuscus*: the shape of target images in echolocation. *J. Comp. Physiol. A* 167:589–616, 1990.

Sinex, D. G., and C. D. Geisler. Auditory-nerve fiber responses to frequency-modulated tones. *Hear. Res.* 4:127–148, 1981. (*Copyright owned by Elsevier Science-NL, Sara Burgerhartstraat 25, 1055 KV Amsterdam, The Netherlands.)

Slaney, M. Auditory Toolbox for Matlab, Apple Computer Technical Report #45, 1994.

Slepecky, N. B. Sensory supporting cells in the organ of Corti: cytoskeletal organization related to cellular function. In: *Active Hearing*, edited by Å. Flock, D. Ottoson, and M. Ulfendahl. Kidlington, UK: Elsevier Science, 1995, pp. 87–101. (*Copyright owned by Elsevier Science Ltd, The Boulevard, Langford Lane, Kidlington OX5 1GB, UK.)

Slepecky, N. Structure of the mammalian cochlea. In: *The Cochlea*, edited by P. Dallos, A. N. Popper, and R. R. Fay. New York: Springer-Verlag, 1996, Chap. 2.

Smith, R. L., M. L. Brachman, and R. D. Frisina. Sensitivity of auditory-nerve fibers to changes in intensity: a dichotomy between decrements and increments. *J. Acoust. Soc. Am.* 78:1310–1316, 1985.

Smith, R. L., and J. J. Zwislocki. Short-term adaptation and incremental responses of single auditory-nerve fibers. *Biol. Cybernet.* 17:169–182, 1975.

Sobkowicz, H. (Ed.) Development and regeneration of the inner ear. *Inter. J. Devel. Neurosci.* 15(4/5), 1997.

Sobkowicz, H. M., S. M. Slapnick, and B. K. August. The kinocilium of auditory hair cells and evidence for its morphogenetic role during the regeneration of stereocilia and cuticular plates. *J. Neurocytol.* 24:633–653, 1995.

Sobkowicz, H. M., B. K. August, and S. M. Slapnick. Post-traumatic survival and recovery of the auditory sensory cells in culture. *Acta Otolaryngol.* 116:257–262, 1996. (*Copyright owned by Scandinavian University Press, Stockholm, Sweden.)

Sobkowicz, H. M., S. M. Slapnick, L. M. Nitecka, and B. K. August. Compound synapses within the GABAergic innervation of the auditory inner hair cells in the adolescent mouse. *J. Comp. Neurol.* 377:423–442, 1997.

Soifer, N., K. Weaver, G. L. Endahl, and C. E. Holdsworth Jr. Otosclerosis: a review. *Acta Otolaryngol. Suppl.* 269:1–25, 1970.

Spoendlin, H. The innervation of the organ of Corti. *J. Laryngol. Otol.* 81:717–738, 1967. (*Copyright owned by Headly Brothers, Ashford, UK.)

Spoendlin, H. The innervation of the cochlear receptor. In: *Basic Mechanisms in Hearing*, edited by A. R. Møller. Orlando, FL: Academic, 1973, pp. 185–230.

Spoendlin, H. Anatomy of cochlear innervation. *Am. J. Otolaryngol.* 6:453–467, 1985. (*Copyright owned by W. B. Saunders, Philadelphia, PA.)

Sridhar, T. S., M. C. Liberman, M. C. Brown, and W. F. Sewell. A novel cholinergic "slow effect" of efferent stimulation on cochlear potentials in the guinea pig. *J. Neurosci.* 15:3667–3678, 1995.

Steel, K. P. The tectorial membrane of mammals. *Hear. Res.* 9:327–359, 1983.

Steel, K. P., and W. Kimberling. Approaches to understanding the molecular genetics of hearing and deafness. In: *Clinical Aspects of Hearing*, edited by T. R. Van De Water, A. N. Popper, and R. R. Fay. New York: Springer-Verlag, 1996, Chap. 2

Stevens, K. N. Constraints imposed by the auditory system on properties used to classify speech sounds: data from phonology, acoustics and psychoacoustics. In: *The Cognitive Representation of Speech*, edited by T. Myers, J. Laver, and J. Anderson. Amsterdam: North Holland, 1981, pp. 61–74.

Stover, L. J., S. T. Neely, and M. P. Gorga. Latency and multiple sources of distortion product otoacoustic emissions. *J. Acoust. Soc. Am.* 99:1016–1024, 1996.

Strube, H. W. Evoked otoacoustic emissions as cochlear Bragg reflections. *Hear. Res.* 38:35–46, 1989.

Stypulkowski, P. H. 3M programmable hearing instruments. In: *Understanding Digitally Programmable Hearing Aids*, edited by R. E. Sandlin. Boston: Allyn & Bacon, 1994, Chap. 6.

Suga, N., and P. H-S. Jen. Peripheral control of acoustic signals in the auditory system of echolocating bats. *J. Exp. Biol.* 62:277–311, 1975.

Suga, N., G. Neuweiler, and J. Müller. Peripheral auditory tuning for fine frequency analysis by the CF-FM bat, *Rhinolophus ferrumequinum. J. Comp. Physiol.* 106: 111–125, 1976.

Sullivan, W. E., and M. Konishi. Segregation of stimulus phase and intensity coding in the cochlear nucleus of the barn owl. *J. Neurosci.* 4:1787–1799, 1984.

Summers, I. R. (Ed.) *Tactile Aids for the Hearing Impaired.* London: Whurr, 1992.

Suzuki, J-I., H. Shono, K. Koga, and T. Akiyama. Early studies and the history of development of the middle ear implant in Japan. *Adv. Audiol.* 4:1–14, 1988.

Talmadge, C. L., and A. Tubis. On modeling the connection between spontaneous and evoked otoacoustic emissions. In: *Biophysics of Hair Cell Sensory Systems.* Singapore: World Scientific, 1993, pp. 25–31.

Talmadge, C. L., G. R. Long, W. J. Murphy, and A. Tubis. New off-line method for detecting spontaneous otoacoustic emissions in human subjects. *Hear. Res.* 71: 170–182, 1993.

Teager, H. M., and S. M. Teager. Evidence for nonlinear sound production mechanisms in the vocal tract. In: *Speech Production and Speech Modelling*, edited by W. J. Hardcastle and A. Marchal. Boston: Academic, 1990, pp. 241–261.

Teoh, S. W., D. T. Flandermeyer, and J. J. Rosowski. Effects of pars flaccida on sound conduction in ears of Mongolian gerbil: acoustic and anatomical measurements. *Hear. Res.* 106:39–65, 1997.

Thurm, U. Mechano-electric transduction. *Biophys. Struct. Mech.* 7:245–246, 1981.

Tonndorf, J., A. J. Duvall, and J. P. Reneau. Permeability of intracochlear membranes to various vital stains. *Ann. Otol. Rhinol. Laryngol.* 71:801–841, 1962.

Trahiotis, C., and D. N. Elliot. Behavioral investigation of some possible effects of sectioning the crossed olivocochlear bundle. *J. Acoust. Soc. Am.* 47:592–596, 1968.

Tricas, T. C., and S. M. Highstein. Visually mediated inhibition of lateral line primary afferent activity by the octavolateralis efferent system during predation in the free-swimming toadfish, *Opsanus tau. Exp. Brain Res.* 83:233–236, 1990.

Tucker, R., and R. Fettiplace. Confocal imaging of calcium microdomains and calcium extrusion in turtle hair cells. *Neuron.* 15:1323–1335, 1995.

Tyler, R. S., and N. Tye-Murray. Cochlear implant signal-processing strategies and patient perception of speech and environmental sounds. In: *Cochlear Implants: A Practical Guide*, edited by H. Cooper. San Diego: Singular Publishing Group, 1991, Chap. 4.

Ulfendahl, M., S. M. Khanna, and Å. Flock. A temporal bone preparation for the study of cochlear micromechanics at the cellular level. *Hear. Res.* 40:55–64, 1989.

Van Beethoven, L. The Heiligenstadt testament, 1802. English translation in: *The Beethoven Compendium: A Guide to Beethoven's Life and Music*, edited by B. Cooper. New York: Thames & Hudson, 1991.

Van Dijk, P., and H. P. Wit. Amplitude and frequency fluctuations of spontaneous otoacoustic emissions. *J. Acoust. Soc. Am.* 88:1779–1793, 1990.

Van Dijk, P., P. M. Narins, and J. Wang. Spontaneous otoacoustic emissions in seven frog species. *Hear. Res.* 101:102–112, 1996.

Van den Hornert, C., and P. H. Stypulkowski. Single fiber mapping of spatial excitation patterns in the electrically stimulated auditory nerve. *Hear. Res.* 29:195–206, 1987a.

Van den Hornert, C., and P. H. Stypulkowski. Temporal response patterns of single auditory nerve fibers elicited by periodic electrical stimuli. *Hear. Res.* 29:207–222, 1987b.

Van Hengel, P. W. J., H. Duifhuis, and M. P. M. G. van den Raadt. Spatial periodicity in the cochlea: the result of interaction of spontaneous emissions? *J. Acoust. Soc. Am.* 99:3566–3571, 1996.

Vernon, J. Attempts to relieve tinnitus. *J. Am. Audiol. Soc.* 2:124–131, 1977.

Vetter, D. E., J. C. Adams, and E. Mugnaini. Chemically distinct rat olivocochlear neurons. *Synapse* 7:21–43, 1991.

Vetter, D. E., E. Saldaa, and E. Mugnaini. Input from the inferior colliculus to medial olivocochlear neurons in the rat: a double label study with PHA-L and cholera toxin. *Hear. Res.* 70:173–186, 1993.

Villchur, E. Stimulation of the effect of recruitment on loudness relationships in speech. *J. Acoust. Soc. Am.* 56:1601–1611, 1974. (*Copyright owned by the American Institute of Physics, Woodbury, NY.)

Voight, H. F., M. B. Sachs, and E. D. Young. Representation of whispered vowels in discharge patterns of auditory-nerve fibers. *Hear. Res.* 8:49–58, 1982.

Von Békésy, G. The variation of phase along the basilar membrane with sinusoidal vibrations. *J. Acoust. Soc. Am.* 19:452–460, 1947. (*Copyright owned by the American Institute of Physics, Woodbury, NY.)

Von Békésy, G. *Experiments in Hearing*. New York: McGraw-Hill, 1960.

Von Gierke, H. E., and W. D. Ward. Criteria for noise and vibration exposure. In: *Handbook of Acoustical Measurements and Noise Control*, 3rd ed., edited by C. M. Harris. New York: McGraw-Hill, 1991, Chap. 26.

Voss, S. E., J. J. Rosowski, and W. T. Peake. Is the pressure difference between the oval and round windows the effective acoustic stimulus for the cochlea? *J. Acoust. Soc. Am.* 100:1602–1616, 1996.

Walsh, E. J., J. McGee, M. C. Liberman, and S. L. McFadden. Long-term physiological consequences of cutting olivocochlear bundle (OCB) in neonatal animals. *Abstr. Assoc. Res. Otolaryngol.* 20:54, 1997.

Wang, M. D., and R. C. Bilger. Consonant confusions in noise: study of perceptual features. *J. Acoust. Soc. Am.* 54:1248–1266, 1973.

Wang, Y., and Y. Raphael. Re-innervation patterns of chick auditory sensory epithelium after acoustic overstimulation. *Hear. Res.* 97:11–18, 1996.

Wangemann, P. Comparison of ion transport mechanisms between vestibular dark cells and strial marginal cells. *Hear. Res.* 90:149–157, 1995.

Wangemann, P., and J. Schacht. Homeostatic mechanisms in the cochlea. In: *The Cochlea*, edited by P. Dallos, A. N. Popper, and R. R. Fay. New York: Springer-Verlag, 1996, Chap. 3.

Ward, W. D. Noise-induced hearing loss. In: *Noise and Society*, edited by D. M. Jones and A. J. Chapman. Chichester, UK: Wiley, 1984, Chap. 4.

Warr, W. B. Organization of olivocochlear efferent systems in mammals. In: *Mammalian Auditory Pathway*: *Neuroanatomy*, edited by D. B. Webster, A. N. Popper, and R. R. Fay. New York: Springer-Verlag, 1992, pp. 410–448. (*Copyright owned by Springer-Verlag, New York, NY.)

Warr, W. B., J. Beck Boche, and S. T. Neely. Efferent innervation of the inner hair cell region: origins and terminations of two lateral olivocochlear systems. *Hear. Res.* 108:89–111, 1997.

Warren III, E. H., and M. C. Liberman. Effects of contralateral sound on auditory-nerve responses. II. Dependence on stimulus variables. *Hear. Res.* 37:105–122, 1989.

Webster, D. B., and M. Webster. Adaptive value of hearing and vision in kangaroo rat predator avoidance. *Brain Behav. Evol.* 4:310–322, 1971.

Webster, D. B., and M. Webster. Kangaroo rat auditory thresholds before and after middle ear reduction. *Brain Behav. Evol.* 5:41–53, 1972.

Weiss, T. F. A model of the peripheral auditory system. *Kybernetik* 3:153–175, 1966.

Westerman, L. A., and R. L. Smith. Conservation of adapting components in auditory-nerve responses. *J. Acoust. Soc. Am.* 81:680–691, 1987. (*Copyright owned by the American Institute of Physics, Woodbury, NY.)

Westermann, S. Principles and application of the Widex multiprogrammable hearing aid system. In: *Understanding Digitally Programmable Hearing Aids*, edited by R. E. Sandlin. Boston: Allyn & Bacon, 1994, Chap. 3.

Wever, E. G. *The Reptile Ear*. Princeton, NJ: Princeton University Press, 1978.

Whitehead, M. L., B. L. Lonsbury-Martin, G. K. Martin, and M. J. McCoy. Otoacoustic emissions: animal models and clinical observations. In: *Clinical Aspects of Hearing*, edited by T. R. Van De Water, A. N. Popper, and R. R. Fay. New York: Springer-Verlag, 1996, Chap. 7.

Wiederhold, M. L., and N. Y. S. Kiang. Effects of electric stimulation of the crossed olivocochlear bundle on single auditory-nerve fibers in the cat. *J. Acoust. Soc. Am.* 48:950–965, 1970.

Wiederhold, M. L., and W. T. Peake. Efferent inhibition of auditory-nerve responses: dependence on acoustic stimulus parameters. *J. Acoust. Soc. Am.* 40:1427–1430, 1966.

Wier, C. C., E. G. Pasanen, and D. McFadden. Partial dissociation of spontaneous otoacoustic emissions and distortion products during aspirin use in humans. *J. Acoust. Soc. Am.* 84:230–237, 1988.

Wightman, F. L., and D. J. Kistler. The dominant role of low-frequency interaural time differences in sound localization. *J. Acoust. Soc. Am.* 91:1648–1661, 1992.

Wightman, F. L., and D. J. Kistler. Sound localization. In: *Human Psychophysics*, edited by W. A. Yost, A. N. Popper, and R. R. Fay. New York: Springer-Verlag, 1993, pp. 155–192.

Wiley, T. L., and M. G. Block. Acoustic and nonacoustic reflex patterns in audiologic diagnosis, In: *The Acoustic Reflex*, edited by S. Silman. Orlando, FL: Academic, 1984, Chap. 11.

Willott, J. R. *Aging and the Auditory System: Anatomy, Physiology, and Psychophysics*. San Diego: Singular Publishing Group, 1991.

Wilson, P. J. Otoacoustic emissions and tinnitus. *Scand. Audiol. Suppl.* 25:109–119, 1986.

Winslow, R. L., and M. B. Sachs. Effect of electrical stimulation of the crossed olivocochlear bundle on auditory nerve response to tones in noise. *J. Neurophysiol.* 57:1002–1021, 1987.

Winslow, R. L., and M. B. Sachs. Single-tone intensity discrimination based on auditory-nerve rate responses in backgrounds of quiet, noise, and with stimulation of the crossed olivocochlear bundle. *Hear. Res.* 35:165–190, 1988.

Wit, H. P., and R. J. Ritsma. Sound emission for the ear triggered by single molecules? *Neurosci. Lett.* 40:275–280, 1983.

Woolf, N. K. The role of viral infection in the development of otopathology: labyrinthitis and autoimmune disease. In: *Clinical Aspects of Hearing*, edited by R. R. Van De Water, A. N. Popper, and R. R. Fay. New York: Springer, 1996, Chapter 6.

Working Group on Communication Aids for the Hearing-Impaired. Speech-perception aids for hearing-impaired people: current status and needed research. *J. Acoust. Soc. Am.* 90:637–684, 1991.

Wotton, J. M., T. Haresign, and J. A. Simmons. Spatially dependent acoustic cues generated by the external ear of the big brown bat, *Eptesicus fuscus. J. Acoust. Soc. Am.* 98:1423–1445, 1995.

Wu, Y-C., J. J. Art, M. B. Goodman, and R. Fettiplace. A kinetic description of the calcium-activated potassium channel and its application to electrical tuning of hair cells. *Prog. Biophys. Mol. Biol.* 63:131–158, 1995.

Wu, Y-C., T. Tucker, and R. Fettiplace. A theoretical study of calcium microdomains in turtle hair cells. *Biophys. J.* 71:2256–2275, 1996.

Xue, S., D. C. Mountain, and A. E. Hubbard. Acoustic enhancement of electrically evoked otoacoustic emissions reflects basilar membrane tuning: experimental results. *Hear. Res.* 70:121–126, 1993.

Xue, S., D. C. Mountain, and A. E. Hubbard. Acoustic enhancement of electrically-evoked otoacoustic emissions reflects basilar membrane tuning: a model. *Hear. Res.* 91:93–100, 1995.

Xue, S., D. C. Mountain, and A. E. Hubbard. Electrically-evoked otoacoustic emissions: direct comparisons with basilar membrane motion. *Auditory Neurosci.* 2: 301–308, 1996.

Zagaeski, M., A. R. Cody, I. J. Russell, and D. C. Mountain. Transfer characteristic of the inner hair cells synapse: steady-state analysis. *J. Acoust. Soc. Am.* 95: 3430–3434, 1994. (*Copyright owned by the American Institute of Physics, Woodbury, NY.)

Zenner, H-P. Motility of outer hair cells as an active actin-meditated process. *Acta Otolaryngol.* 105:39–44, 1988.

Zheng, X-Y., D. Henderson, S. L. McFadden, and B-H. Hu. The role of the cochlear efferent system in acquired resistance to noise-induced hearing loss. *Hear. Res.* 104:191–203, 1997a.

Zheng, X-Y., D. Henderson, B-H. Hu, D-L. Ding, and S. L. McFadden. The influence of the cochlear efferent system on chronic acoustic trauma. *Hear. Res.* 107: 147–159, 1997b.

Zidanic, M., and W. E. Brownell. Fine structure of the intracochlear potential field. I. The silent current. *Biophys. J.* 57:1253–1268, 1990.

Zweig, G. Finding the impedance of the organ of Corti. *J. Acoust. Soc. Am.* 89: 1229–1254, 1991.

Zweig, G., and C. A. Shera. The origin of periodicity in the spectrum of evoked otoacoustic emissions. *J. Acoust. Soc. Am.* 98:2018–2047, 1995.

Zweig, G., R. Lipes, and J. R. Pierce. The cochlear compromise. *J. Acoust. Soc. Am.* 59:975–982, 1976.

Zwicker, E. ''Otoacoustic'' emissions in a nonlinear cochlear hardware model with feedback. *J. Acoust. Soc. Am.* 80:154–162, 1986.

Zwicker, E., and E. Schloth. Interrelation of different oto-acoustic emissions. *J. Acoust. Soc. Am.* 75:1148–1154, 1984.

Zwislocki, J. Theorie der Schneckenmechanik. *Acta Otolaryngol. Suppl* 72:1–76, 1948.

Zwislocki, J. J., and E. J. Kletsky. Tectorial membrane: a possible effect on frequency analysis in the cochlea. *Science* 204:639–641, 1979.

Zwislocki, J. J., and L. K. Cefaratti. Tectorial membrane. II. Stiffness measurements in vivo. *Hear. Res.* 42:211–228, 1989.

INDEX

Note: Bold type indicates the central focus of an important topic, usually a full chapter.

Acetylcholine (ACh), 110, 187, 264–265
Acoustic axis (of pinna), 33, 48
Acoustic fovea, 197
Acoustic impedance, 27, 43–45, 48, 50, 52–53, 59–60, 62–64, 71, 131, **330–337**
Acoustic reflex, 49–50, 52–53
Acoustic resonance, 31, 48, **328–329**
Acousticolateralis system, 91, 106, 172, 179, 256, 271–272, 313
Acoustics (see Sound)
Actin, 79, 92–93, 95, 99, 119
Adaptation
  hair cell, 98–100
  neural, 184–187, 261
  psychoacoustic, 269
Afferent innervation, **169–182** (see also Primary auditory neurons)
Aging, effects of, 276–277, 285–292
''Air-bone'' gap, 279
Amplification of Signal Power, in
  external ear, 30–32
  middle ear, 39, 42, 53

inner ear, 100–101, 127, 135–138, 163, 192
  suppression of, 143, 145–151, 218–219, 221, 225, 227, 282
  hearing instruments (aids), 301–307
Amplitude histogram, 157
Animations, 6, 41, 57, 83, 93, 197, 201, 276
Anastomosis of Oort, 250–251
Articulation index, 316
Aspirin, 122, 153, 158, 162, 293
Attentive state, 269
Audiograms, 44, 153, 276, 284–287, 294, 298–299
Automatic gain (volume) control, 52, 54, 183, 187, 216, 225, 233, 238, 243, 304–305, 317
Azimuth (of sound source), 24, 30–34, 47–48

Barn Owl
  acoustic fovea, 197

Barn Owl (*Continued*)
  otoacoustic emissions, 158, 160
  phase synchrony (neural), 202
  sound-source localization, 3, 23,
      34–35
Basilar membrane (mammal)
  acoustically induced movements,
      57–71, 141–156, 160–163
  electrically induced movements, 128
  structure, 74–75, 129
Basilar papilla (lizard), 83–85,
      103–104
Bats
  acoustic fovea, 197
  audible frequency range, 20, 41, 52,
      119
  efferent effects, 263
  frequency tuning (cochlea), 67, 195
  location/characteristic-frequency
      ''map,'' 196
  middle-ear contractions, 51–52
  ossicles, 46
  otoacoustic emissions, 157, 162
  outer hair cells, 111
  pressure level of cries, 51
  pressure transformations (external
      ear), 32
  sound-source localization, 3, 23
  temporal acuity, 36
Behavioral effects of
  deefferentation, 269–270
  hearing impairment, 275
Bird ears
  audible frequency range, 106
  ear canal, 38
  efferent and ACh effects, 264
  frequency tuning, 106
  middle-ear contractions, 52
  neural encoding of sounds, 202
  otoacoustic emissions, 158, 160
  regrowth, 313–315
  suppression, 226
Blood supply (see vascular system)
Brownian motion, 11, 97, 194

Calcium ions (Ca^{2+}), in hair cells
  extrustion, 112

flow into cilia, 95–96, 112
  roles in
    adaptation, 99–100
    efferent effects, 261, 264–265
    electrical frequency tuning,
        105–107
    exocytosis, 174, 179, 187
    motility, 119, 123
Calcium-activated K$^+$ channels,
    105–106, 265
Capacitance (hair-cell), 117–118
  voltage-dependent changes, 137, 174
Characteristic frequency
  definition, 102, 192–193
  ''map'' vs. cochlear location, 196,
      202, 281, 284
Characteristic place (definition), 138
Chick cochlea (see bird ears)
Cilia (see Stereocilia)
Clipping, 146, 303
Cochlea (mammalian), 29, 56, **72–83**
  blood supply, 76, 86, 111, 294
  components (see also individual
      listings)
    basilar membrane, 74, 128–129
    bony spiral lamina, 74–75
    cochlear partition, 73–74
    Deiters' cells, 76–80, 110, 129,
        132, 294, 315–316
    endolymphatic system, 56–57
    habenula perforata, 171
    helicotrema, 56, 135
    Hensen's cells, 76–78
    Hensen's stripe, 79, 82
    inner hair cells, 76, 110
    marginal (dark) cells, 86, 111
    modiolus, 73–74, 309
    organ of Corti, 74–79, 283
    outer hair cells, 76–81
    oval window, 29, 38–41, 56–57
    perilymphatic system, 55–57
    pillar cells, 75–78, 80–82
    Reissner's membrane, 56, 60–61,
        71, 74
    reticular lamina, 77–80, 82, 84
    round window, 29, 38–41, 56–57,
        278
    scala media, 56, 61, 74, 85
    scala tympani, 56, 61, 74, 85

Cochlea (mammalian) (*Continued*)
  scala vestibuli, 56, 61, 74, 85
  spiral gangion, 74–75, 170
  spiral ligament, 74–75, 137
  spiral limbus, 74–75, 81
  stria vascularis, 74–75, 86, 111, 113
  tectorial membrane, 74–84
  tunnel of Corti, 75–76
  coordinate system (definition), 87
  deefferented, 268–271
  development, 271
  dimensions, 72–73
  electrical excitation, 130–131, 163–164, 308–311
  frequency-tuning mechanisms (model), 60–64
  processing "window," 205, 215
  repair and regeneration, 315–316
  sound propagation within, 56–59, 200–201, 296
Cochlear amplifier, 66, 68, **125–138**
  compressive nature, 134–135, 138
  damage to, 282, 301
  dependency on stria vascularis, 290–291
  efferent effects, 257
  "gain," 65, 146, 257, 267
  model of, 133–136
  spatial localization, 135, 150, 221, 282
  suppression effects, 144–147
Cochlear implants, 308–311
Cochlear microphonic potential, 116, 263, 267
Cochlear nucleus (brainstem), 170, 201–202, 252–253, 311
Cochlear partition, 73–74
  models of, 60–64, 127, 133, 142–150, 154–156, 158, 239, 296
  vibrations of, 56–60, 65–71, **125–138**, 296
  nonlinear nature, 65–69, **139–165**
Compression (see element involved)
Compound action potential, 270, 288–289
Conductive hearing loss, 277–279
Crocodilian ears, 38, 106–107

Crossed olivocochlear bundle (COCB), 127, 158, 250, 253, 257–259, 262–263, 267, 269
Cubic distortion tone (see Distortion)
Cytocochleogram, 281, 284

d', 262–263
Damping
  acoustic impedance of, 332, 334–336
  in hair cell tuft, 101
  in middle ear, 46–47
  in inner ear, 82–83, 126, 132
  negative, 127, 132–138
Deafness, 295, 316
decibels, dB SPL (definition), 16–17
Deiters' cells, 76–80, 110, 129, 132, 294, 315–316
Displacusis, 269
Distortion-product emissions (see otoacoustic emissions)
Distortion products (definition), 165
  cubic distortion product, 152–153, 165, 304
Dominance (by one component), 142–143, 216, 236, 244
Doppler shift, 64, 125
Dynamic range, of
  efferent (MOC) neurons, 254
  hearing instruments, 298–301, 317
  human hearing, 21, 298–301
  primary auditory neurons, 187–191, 225, 233, 237, 245, 262
  sounds, 4, 16–17, 21

Eardrum, 26, 29, 40–41
  input impedance, 44–47, 52, 328
  pars flaccida, 40
  perforation, 277–278, 296
  pressure measurements, 29–33
Efferent innervation, **249–272**
  anatomy, 250–253
  effects on perception, 268–270
  effects on primary neuron responses, 127, 258–263

Efferent innervation (*Continued*)
  ''slow'' effects, 261, 271
  systems (see Medial and Lateral
    olivocochlear systems)
Efferent neurons
  neurotransmitters, 264–265
  responses to sound, 253–256
''Effective'' area of external/middle
    ear, 47–48
Endocochlear potential, 85–86, 136,
    289–290
Endocytosis (definition), 182
Endolymph (composition), 85, 112
Endolymphatic system, 38–39, 55–56,
    85–86, 111–112
Energy density, 15, 28
English language
  consonants, 233, 237–238, 241, 246
  frequency range, 21, 237, 299
  primary neuron responses to, **229–
    248**
  vowels, 230–236, 241, 245–247
Equal-loudness contour, 298–299
Excitatory postsynaptic potential
    (EPSP), 172–174, 177–179,
    181, 191
Exocytosis (definition), 182
External ear, **23–36**, 277
  cues for sound localization, 28–35
  impairment, 277
Extracellular potentials, 224, 256, 267

Feedback
  from central nervous system 49–53,
    171–172, **249–272**
  in hearing instruments (aids), 304–
    305, 307
  in cochlear-amplifier theory, 127,
    132–133, 137, 158–163
Feedforward (cochlear-amplifier
    theory), 133–136
Filters
  band-pass (tuned), 103–107, 137,
    204–205, 238
    frequency-time interconnections,
    204–205

  in hearing instruments (aids), 302,
    306, 310
  low-pass, 102, 117, 136, 202
    corner frequency, 42, 117, 202
Fimbrin, 93
Firearms, effects on hearing, 21, 52,
    285–286
Fish acousticolateralis system
  efferent effects (lateral line), 256,
    271
  continual hair-cell generation, 313
  sacculus, 172, 191
Formants (see vowels)
Forward masking, 187
Fourier Analysis, 17–20, 70, 165, 184,
    205, 208, 221, 231, 239, 247,
    318–327
  fast Fourier transform (FFT), 325–
    326
  frequency-time transformations, 204–
    205
Fractal processes, 182
Frequency (definitions), 14, 21, 228
Frequency spectrum (definition), 24,
    152, 165
Frequency tuning curve (definition),
    65–66, 192
Frequency tuning mechanisms, 101–
    107 (see also Cochlea)
Friction (see Damping)
Frog ear
  amphibian papilla, 106–107, 226
  basilar papilla, 104, 107, 226
  efferent effects, 256, 271
  middle ear, 49
  otoacoustic emissions, 158, 160,
    162
  saccular hair cells, 93, 101, 106–
    107, 137, 256
  suppression (neural), 226
Furosemide, 153, 179, 289–290

γ-aminobutyric acid (GABA), 265
Gain (see cochlear amplifier)
Genetic factors, 275, 285
Gentamicin, 153

Glottal pulses, 231, 235
Glutamate, 174–175, 187
Guns (see firearms)

Hair cells (general)
    afferent innervation, 92, 172–175
    components, 92–96, 315–316 (see
        also individual listings)
    degeneration, 51, 281–284
    efferent innervation, 92, 271
    exocytosis, 174
    frequency-tuning mechanisms, 101–
        107
    functional axis, 93
    regrowth and repair, 312–315
    receptor (transduction) potential (see
        individual listing)
    resistance, 97
    transduction current, 95–99, 113,
        116–117, 132–133, 136, 138,
        202, 267, 290
    transduction processes, **91–108**
Hearing (see also individual species)
    frequency/sound-pressure range, 21,
        299
    importance, 3, 45, 229, 275
    thresholds (tonal), 16, 21, 44, 299
Hearing impairment
    causes, 51–52, **275–294**
        acoustic trauma, 51–52, 280–285
        aging, 276–277, 285–291
        genetic, 275, 285
        ototoxic drugs, 275, 282–283
    conductive losses, 277–279
    sensorineural losses (categories), 277
    treatments, **295–317**
Hearing Instruments (aids), 296–311
    compression, 299–306, 317
    digital, 306–307
    distortion in, 303–304, 306
    expense, 307
    for middle-ear impairment, 296–
        297
    historical development, 302
Hensen's cells, 76–78
Hensen's stripe, 79, 82
Histogram (see individual type)

Horns, acoustic, 28
Horseradish peroxidase (HRP), 170,
    175, 181, 195
Human ear, 28–29, 73
    anatomy, 28–29, 73, 171, 175
    eardrum pressures, 29–33
    intracochlear pressures, 60
    middle-ear muscles, 51–52
    otoacoustic emissions, 126, 152–
        154, 156–163
    vibrations (basilar membrane), 57–
        59
Human hearing
    frequency/sound-level range, 20–21
    impairment, 275–279, 283–287,
        291–294
        treatments, **295–317**
    importance of, 229, 275
    perceptions, 3, 17, 236, 246, 268–
        269, 298–301, 308–310, 321
        with defferented ears, 268–269
    sound-source localization, 33–34, 36
    thresholds (tonal), 16, 20–21, 299

Impedance, 26–28, **330–337**
    acoustic, 27–28, 44–46, 62, 328
    reactive component, 62, 336
    resistive component, 62, 336
Impulse response, 205–206, 210, 227
Inertia, 82–84, 91
Inner hair cells, 76, 110
    afferent innervation, 171–175
    anatomy, 109–110
    effects of damage, 280–284
    efferent effects, 256–257, 268
    efferent innervation, 171–172
    electrophysiology, 113–116
    excitation, 82–83
    frequency tuning, 102
    input-output (I/O) curve, 114–116,
        206
    neurotransmitter, 174–175
Intensity, of sound (definition), 17
Interaural (definition), 25
    pressure differences, 24, 30–34
    spectral differences, 24, 34
    timing differences, 33–34, 36

Interspike interval histogram, 177, 179
Isoresponse curve (see frequency
    tuning curve)

Jitter, of neurotransmitter release, 202

Kinocilium, 92–93, 95, 97, 109, 315

Laser interferometer, 65, 126
Lateral line organ, 91, 256, 271
Lateral superior olivary (LOC) systems,
    250–253, 265, 270
Linear responses
  of cochlea, 66, 70, 190
  of middle ear, 19, 37, 41
Linear system, 19
  definition, 22
  impulse response, 205, 227
  properties, 22, 36, 67, 71, 140, 210,
      227, 247
Line-busy effect, 246
Lizard ears
  basilar papilla, 83–85
  frequency range, 42, 202
  frequency selectivity, 103–104, 107
  middle ear, 37–40
  otoacoustic emissions, 158, 160
  phase synchrony (neural), 202
  stapes vibrations, 42–43
  suppression (two-tone), 226
  tectorial structures, 104
Loudness (perceptual), 298–301

Mammalian ear, 29
  external, 28–33, 277, 302
  inner (see cochlea)
  middle (see middle ear—mammal)
"Masking"
  of primary neuron responses, 244–
      246, 261–263, 270
  of tinnitus, 293, 311–312

Mass
  acoustic impedance of, 331–336
  of endolymph, 104
  of cochlear partition, 60–64
  of middle-ear ossicles, 45–46
  of tectorial structures, 104
Medial superior olivary (MOC) system,
    250–253, 264–265
  effects on outer hair cells (model),
      265–268
Ménière's disease, 268, 285
Microtubules, 75, 78, 92–93, 132
Middle ear, 26–27, **37–54**
  basic function, 26–27
Middle ear (lizard), 37–43
Middle ear (mammal), **40–54**
  axis of rotation, 40–41, 48
  center of mass, 48
  components, 40–41
    eardrum, 40–41 (see also
      Eardrum)
    Eustachian tube, 29, 40, 48, 278
    incus and malleus, 40–41
    stapedius muscle, 40, 49–51
    stapes, 29, 42, 49, 277–279, 296
    tensor tympani, 49, 51
  disorders, 53, 277–279
  efficiency, 46–48
  lever ratio, 42
  models of, 44
  muscles, 49–53
  treatments for disorders, 296–297
  volume, 45, 49
Mitochondria, 52, 92, 110, 173, 180–
    181
Models, of
  cochlear vibrations, 60–64, 71, 87,
      127, 133–137, 142–150, 154–
      156, 159, 296
  efferent (MOC) activity, 265–268
  hair-cell
    adaptation, 95, 99–100
    electrophysiology, 112–114
    excitation, 95–96
    frequency tuning, 103–107
    tip-link and tip-junction stretch, 96
  middle-ear processes, 44
  neural responses to speech, 238–239
  neural spike generation, 177–179,
      181

Models, of (*Continued*)
    otoacoustic emissions, 154–156, 158
    suppression (two-tone), 142–150
    transmitter release, 185–188
Modulation
    amplitude, 211–214
    frequency, 214–216, 243
Mössbauer effect, 64, 125
Myosin, 79, 93, 99, 119

Nernst potential, 111–113, 124, 265–
    266
Neurotransmitters
    afferent, 174
    efferent, 110, 264–265
Newton's second law, 108, 331
Noise
    broadband (wide-band), 227
        (definition), as
        masker of primary stimulus, 244–
            247, 261, 269–270
        primary stimulus, 33–34, 36, 157,
            159, 183, 208–210, 226, 275,
            280–289
        tinnitus treatment, 311–312
        unmasker of masked stimuli, 261–
            263, 272
    inherent, 153, 194
    white, 228, 248
Nonlinear
    analytical methods, 165, 209–210
    cochlear partition responses
        compression, 65–69
        otoacoustic emissions, **152–164**
        suppression (two-tone), **139–151**
    instrument processing, 303–306

Ohm's law, 113 (definition), 116, 267
Olivocochlear bundle (OCB), 127, 158,
    250–251, 253, 256–259, 262–
    263, 267, 269
Organ of Corti, 75–83, 85–87, 109–
    110, 281–283, 309, 316
    damage to, 281–283
    deformation, 127–132

electrochemical milieu, 85–86
innervation, 74–76, 170–172, 180–
    182, 252
potentials (extracellular), 116, 224,
    266–268
"Orienting" response, 34
Ossicles, 29, 38, 40–48, 53, 154, 278,
    296–297
Otitis media, 278
Otoacoustic emissions, 126–127, **152–
    164**
    "distortion product," 152–156
        diagnostic use, 285–286
        of cochlear model, 154–156
    efferent effects, 126–127, 264
    electrically evoked, 163–164
    "spontaneous," 127, 156–161
        frequency spectrum, 159
        relation to pathology, 159
        source(s), 158–160
    "stimulus frequency," 163
    "transiently evoked," 160–163
        frequency spectrum, 161
        relation to pathology, 163
        source(s), 162–163
Otosclerosis, 278–279, 296
Ototoxic drugs, 127, 153, 275, 280,
    282, 314
Outer hair cells, 76–82, 110–111
    afferent innervation, 110, 171–172,
        175–176
    capacitance changes, 122, 137
    cochlear microphonic contribution,
        116
    effects of damage, 280–285
    efferent effects, 256, 258
    efferent innervation, 171–172, 175–
        176, 250–252
    excitation, 80–82
    input-output curve (I/O), 114–116,
        145–147
    length, 110–111
    longitudinal tilt, 77, 129
    motility ("reverse transduction"),
        118–123
    protein constituents, 79
    receptor potentials (see Receptor
        potentials)
    specific capacitance, 118

Outer hair cells (*Continued*)
  specific conductance, 117–118
  transduction current, 111–114, 133, 267, 290
  turgor, 122–123
  ultrastructure, 110, 120–123
Oval window, 29, 38–41, 48–49, 53, 56–57, 59, 73–74, 278, 296–297

Pathology, 51, 159–160, 163, **275–294**
Perilymphatic system, 38–39, 55–57, 85–86, 111–112
Period histogram, 197–199, 203, 212, 223
Piano (analogy), 69–70, 196
Pigs, sound localization, 34
Phase
  lags and leads, 319
  of traveling waves, 58–59, 61–62, 67, 154–155
Phase locking (synchrony), 197–202, 211–216, 234–237
Pillar cells, 75–78, 80–82, 128, 132
Pillars (OHC constituent), 120–121
Pinna, 29–34, 48, 302
Poisson process, 177
Poststimulus time histogram 184, 197, 203, 206, 208, 214–215
Potassium ions (K^+)
  Ca^{+2}-activated K^+ channels, 105–107, 265–266
  concentrations in lymphs, 85–86
  flow into stereocilia, 105–107, 110
  flow through hair cell, 111–114, 266
  Nernst potential, 112–113, 124, 265
Power, 17, 47, 100–101, 108, 138, 227, 302
Power series, 165
Pressure
  acoustic, 11–17, 26, 29
  amplification, 26–28, 30–31, 42, 53, 59–60
  decibel scale (dB SPL), 16–17
  gradient reception, 49
  hydrostatic (turgor), 122–123
  intracochlear, 59–60
Presbycusis, 276

Primary auditory neurons (Type I), 171, 251–252
  afferent innervation, 170–175
  effects of deefferentation, 270–271
  effects of depletion, 291
  effects of hair cell damage, 280–283
  efferent effects, 127, 258–263, 270
  efferent innervation, 171, 251–252
  ''masking'' of responses, 244–247, 261–263
  processing ''window,'' 215
  refractoriness, 173–174, 178–179, 181, 185, 199, 207–208, 246
  responses to tones, **183–203**
    adaptation, 184–187, 199, 211
    characteristic frequency (definition), 192–193
    characteristic place, 220
    compression, 185, 189–192
    dynamic range, 188–191
    efferent effects, 127, 258–263, 270
    frequency tuning curve (construction), 189
    phase locking (synchrony), 197–202
    response area, 215, 217
    saturation of rate, 188–190
    suppression of, 216–227
    threshold, 21, 188–190, 193–194, 203, 288
  responses to clicks (impulses), 206–209
  responses to AM tones, 211–214
  responses to FM tones, 214–216
  responses to noise, 208–210
  responses to pairs of tones, 216–227
  responses to speech, **229–248**
  specializations of ''low-spontaneous'' neurons, 191, 212–213, 223–224, 233–234, 236–237, 243–246, 260–261
  spontaneous discharges, 176–182, 226
    categories (definition), 180
  suppression (two-tone), 216–227, 246
    as automatic gain control, 225
    high-side, 218–221
    low-side, 218, 221–226, 246
  ultrastructure, 173, 181

Primary auditory neurons (Type II),
    171–172, 175–176, 252–253
Primate cochleas
    anatomy (irregular), 159
    primary neuron responses, 189, 198–
        200
    otoacoustic emissions, 152, 154, 157,
        159, 162
Probe tone, 141

Quality factors
    Q (for electronic filters), 205, 227
    Q_{10} (for cochlea), 67, 194–195, 207,
        227
    Q_{20} (for cochlea), 259
Quanta (neurotransmitter), 173–174,
        178, 202
    uniquantal (EPSP), 173–174, 177–
        179, 181, 191

Receptor (transduction) potentials
    efferent effects, 257, 265–267
    generation, 100, 108, 113–118
    role in electromotility, 132–133,
        136–138, 145–150
    as synaptic drive, 169, 185–186,
        189–191, 197, 199–201, 206–
        208
Recruitment, 300
Refractory period, 173–174, 178–179,
        181, 185, 198–199, 207–208,
        246
Reissner's membrane, 56, 60–61, 71,
        74
Reptile (see also lizard ears)
    inner ear, 38–40, 55, 83–85
        endolymphatic system, 39–40
        oval window, 38–39
        perilymphatic system, 39–40
        round window, 38–39
        sensory surface, 38, 83–85
        vibrations, 56–57
    middle ear, 37–40, 42–43
        lever function, 39
        muscles, 52

    ossicles, 38–39, 43, 52
    pressure-gradient operation, 38,
        49, 277–278
    vibrations, 42–43
Reservoir models, 185–188, 198–199,
        208, 211, 238–239
Resistance (see also Damping)
    acoustic, 43, 53, 334–336
    electrical, 97, 101, 112–116, 256,
        265–267
    mechanical, 337
    psychological, 307
Resonance
    electrical, 104–107
    quarter-wave-length, 31, 48, **328–
        329**
    spring-mass-damper system, 62–64,
        69–70, 103–104, 131, 337
Rest point (of hair-cell I/O curve), 99–
        100, 114, 116, 146
Reticular lamina, 77–80, 82, 84
    composition, 129
    movements within organ of Corti,
        128–130, 132
    role in lymph separation, 85–86, 294
Reverse correlation (revcor), 209–210
Reverse transduction (OHC), 118–123,
        164
Rock music, 21, 51, 282, 287, 315
Round window, 29, 38–41, 56–57,
        278

Salycilate (see aspirin)
"Second messengers," 98, 265
Selective attention, 269
Sensorineural impairment, 277, **280–
        292**
Signal-to-noise ratio, 244–246, 248
Silent current, 114, 198
Sodium ions (Na^+), 85, 86, 112, 181
Sound waves, **11–22**
    basic properties, 11–17
    pressure
        amplification, 26–28, 30–31, 53
        scale, 16–17
        sensors, 25–28
        transformations by external ear,
            28–33

Sound waves (*Continued*)
    transformations by middle ear, 44–48
    propagation
        in air, 12–16, 19, 23–24
        in cochlea, 56–59, 70, 296
        in cochlear models, 62, 155
    source location
        azimuth, 24, 30–34, 47–48
        elevation, 31–32
        estimation of, 33–36
        plane of equal intensity, 35
        virtual, 32
    transmission across boundaries, 25–26
Spectrogram, 239–243, 245
Spectrotemporal receptive fields, 210
Speech (see also Vowels)
    comprehension, 291–292, 301
    importance of, 229, 275
    sounds, 230–235, 241, 245
    theory of production, 230–233
Spiral ganglion neurons
    type I (see Primary auditory neurons—Type I)
    type II, 171–172, 175, 252–253
Spontaneous otoacoustic emissions, 127, 156–161
Springs, 43, 60–64, 104, 122, 282
Stapes, 29, 40–43, 73
    effect of otosclerosis, 278–279
    effect of stapedius muscle, 49
    mobilization, 296
    vibrations, 42–43, 56–57, 65–66, 278–279
Stereocilia (''cilia''), 76–80, 92–93
    arrangement on cuticular plate, 93–94
    damage to, 280–281, 294
    free-standing, 83–84
    movements produced by sound, 80–85
    oscillations, 137
    protein constituents, 79, 92–93
    role in hair-cell excitation, 94–100, 110–112
    tip junctions, 96
    tip links, 92–96
    ultrastructure, 92–93

Stiffness, of
    air, 45, 332–336
    cilia (rotational) 81, 96, 104, 137
    cochlear partition (model), 60–64, 131, 282
    middle-ear, 44–45, 48–52, 59, 278–279, 296
    tectorial structures, 81, 87
Stria vascularis, 74–75, 86, 111, 113
    effects of impairment, 277, 283, 289–291
Stroboscopic illumination, 58
Synapses (ultrastructure)
    afferent, 171–173
    efferent, 171–172, 251–252
    complex, 181
    reciprocal, 175, 252
Synaptic bar, 172–173, 175
Synchrony coefficient, 201–203, 211–213
Summating potential, 116
Superposition, 140 (definition)
Suppression
    of cochlear partition vibrations, **141–151**
        high-side, 147–151
        low-side, 143–147
        mutual, 141–143
    of primary neuron responses, **216–225**
        effects of aging, 288
        rate suppression (definition), 218
        synchrony suppression (definition), 218
        two-tone, 216–225, 244
        single-tone, 226
        unknown factor(s), 224, 261
Suppressibility, 217–218

Tactile aids for hearing impaired, 308
Tectorial membrane, 74–84
    mass (inertia), 83, 104
    regrowth, 314
    role in hair-cell transduction, 80–84
    viscoelastic properties, 87
Tension fibroblasts, 75, 137

Tinnitus, 160
  causes, 292–294,
  treatments, 311–312
Tip junctions, 96
Tip links, 92–96
Tones (pure)
  audibility range (frequency), 20–21,
    41–42, 52, 106, 119, 202
  audibility range (pressure), 4, 21
  basic parameters, 21, 318–321
  perception of, 269, 298–299, 321
Tonotopic organization, 170
Transduction (hair cell), **91–108**
  adaptation, 95, 98–100
  currents, 95–99, 113, 116–117,
    132–133, 136, 138, 202, 267,
    290
  potentials, 100, 113–115, 132–133,
    146, 179, 190–191, 265–266
  sites, 94–96
  trapdoor model, 95–96
  sensitivity, 97
  speed, 98
Traveling wave, 57–62, 68, 154–156,
    296
Traveling-wave amplifier, 133
Treatments for damaged ears, **295–317**
  middle-ear disorders, 296–297
  sensorineural disorders, 297–311
  tinnitus, 311–312
Tumors, 53, 275, 292
Turtle ear
  hair cells, 92–94
    calcium extrusion, 112
    efferent effects, 256, 264
    frequency tuning, 104–107
    oscillations, 137
    ''hotspots'' (Ca^{2+}), 107
    transduction currents, 97–100
  phase synchrony (neural), 202

vestibular system, 271
Two-tone suppression (see Suppression)
Tympanometry, 52–53, 279

Uniquantal (EPSP), 173–174, 177–
    179, 181, 191
Usher's syndrome, 285

Van der Pol oscillator, 158
Vascular system, 76, 86, 111, 115, 275,
    294
Vesicles, 172, 175, 178, 182
Vestibular system, 56, 86, 91, 268, 271,
    285, 315
Vibrations
  cochlear partition
    pure tone, **56–70**
    two-tone, 141–151, 154–156
    stapes, 42–43, 56–57, 65–66, 278–
    279
Vocal folds (cords), 230
Volition, 271
Voltage clamp, 97, 108
Vowels
  formants, 232–235, 241–242, 245
  production of, 230–233
  neural responses to, 233–236, 240–
    247
Vocalization, effects on middle ears,
    51–52

Wavelength (definition), 12, 14
Wavelets, 327
World Wide Web, 6 (see Animations)